Dyslexia in Different Languages
Cross-linguistic Comparisons

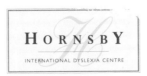

WYE STREET   LONDON SW11 2HB

TELEPHONE 020 7223 1144   FAX 020 7924 1112   E-MAIL dyslexia@hornsby.co.uk

This book is dedicated to my beloved family,
Yianni, Dimitri, Milto and Alexander,
and in loving memory of my dear parents
Milto and Maria Kyrtsis.

Dyslexia in Different Languages

Cross-linguistic Comparisons

Edited by

Nata Goulandris, PhD

University College London

Consultant in Dyslexia

Professor Margaret Snowling

University of York

W

WHURR PUBLISHERS

LONDON AND PHILADELPHIA

© 2003 Whurr Publishers

First published 2003 by
Whurr Publishers Ltd
19b Compton Terrace, London N1 2UN, England and
325 Chestnut Street, Philadelphia PA 19106, USA

British Library Cataloguing in Publication Data

A catalogue record for this book is available from the British Library.

ISBN 1 86156 153 9

Printed and bound in the UK by Athenaeum Press Limited, Gateshead, Tyne & Wear.

Contents

Contributors

Maggie Bruck, John Hopkins University, Baltimore, USA

Markéta Caravolas, Department of Psychology, Liverpool University, UK

Estelle Ann Lewin Doctor, Institute of Education, University of London, UK

Fred Genesee, Department of Psychology, McGill University, Montreal, Canada

Nata Goulandris, Department of Human Communication Science, University College London, UK

Elena L Grigorenko, Yale University, USA and Moscow State University, Russia

Bente E Hagtvet, Institute of Special Needs Education, University of Oslo, Norway

Peter F de Jong, Department of Education, University of Amsterdam, The Netherlands

Denise Klein, Cognitive Neuroscience Unit, Montreal Neurological Institute, McGill University, Montreal, Canada

Karin Landerl, Department of Psychology, University of Salzburg, Austria

Solveig-Alma Halaas Lyster, Institute of Special Needs Education, University of Oslo, Norway

Sonali Nag-Arulmani, The Promise Foundation, Karnataka, India

Åke Olofsson, Center for Reading Research, Stavanger, Norway

Dimitri Nikolopoulos, University of Patras, Greece

David L Share, Haifa University, Israel

Margaret Snowling, Department of Psychology, University of York, UK

Marcin Szczerbiński, University College London and University of Sheffield, UK

Connie Suk-Han Ho, University of Hong Kong, China

Taeko Nakayama Wydell, Department of Psychology, Brunel University, UK

Acknowledgements

I would like to thank Margaret Snowling for her generous and invaluable support and encouragement. I am also grateful to my colleagues in the Department of Human Communication Science and the members of the Developmental Reading Group who have contributed to this book either directly or indirectly through many interesting and challenging discussions. In particular I would like to thank Joy Stackhouse, Liz Nathan, Bill Wells, Marcin Szczerbiński, Mike Coleman and Dimitri Nikolopoulos – it has been an honour and a pleasure to work with you. Finally, I would like to thank the contributors for their stimulating chapters and Whurr Publishers for their enthusiastic help and their perseverance with numerous troublesome non-English fonts.

CHAPTER 1

Introduction: developmental dyslexia, language and orthographies

NATA GOULANDRIS

Until recently most of the research on developmental dyslexia has been conducted in the English language. Consequently, our understanding of dyslexia was confined to the characteristics of dyslexia in English. With the emergence of cross-linguistic studies of dyslexia, it has become increasingly evident that it is essential to consider developmental dyslexia in terms of the specific language of instruction because the behavioural manifestations of the disorder cannot be identified without reference to the core characteristics of the spoken and written language in use. To identify the presenting signs of dyslexia in a specific language, it is necessary first to appreciate the relevant linguistic features of that language and secondly to understand how normal reading and spelling acquisition develops and what cognitive skills underpin this development. Such a framework can then be used by researchers and practitioners to identify individuals whose performance differs markedly from the norm on tasks involving literacy, language, speed of processing and short-term memory.

The linguistic properties of each language, in particular the phonological, morphological and orthographic characteristics, will influence the ease or degree of difficulty with which young children learn to read and spell. Existing evidence points to important differences between writing systems in terms of the linguistic units represented graphically (logographic, syllabic or alphabetic). Logographic scripts represent units of meaning such as words or morphemes. Chinese (see Chapter 14) and Japanese Kanji (see Chapter 13) are examples of logographic scripts. In syllabic scripts such as Japanese Katakana (see Chapter 13), Hindi and Kannada (see Chapter 12) the symbols represent syllables. Alphabetic scripts such as English and the other European languages represent phonemes (speech sounds). The level of transparency (how reliably a letter maps onto a speech sound) measured on a continuum with 'transparent' or 'shallow' at one end and 'opaque' or 'deep' at the other, has been shown to determine how easily children learn to read. In a transparent orthography the mappings between a grapheme (the letter or letters used to represent a speech sound) and phonemes (speech sounds) are reliable and children can use this information to sound out unfamiliar words. In 'opaque' orthographies there are numerous mappings between letters and sounds (consider the spelling of the long *o* /əʊ/ in the words 'hole', 'road', 'low', 'so', 'though' and 'toe') and phoneme–grapheme correspondence rules are much less reliable. The degree of consistency of sound-letter mappings may also vary according to word position. In highly consistent orthographies, a grapheme is pronounced the same when it occurs in any position in a word. Transparent languages are much more consistent than opaque languages.

Existing cross-linguistic research (e.g. Wimmer, 1993) indicates that for alphabetic languages the most important linguistic characteristic for ensuring success in learning to read is the consistency of the orthography, defined as the extent to which learners can rely on phoneme–grapheme mappings to help them identify unfamiliar words. Transparent orthographies, those that represent the phonological or sound features of the language, such as Italian, Spanish and Greek, present few problems for young readers and most children can read the majority of written words after only one year of schooling (Seymour, 1998). Opaque and inconsistent orthographies, on the other hand, such as English (and to a lesser extent French, Polish and Danish), which give precedence to the morphemic level of language over the phonological level (Albrow, 1972), are far more diffi-cult to master and reading difficulties are more prevalent. Moreover, whereas measures of reading accuracy are a useful diagnostic tool in English, they are of limited value when assessing poor readers of transparent languages who are often as accurate as good readers. In highly transparent orthographies, many studies report that only reading rate differentiates poor and good readers (see Wimmer, 1993, 1996; Chapter 4). In moderately trans-parent orthographies, reading error differences are also in evidence (see Chapter 5 – but note that Chapter 2 also reports accuracy deficits in German-speaking dyslexics).

However, other linguistic abilities, such as grammatical awareness and knowledge, are important for learning to read and write. Rego and Bryant (1993), for example, demonstrated that grammatical sensitivity also contributes to reading success and that it enabled children to make use of context to predict unfamiliar words. Grammatical sensitivity is, however, likely to play a more critical role in inflected languages such as French, Greek and Polish than in relatively uninflected languages such as English. Other factors that might affect the acquisition of phonological awareness and learning to read include the complexity of the syllabic structure, and ortho-graphic 'peculiarities' (Morais, 1995). Languages that are composed of short, simple, staccato-like consonant-vowel (CV) syllables, such as Greek and Italian, enable children to appreciate the phonemic components of words more easily than languages that contain many complex clusters. Similarly, orthographies that incorporate numerous irregular words, such as English, confuse the learner and render the task of extracting rule-based regularities more difficult and prolonged. Visual complexity of the script may also contribute to reading difficulties in languages demanding high levels of visual discrimination and memory skills (see, for example, Share, Chapter 11).

The influence of instructional methods on the cross-linguistic manifestations of dyslexia must not be overlooked. The majority of languages with shallow, transparent and consistent orthographies are taught using highly structured phonics methods that explicitly teach letter–sound mappings and consonant–vowel (CV) syllables that can be combined into familiar words. Considering the reliability of the mappings, this teaching method is extremely effective because learners receive positive feedback throughout the learning process.

The age at which children begin formal schooling is another plausible influential factor. In England, children begin formal schooling at 5-years of age, whereas in many other European countries schooling begins at 6 or 7, when children have a more developed and sophisticated oral language system and more proficient cognitive skills.

This book sets out to explore these issues by presenting current research into dyslexia in non-English languages, including: alphabetic languages such as Afrikaans, French, German, Greek, Hebrew, Norwegian, Swedish and Polish; semi-syllabic and semi-alphabetic scripts, such as Kannada, Tamil, Hiragana and Katakana; and logographic scripts, such as Chinese and Kanji. Its objective is to explore a variety of languages and to identify both the typical reading and spelling difficulties characteristic of each language, considering its unique linguistic properties, and the common core or universal deficits that can be considered to be the defining characteristics of developmental dyslexia regardless of language. Each chapter begins with a description of the linguistic features of the language in question, how that language differs from English and what problems beginners may face acquiring literacy. We begin by examining the more transparent languages and proceed through the less regular to the opaque orthographies. Logographic scripts are considered at the end of the volume.

I will begin with a brief summary of developmental dyslexia in English. (A comprehensive and highly readable account of developmental dyslexia in English-speaking children can be found in Snowling, 2000.) Developmental dyslexia is a disorder that generally persists through life (Bruck, 1990). The presenting symptoms differ according to an individual's age, the severity of the disorder and the compensatory strategies available. A child is usually referred for assessment because of reading and spelling difficulties. However, these presenting symptoms are invariably the tip of an iceberg. The reading and/or spelling difficulties are generally accompanied by subtle spoken-language difficulties, and some researchers consider dyslexia to be primarily a language disorder (Vellutino, 1979; Scarborough, 1991; Hohnen and Stevenson, 1999).

The most influential and generally accepted theory to date is the phonological deficit hypothesis. This hypothesis states that dyslexics have impairments in phonological processing as demonstrated by deficits in short-term memory processing, word and nonword repetition, rapid automatized naming and in phonological awareness tasks such as sound categorization, phoneme and syllable segmentation, deletion and spoonerisms. Snowling (2000) contends that dyslexics have difficulties storing and retrieving fully specified phonological representations and that this difficulty underlies all the other behavioural manifestations. For example, phonological awareness difficulties prevent dyslexics from extrapolating letter–sound mappings when learning to read, and they are consequently impaired in their use of phonological recoding strategies when sounding out unfamiliar words or nonwords (Rack et al., 1992). Spelling impairments persist even when the initial reading difficulties appear to be resolved and are invariably still present in adulthood (Bruck, 1990). There is now also considerable evidence that proficient phonological processing is equally as important for learning to read and spell non-English languages as it is for acquiring literacy skills in English (see Chapters 4, 10 and 14).

Research on the biological bases of dyslexia indicates that it is familial, heritable and genetic (Smith et al., 1983). The offspring of dyslexic parents are significantly more likely to be dyslexic than the offspring of unaffected parents, as dyslexia runs in families and family history is one of the most significant risk factors, with between 25% and 65% of children with a dyslexic parent being affected (Scarborough, 1990). However, what reading component skills are inherited? Whereas initially it appeared that only phonological coding (measured using a nonword reading task) was heritable (Olson et al., 1989), more recent evidence suggests that both the phonological and the orthographic components of reading are heritable (Hohnen and Stevenson, 1999). Moreover, DeFries et al. (1997) demonstrated that reading and spelling skills are differentially heritable; reading skills are heritable early in development but spelling skills become more heritable as children grow older.

Numerous studies using imaging technology have provided a clearer understanding of the localization of language and phonological processing in the brain and will enable researchers to investigate the neural substrate of dyslexia. For example, Shaywitz et al. (2001) report that the performance of dyslexic readers on a nonword rhyming task differed markedly from controls.

The adult dyslexics showed abnormal activation in the left hemisphere posterior cortex, including both visual and language regions, as well as the angular gyrus, an area considered important for cross-modal integration. For normal readers there was more activation in the left hemisphere whereas for dyslexics greater activation occured in the right hemisphere.

Further evidence that dyslexia is a neurocognitive disorder was provided by a cross-linguistic study undertaken by Paulesu et al. (2001), who compared the brain activity of Italian, French and English dyslexics while they were reading. The reading and phonological skills of all the dyslexic groups were impaired compared to controls. Moreover, positron emission tomography (PET) scans showed reduced activity in the same region of the left hemisphere for all three dyslexic language groups. However, differences in the comparative reading performance of the 3 groups were reported with Italian dyslexics attaining higher levels of accuracy on word and nonword reading than French and English dyslexics as expected, considering the differences in the transparency of the respective languages. The researchers argue that the same neurocognitive basis underlies dyslexia but that differences in the orthographies of the languages influence the severity of the reading, spelling and phonological deficits.

The biological and neurocognitive evidence strongly suggests that dyslexia is a biological disorder and a universal one. The authors in this book investigate the behavioural level of dyslexia and how the spoken language and orthography under consideration interact with the deficits resulting from the biological susceptibility.

Dyslexia in different languages

One of the first challenges to the then widely held assumption that the course of reading development was similar in all languages, was made by Heinz Wimmer (1993). Instead, he, Karin Landerl, Uta Frith and his research group demonstrated that German, a transparent language, posed fewer problems for learners than deep languages and that the acquisition of literacy skills was quicker and smoother for all German learners, even dyslexics, than for English-speaking children.

Karin Landerl (Chapter 2) reviews the seminal work emanating from this Austrian group and then considers how a phonological deficit may affect children learning to read a consistent language such as German. She proposes that the orthographic structure of a language may be a crucial factor in determining the types of difficulty demonstrated by children with phonological deficits. For example, it is easier for children with phonological deficits to learn to read consistent languages such as German, because the grapheme–phoneme correspondences are so reliable. A comparison of

English and German dyslexic children reported in Chapter 2 provides strong support for this view (Landerl et al., 1997). Not only did the German dyslexics outperform their English counterparts on accuracy of word and nonword reading, but they also made far fewer errors on vowels than the English dyslexics. However, both dyslexic groups produced significantly more nonword reading errors than reading-age controls, in line with the nonword reading deficit hypothesis (Rack et al., 1992). This is a particularly important finding because, hitherto, only speed deficits had been reported for German dyslexics. In addition, both dyslexic groups displayed a reading speed impairment for both words and nonwords, although the English dyslexics were more seriously impaired than the German dyslexics. Landerl et al. also reported that the German dyslexics had deficits on automatized rapid naming and spoonerism tasks, indicating that the phonological deficit hypothesis is equally applicable for German-speaking dyslexics even though their difficulties are more circumscribed than those of their English counterparts. This study also investigated, but did not find evidence for, visual processing difficulties or general automatization impairments.

In Chapter 3, Peter de Jong emphasizes that there are substantial similarities between the German and Dutch orthographies and that dyslexic children in both countries experience similar problems in spite of the fact that all children are taught using explicit phonics methods. Dutch-speaking dyslexics have few problems reading words and decoding nonwords, but they are severely impaired compared to controls on reading rate. This phonological decoding speed impairment is especially severe when they are asked to decode nonwords. Dutch dyslexics also display difficulties with tasks requiring phonological processing and manipulation. The literature provides evidence of deficits on consonant deletion, serial rapid naming and working memory tasks. De Jong concludes that for Dutch learners the core deficit presented by dyslexics is impaired rapid decoding of nonwords but that phonological processing deficits underpin Dutch children's inability to decode quickly and automatically. Whereas a number of intervention studies have been undertaken to speed up word and nonword recognition in Dutch, improvements have been disappointing and transfer effects on untrained stimuli short-lived.

Greek is a transparent, consistent language. Systematic phonics instruction is given from the outset and is accompanied by syllable and phoneme segmentation exercises. Greek is also a highly inflected language requiring extensive knowledge of grammar and syntax in order to spell correctly. In Chapter 4, Dimitris Nikolopoulos, Maggie Snowling and I set out to investigate whether the orthographic transparency of the Greek language would enable poor readers to attain reading competence in line with German dyslexics. The 28 Greek-speaking poor readers were tested on a battery of phonological and syntactic awareness tasks, and on single-word reading and spelling performance. The dyslexics attained high scores on the word and nonword reading tasks. When reading errors occurred they were provoked by a combination of factors, including orthographic complexity, low word frequency and a large number of syllables. The dyslexics' spelling performance showed that their alphabetic skills were proficient. All their spellings were phonologically plausible but contained incorrect graphemes. The dyslexics also attained high scores on most of the phonological awareness tasks. The only tasks that differentiated them from controls were spoonerisms, phoneme substitution and consonant segmentation. However, deficits in reading rate were uncovered, with the dyslexics taking approximately twice as long to read words and nonwords as the same-age controls. The dyslexics were also impaired when spelling less-frequently occurring inflectional morphemes, suggesting that their ability to extrapolate orthographic spelling patterns requiring syntactical knowledge was imperfect. This evidence points to an underlying phonological processing deficit in line with that reported for English-speaking dyslexics. Moreover, the majority of Greek dyslexics resemble surface dyslexics as they do not show the pervasive phonological deficits characteristic of phonological dyslexics and produce primarily orthographic spelling errors.

In Chapter 5, Marcin Szczerbiński presents an overview of research on reading difficulties in Polish. Polish orthography is highly consistent for reading but much less consistent for spelling, as the morphological principle is adhered to and words that contain the same morpheme are spelled identically. Consequently, knowledge of morphemes comprising both the spelling of roots and of inflectional endings is essential for producing orthographically correct spellings. Polish is also a highly inflected language and Marcin Szczerbiński emphasizes that readers must learn to recognize the rapidly alternating visual and phonological forms of the same root word, unlike in English where only slight variations occur.

Although it is generally thought in Poland that spelling disorders are the dominant form of learning difficulty, empirical studies show that children referred for spelling difficulties invariably have additional reading problems, especially slow rate of reading. Younger children also have considerable difficulties with decoding. The close links between spoken-language deficits and dyslexia are generally recognized. In a recent small-scale study undertaken by Szczerbiński, dyslexics were subdivided according to whether they differed from chronological-age controls on reading accuracy or reading rate. Both groups had double deficits on phonological awareness and rapid naming measures, but accuracy dyslexics had more difficulty with phonological awareness tasks and had a profile comparable to classic phonological dyslexics, whereas low-speed dyslexics were more impaired on the rapid naming tasks.

Russian is also halfway along the transparency/opacity continuum. Elena Grigorenko explains in Chapter 6 that Russian is basically consistent for reading, but sound-spelling correspondence rules are much less reliable for spelling. As the Russian spelling rules are numerous and complex, spelling poses far greater difficulties for learners than reading. In addition, the morphological principle is generally adhered to, but there are also numerous exceptions to it.

Grigorenko reports that the incidence of reading and spelling difficulties in a large sample of over 1000 1st- to 4th-grade schoolchildren was small. Boys made more spelling errors and their spelling performance was more variable than that of girls. When criteria of specific reading or spelling difficulties were applied by selecting children who performed within the normal range on the arithmetic task but poorly on spelling, approximately 7.5% were identified. Reading difficulties did not always entail spelling difficulties. Some children had only reading impairments and others only spelling deficits.

In another large-scale study of high school students' spelling skills, an error analysis was undertaken. The results demonstrated that Russian high school students still make a large number of spelling errors. Second, and somewhat surprisingly considering that Russian is quite consistent, there were a large number of phonology-based errors. However, the predominant types of spelling errors were morphological, comprising both inflectional and derivational errors.

In Chapter 7, Klein and Doctor examine how the orthographic structure and the consistency of sound–letter mappings shape the difficulties encountered by bilingual children. Three case studies of bilingual Afrikaans-English are presented using a comprehensive psycholinguistic battery. The contrast between the highly consistent orthography of Afrikaans and the unpredictable English orthography is of particular interest. These case studies demonstrate that although a shallow orthography such as Afrikaans is easier for children who can use phonological recoding skills, readers who adopt partial visual strategies will make many errors because there are so many visually similar words.

Swedish is yet another relatively shallow orthography taught initially by the systematic introduction of letters in tandem with phonics-based instruction. Although Swedish has almost perfect 1-1 mapping between letters and sounds, most consonants have at least two or more orthographic representations. In certain instances, phonological discriminations involving vowel length and syllable stress are required in order to spell correctly. The presence of compound words and complex phoneme–grapheme relationships may pose particular problems for the dyslexic.

In Chapter 8, Åke Olofsson describes several investigations of pupils' ability to use orthographic and phonological information. He reports that phonological skills are fully developed by the end of primary school, whereas orthographic processing skills continue to develop up to adulthood. However, adults with childhood diagnoses of dyslexia were impaired on orthographic and phonological decoding tasks as well as on a spelling test requiring orthographic knowledge. Self-report data revealed that the dyslexic adults considered themselves inferior to controls on spelling and second-language learning. He concludes that when reading speed is taken into account, Swedish dyslexics continue to demonstrate impaired phonological and orthographic processing.

In Chapter 11, David Share provides an overview of the literature on reading acquisition and disabilities in Hebrew. Hebrew is characterized by its derivational orthography in which content words are represented by a conso-nantal 'root' and vocalic 'pattern'. The vocalic 'pattern' comprises infixes, prefixes and suffixes. In the more common form of Hebrew text (unpointed text), vowels are not represented. Lexico-morphological knowledge is there-fore a crucial factor in word recognition and contextual processing is often needed to disambiguate the text. To facilitate the learning task, beginning readers are taught pointed text in which both consonants and vowel diacritics map on to phonemes perfectly.

Phonological awareness is an important predictor of reading in Hebrew but is weaker than in English. Hebrew dyslexics perform poorly on nonword reading accuracy and speed measures and on phonological awareness tasks, but also have deficits in morphological knowledge when compared to vocabulary age-matched controls. This indicates that in order to read Hebrew successfully, access to both phonological and morphological information is essential.

Moreover, in subtype analyses of diagnosed dyslexics (Lamm and Epstein, 1994), very few were classified as phonological dyslexics. The majority were labelled surface/lexical dyslexics and the next largest group (approximately 25% of the sample) were categorized as having visuo-motor deficits. David Share argues that visuo-spatial factors play an important role in the early stages of reading acquisition, when visual discrimination is vital, and that this accounts for the existence of a large number of disabled readers whose diffi-culties are due to visuo-spatial deficits. However, he suggests that the individ-uals who have been labelled as surface dyslexics may actually have a mild form of phonological deficit, which shows up only as an orthographic repre-sentation deficit. The ease with which children learn to read a regular orthog-raphy taught by systematic instruction may mask underlying phonological problems in children presenting the characteristics of surface dyslexics.

Difficulties with phonological processing tasks such as spoonerisms, rapid naming, digit- and word-span tasks, and spelling impairments are characteristic of dyslexic children regardless of the language spoken. It is therefore surprising that so few cross-linguistic studies of dyslexics' spelling difficulties have been undertaken. The next 2 chapters focus on children with spelling difficulties.

Markéta Caravolas, Maggie Bruck and Fred Genesee present a study in Chapter 9 investigating the spelling performance of English- and French-speaking poor spellers and comparing their performance to same-language children of the same age. They were particularly interested in whether the greater inconsistency of phoneme–grapheme mappings in English would cause English dyslexics to have more difficulties than their French counterparts. They predicted that the difference in the degree of transparency of the two languages would influence the types of errors produced based on their phonological input hypothesis. This states that language-specific differences in phonology will influence children's ability to form phonological representations. As predicted, both French groups spelled words and nonwords more accurately than their English counterparts, but in addition the French poor spellers were less impaired on vowels than the English poor spellers. Caravolas et al. attribute this difference to the more consistent French writing system. Moreover, although both groups of poor spellers produced fewer phonologically plausible errors (sounding like the target word) than controls, the English poor spellers performed more poorly. Caravolas et al. argue that this provides further support for the hypothesis that phonological processing deficits underlie children's spelling deficits across alphabetic languages.

In Chapter 10, Bente Hagtvet and Sol Lyster compare the spelling performance of Norwegian good and poor decoders. Norwegian is an alphabetic script that falls in an intermediate position on the transparency continuum. Although most phonemes are represented by one grapheme, some have alternative graphemic representations. In addition, Norwegian orthography adheres to the morphological principle (as does English), so semantically related words retain the same spelling even when their pronunciation differs. These morphemic constraints consequently result in a number of exceptional spellings. Despite the fact that Norwegian has numerous spelling anomalies, poor readers were able to spell most regular words and nonwords and demonstrated relatively proficient use of sound-spelling rules. Overall, the same factors, namely lack of familiarity, orthographic complexity, presence of consonant clusters, word length and irregularity, proved difficult for all the young spellers but posed greater problems for the poor reader group. The poor readers' errors were primarily confined to low-frequency, irregularly spelled words and words containing complex graphemes. However, qualitative error analysis demonstrated that poor readers were less likely to represent the sound structure of the words they were spelling than the good readers, and produced many more multiple errors in their spelling attempts.

The final three chapters investigate dyslexia in non-alphabetic languages. In Chapter 12, Sonali Nag-Arulmani considers learning to read and reading difficulties in India. This truly multilingual environment poses many difficulties for young readers, who frequently are obliged to learn the orthography of a language that is not their mother tongue. Currently the three-language policy promotes literacy in three languages selected by the parents – a daunting task for any learner!

Most Indian orthographies are based on the Brahmi script and are transparent. Syllabographs are the primary orthographic unit used in conjunction with some alphabetic symbols. Sonali Nag-Arulmani argues that children learning to read semi-syllabic and semi-alphabetic scripts used for Indian languages may experience difficulties with phonological or orthographic processing and with linking phonological to orthographic representations. Mastery of the large number of syllabographs extends over the first four years of schooling. Children who fail to master these syllabographs, many of which are visually confusing, become poor readers. Intervention comprising instruction in syllable names and sequences resulted in significant improvements in syllabograph naming skills as well as in reading accuracy and speed.

In Chapter 13, Taeko Wydell provides a detailed account of the two scripts that are used simultaneously when writing in Japanese. The syllabic script Kana, with its transparent print-to-sound mappings, ensures fast and accurate learning. Kanji symbols are then learned by rote and each character's pronunciation is concurrently given in Kana. She contends that learning to read in Japanese is rarely problematic and that the incidence of reading difficulties is very low. By grade 6 only 1% of Japanese children were reading delayed or impaired.

Wydell presents a case study of a bilingual English/Japanese dyslexic whose literacy skills are perfect in Japanese but extremely poor in English. She introduces the hypothesis of granularity and transparency (Wydell and Butterworth, 1999) to explain why an individual may demonstrate reading and spelling problems in one language and not in the other. According to this hypothesis, there will be a low incidence of developmental dyslexia in orthographies that utilize large sound units at the level of the whole character or of words, and in languages that are consistent and transparent. As both Japanese orthographies fall within these categories, there will be a low incidence of phonological dyslexia in individuals learning those scripts. In contrast, as English is inconsistent and opaque and the mappings between phonology and orthography are at the level of the phoneme, phonological developmental dyslexia will arise.

Wydell's study of AS demonstrates the striking dissociation between his severe phonological difficulties and his reading and spelling impairments in English, as opposed to his competent literacy skills in Japanese. Interestingly, he had no difficulties reading Kana nonwords despite the fact that his performance on phonological lexical decision tasks was poor compared to Japanese controls. Wydell concludes that working memory deficits are more detrimental when reading an inconsistent orthography such as English than when reading a consistent script that can be decoded on-line, syllable by syllable.

Contrary to the position argued by Wydell, Connie Ho in Chapter 14 argues that recent studies suggest that dyslexia is equally as prevalent among readers of Japanese and Chinese as of English. In this chapter, Ho considers the evidence that phonological skills are universally important for reading, regardless of the type of script used. Citing a four-year longitudinal study (Ho and Bryant, 1997) she provides evidence that, whereas visual processing and memory skills are predictive of reading performance in year 1 and 2, phonological processing skills become predictive in grades 2 and 3. According to Ho, Chinese children use wholistic whole-word recognition for familiar characters but apply information derived from the phonetic and semantic radicals when confronted with unfamiliar characters. Phonological awareness enables Chinese beginners to learn OPC (orthographic–phonology correspondence) rules in the same way as it provides the foundation for learning grapheme–phoneme correspondences in alphabetic languages.

Recurrent themes

Certain recurrent themes appear throughout the text and are worth highlighting. First, there is general agreement that language-specific differences account for significant individual differences in performance in phonological awareness and reading and spelling ability (Caravolas, 1993). In all cases, the degree of transparency and the relative importance of linguistic features, such as the importance of morphology in Hebrew and Russian, or timing (e.g. stress or syllable; see Chapter 9), influences the types of problems encountered while becoming literate in each language.

Second, virtually all the authors in this book ascribe the reading and spelling difficulties of the dyslexics to phonological processing difficulties, in spite of the fact that in a number of languages, such as German, Greek and Dutch, dyslexics were able to perform many of the more simple phonological tests with ease. However, when faced with more challenging tasks such as spoonerisms, phonological memory tasks or rapid naming, performance deficits were reported. The only exception is Taeko Wydell, who argues that phonological processing deficits do not impede the acquisition of reading competence in Japanese because the units of writing are larger than the phoneme, and because Kana has perfect symmetry between letters and sounds, it is easily learned.

Third, the predominance of spelling impairments is a common theme. All the authors report that writing impairments are more severe in their language regardless of language or type of script. This is ascribed to a general imbalance in the relationships between grapheme-to-phoneme and phoneme-to-grapheme mappings. Even in highly consistent languages such as German, several graphemes can represent the same phoneme. The inevitable introduction of foreign loan words and the retention of the original spellings for historical reasons also produce more ambiguity for spelling across languages.

Finally, the overall picture provided by the studies in this book concurs with the strong evidence made available by recent imaging studies (e.g. Paulesu et al., 2001; Shaywitz et al., 2001). Children who are at risk of dyslexia have underlying phonological processing impairments. The extent to which this biological substrate of deficits will affect their literacy skills is dependent on the linguistic demands of the orthography they will encounter. If they are required to learn an irregular language such as English or French, reading, spelling and phonological processing difficulties will be evident. If they are only exposed to regular orthographies such as Italian or Spanish, their underlying impairments will be masked by their apparently proficient literacy skills. The only tasks likely to uncover these hidden deficits are speed of processing tasks, complex phonological processing tasks such as spoonerisms, and spelling. In conclusion, neurobiological evidence demonstrates that the pattern of brain organization differs in dyslexics when compared to controls. However, the orthography (or orthographies) that dyslexic individuals are exposed to determines the severity and extent of the behavioural manifestations.

In conclusion, studies of dyslexia in non-English languages are collected here to permit us to make more informed generalizations about the nature of developmental dyslexia and the universal properties of the disorder that transcend languages. Concurrently such studies will enable practitioners to arrive at language-specific recommendations for the identification and remediation of developmental dyslexia. An appreciation of language-specific factors is critical because in many countries there are as yet few test instruments available to assess and identify children with specific learning difficulties. Often the teaching programmes available are simply translations of existing materials designed for instructing English-speaking dyslexics. These are frequently unsuited to the foreign language because they do not take into account the language's specific linguistic features and the type of difficulties experienced by the dyslexic child when trying to learn to read and write that particular language. It is hoped that this book may form a bridge from theory to practice and facilitate the development of better models for the identification, assessment and remediation of reading disorders in an increasingly global society.

References

Albrow KH (1972) The English Writing System: Notes towards a description. London: Longman.

Bruck M (1990) Word recognition skills of adults with childhood diagnosis of dyslexia. Developmental Psychology 26: 439–454.

Caravolas M (1993) Language-specific influences of phonology and orthography on emergent literacy. In J Altarriba (ed) Cognition and culture: a cross-cultural approach to psychology. Netherlands: Elsevier Science Publishers.

DeFries JC, Alarcon M, Olson RK (1997) Genetic etiologies of reading and spelling deficits: developmental differences. In C Hulme, MJ Snowling (eds) Dyslexia: biology, cognition and intervention, pp 20-37. London: Whurr.

Ho CS-H, Bryant PE (1997) Learning to read Chinese beyond the logographic phase. Reading Research Quarterly 32: 276-289.

Hohnen B, Stevenson J (1999) The structure of genetic influences on general cognitive, language and phonological reading abilities. Developmental Psychology 35: 590-603.

Lamm O, Epstein R (1994) Dichotic listening performance under high and low lexical work load in subtypes of developmental dyslexia. Neuropsychologia 32: 757-785.

Landerl K, Wimmer H, Frith U (1997) The impact of orthographic consistency on dyslexia: a German-English comparison. Cognition 63: 315-334.

Morais J (1995) Introduction: do orthographic and phonological peculiarities of alphabetically written languages influence the course of literacy acquisition? Reading and Writing 7(1): 1-7.

Olson RK, Wise B, Conners F, Rack J, Fulker D (1989) Specific deficits in component reading and language skills: genetic and environmental influences. Journal of Learning Disabilities 22: 339-348.

Paulesu E, Demonet J-F, Fazio F, McCrory E, Chanoine V, Brunswick N, Cappa SF, Cossu G, Habib M, Frith CD, Frith U (2001) Dyslexia: cultural diversity and biological unity. Science 291: 2165-2167.

Rack J, Snowling M, Olson R (1992) The nonword reading deficit in developmental dyslexia: a review. Reading Research Quarterly 27: 29-53.

Rego LL, Bryant PE (1993) The connection between phonological, syntactic and semantic skills and children's reading and spelling. European Journal of Psychology of Education 8(3): 235-246.

Scarborough HS (1990) Very early language deficits in dyslexic children. Child Development 61: 1728-1743.

Scarborough HS (1991) Antecedents to reading ability: pre-school language development and literacy experiences of children from dyslexic families. Reading and Writing 3: 219-233.

Seymour P (1998) Conference presentation, EPS Conference, Cambridge, 4 April.

Shaywitz BA, Shaywitz SE, Pugh KR, Fulbright RK, Mencl WE, Constable RT, Skudlarski P, Fletcher JM, Lyon GR, Gore JC (2001) The neurobiology of dyslexia. Clinical Neuroscience Research 1: 291-299.

Smith SD, Kimberling WJ, Pennington BF, Lubs HA (1983) Specific reading disability: identification of an inherited form through linkage science. Science 219: 1345-1347.

Snowling M (2000) Dyslexia. Oxford: Blackwell Publishers.

Vellutino FR (1979) Dyslexia: research and theory. Cambridge, MA: MIT Press.

Wimmer H (1993) Characteristics of developmental dyslexia in a regular writing system. Applied Psycholinguistics 14(1): 1-33.

Wimmer H (1996) The early manifestation of developmental dyslexia: evidence from German children. Reading and Writing 8: 171-188.

Wydell TN, Butterworth BL (1999) A case study of an English-Japanese bilingual with monolingual dyslexia. Cognition 70: 273-305.

CHAPTER 2

Dyslexia in German-speaking children

KARIN LANDERL

The central finding with respect to dyslexia in the past few decades is that specific difficulties in reading acquisition are typically caused by a deficit in phonological processing. Phonological abilities play an important role in reading acquisition because alphabetic spelling systems depict the sounds of spoken words. The assumption is that phonologically impaired children have difficulties in accessing the abstract phonemic speech segments and consequently in mapping alphabetic print on to spoken language (Gleitman and Rozin, 1977; Liberman, 1982).

The evidence for this theory has so far come largely from children with difficulties learning to read English. However, this universal account of dyslexia needs to be reconciled with the fact that different orthographies have different mapping rules. The English orthographic system is in fact quite distant from the one phoneme–one grapheme ideal of an alphabetic writing system. Typically, a particular grapheme corresponds to several phonemes (e.g. the *a* in *hand*, *ball*, *garden* and *hate*) and a particular phoneme can be represented by several graphemes (e.g. /u:/ in *two*, *too* or *through*). In addition to the low consistency on the grapheme–phoneme level, English orthography has a high number of irregular or exceptional spellings that cannot be decoded via grapheme–phoneme translation. English was termed a 'deep' orthography (Liberman et al., 1980), because the system represents consistencies on the deeper linguistic level of morphology rather than on the more shallow level of phonology, i.e. words that belong to one word family are spelled similarly, even if their pronunciation is quite different (e.g. *sign–signature*, *heal–health*).

German orthography, on the other hand, although far from having perfect one-to-one correspondences between graphemes and phonemes, is certainly much more on the shallow side of the continuum of orthographic consistency and is therefore a more typical example of an alphabetic writing system

15

than English. With only very few exceptions, each grapheme corresponds to only one phoneme. Only the grapheme *v* usually corresponds to the phoneme /f/ (e.g. *Vater*, English: father), but sometimes is pronounced as /v/ (e.g. *Vase*, English: vase). Grapheme–phoneme correspondences for vowels are as consistent as for consonants.

This stands in marked contrast to English, where grapheme–phoneme correspondences for vowels are especially unreliable. For example, the vowel grapheme *a* is pronounced differently in the English words *hand*, *ball* and *garden*, but in the corresponding German words *Hand*, *Ball* and *Garten*, the vowel is consistently pronounced as /a/. Vowel quality is unequivocally determined by the vowel grapheme, only the representation of vowel length is somewhat more complex. Long vowels are either marked by doubling of the vowel letter (*Tee*), or by a so called 'silent h' after the vowel letter (*Reh*) or simply by not doubling the consonant letter after the vowel, since this normally signals that the vowel is short (e.g. *Ofen* is pronounced as /o:fən/ while *offen* is pronounced as /ofən/ with a short vowel). Even if such complexities of vowel length representation are neglected by the inexperienced reader, there is a good chance that simple left-to-right decoding will lead to the correct word pronunciation, because it is quite exceptional that two words differ solely in vowel length.

The second important difference between reading acquisition in English and German is reading instruction. In German (as in most other consistent orthographies), reading is typically taught via a straightforward phonics teaching regimen fostering word recognition via phonological decoding by heavy emphasis on teaching of letter–sound correspondences and blending and sounding out words. For example, in a reading primer widely used in Austria (Eibl et al., 1996), children playfully learn the letter–sound correspondences for *m*, *o*, *a*, *i* and *l* over the first weeks of reading instruction (complemented by many phonemic awareness games and lessons in which the teacher reads gripping stories to the children and discusses them to awaken their interest in reading). The children then start to practise sounding out simple words like *Oma*, *Mama*, *im* and even short sentences like *Mia malt mit Oma* (Mia paints with granny).

The next two letter sounds that are taught are *t* and *r*, and now the children are able to decode the spell of a mysterious magician (*mora mora mori, mira mira lori, lora lira lot*, etc.). This is the first nonword decoding exercise that the children master with great pleasure. Soon, they are able to answer written questions about a picture in the primer like *Wo ist Uta?* (Where is Uta?) or *Warum ist Timo im Turm?* (Why is Timo in the tower?). Thus, although the children are far from being able to read books, because they know only part of the phonological code, they learn that phonological decoding is a useful technique to work out short but meaningful written texts.

Such a straightforward phonics teaching approach is suitable for consistent orthographies where most graphemes correspond to only one phoneme. Due to the high level of complexity of the phonological code in the English orthographic system, more than one grapheme–phoneme correspondence would have to be taught for many graphemes. In contrast to German, where the consistent orthographic structure plainly suggests that phonics teaching is the most efficient means to introduce children to the alphabetic code, reading instruction programes in English in general put more emphasis on whole-word recognition and less on phonological decoding abilities. This is obviously a consequence of the complexity of the mappings between phonology and orthography in English. However, explicit teaching of the alphabetic code as provided in German might be especially beneficial for children who, due to a phonological deficit, have difficulties cracking the alphabetic code on their own, for example, working out that the letter 'm' represents the same sound /m/ in the word spellings *mother*, *come* or *summer*.

German is an interesting test case for the phonological deficit hypothesis of dyslexia. It seems plausible that orthographic consistency affects both the nature and degree of reading difficulties. If grapheme–phoneme relations are consistent, then even a child with phonological difficulties may, with appropriate phonics instruction, learn to map print on to speech and accordingly show little or no delay in reading acquisition. Conversely, if such a child learned an orthography with opaque and confusing grapheme–phoneme relations, there would be severe problems in reading acquisition. For English dyslexic children, a large number of studies have shown that the phonological decoding of nonwords is excessively difficult (Rack et al., 1992). These specific difficulties have been interpreted as a consequence of the phonological deficit underlying dyslexia. However, the contribution of the high complexity and inconsistency of English orthography to dyslexic children's difficulties is unclear. In principle, it is possible that phonologically impaired children acquiring the consistent German orthography do not show the same difficulties because they are able to acquire the comparably simple mapping rules despite their phonological deficit. Thus, a close examination of the reading difficulties of children acquiring a consistent orthography like German, which is provided in the first part of this chapter, can tell us more about the influence of orthographic structure.

Taking the argument further, one could assume that only in the phonologically complex English orthographic system is dyslexia caused by a phonological deficit, while in a consistent orthography like German, a phonological impairment has no major influence on reading acquisition. The question is, therefore, does the phonological deficit account hold for German as well as for English dyslexic children or do we have to look for other cognitive deficits that might underlie the reading difficulties of German-speaking children? Findings relevant to this question will be reviewed in the second part of this chapter.

Reading and spelling difficulties

What makes German especially appropriate for a comparison with English is that although the two orthographies differ in consistency of grapheme–phoneme correspondences, the two languages are closely related. There are many words that are very similar or even identical in English and German, allowing us to present English and German children with more or less the same reading material. We took advantage of this close relationship between the two languages in a study directly comparing the word and nonword reading abilities of 12-year-old English and German dyslexic children (Landerl et al., 1997). The children of both language groups were severely delayed in their reading development with a mean delay between three and four years. Each of the two groups consisted of 18 dyslexic children and was compared with a group of reading-age control children who were about 8 years old.

The reading abilities of English and German dyslexic children were assessed with a single-item presentation task. The children were presented with a word or nonword spelling on a computer screen. They were asked to read the item as quickly as possible, allowing us to assess both reading accuracy and reading speed. Reading speed was measured from the onset of presentation until the child pressed a reaction-time button before he gave his response. We presented items of one-, two- and three-syllable length. All words had similar spellings and pronunciations and identical meaning in the two languages (e.g. *ball–Ball*, *summer–Sommer*, *discussion–Diskussion*). The one- and two-syllable nonwords were derived from the words by exchanging the consonants at the beginning of the words. For example, the English nonword *hoat* was derived by replacing the first consonant of *b-oat* with the first consonant of the word *h-and*. Similarly, the German nonword *Hoot* was derived from *Hand* and *Boot*. For the three-syllable nonwords the syllables of the three-syllable words were rearranged. For example, the English nonword *ralective* was constructed by combining the first syllable of *radio*, the second syllable of *electric* and the third syllable of *positive*. The German equivalent of this nonword is *Ralektiv*. This method of item construction ensured that both word and nonword items were similar for the two language groups and that no orthographically illegal units occurred.

The mean percentage of errors as well as the mean reading times for correctly read items are presented in Figure 2.1. From the upper section of Figure 2.1 it is obvious that overall, the English dyslexic children made many

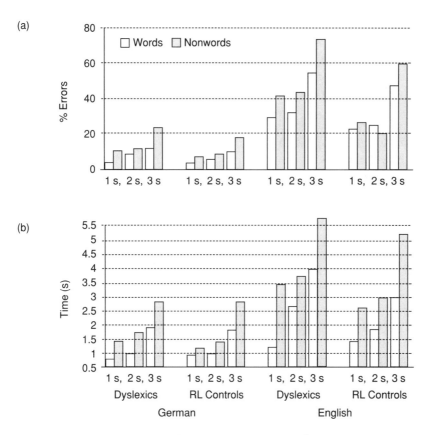

Figure 2.1 Mean percentage of errors and mean reading times for word and nonword reading for German and English dyslexic and reading-level (RL) control children. 1 s, one syllable; 2 s, two syllables; 3 s, three syllables.

more errors than the German dyslexic children. There was no overlap in mean error percentages: the German dyslexic children read the three-syllable nonwords (the most difficult item category) more accurately than the English dyslexic children read the one-syllable words (the easiest category). Figure 2.1 also shows that the increase in errors with increasing syllable length as well as the increase from words to nonwords was larger for the English than for the German dyslexics. Both groups of dyslexic children read the words as accurately as the corresponding reading level control group but showed reliably lower reading accuracy for nonwords, although due to the generally high reading accuracy of the German children the difference is not as marked as for the English children.

A direct consequence of orthographic consistency is the difference in the number of errors where the vowel grapheme(s) of word items was misread, in the sense that a possible but inappropriate grapheme–phoneme relation was used (e.g. /li:θə/ or /liəθə/ for *leather*, /tigə/ for *tiger*). Overall, there were 324 instances of incorrect pronunciations of the first vowel grapheme in the word items among the word reading errors of the English dyslexic children, while only 20 such vowel misreadings were observed among the German dyslexic children. Another typical error type was consonant intrusion like 'blend' or [brind] for the English nonword *biend*, or [breind] for the German nonword *Beund*. Such consonant intrusions occurred 310 times for the English dyslexic children and 67 times for the German dyslexic children.

A frequently occurring error among the English dyslexic children was that a similar word was read for a word item (e.g. *friend* ➔ *'find'*) or a nonword item (e.g. *brined* ➔ *'blind'*). For the three-syllable word *character*, five different erroneous word responses occurred ('chancellor', 'calendar', 'calculator', 'charger' and 'tractor'). Overall, the English dyslexic children produced erroneous word responses to 14% of all word items and 6% of all nonword items. Due to the comparatively few errors of the German dyslexic children, only 2% of the word and 1% of the nonword items led to wrong word responses. Another observation was that many different readings were produced by the English dyslexic children for the same item. For the three-syllable nonwords, English dyslexic children produced, on average, 14 different pronunciations. This means that most of the 18 children created a novel pronunciation.

In summary, the German dyslexic children showed much better reading accuracy than the English dyslexic children and were less affected by increasing item length and by word–nonword variation. However, dyslexic readers of both language groups showed more reading errors for nonwords than much younger reading-level controls. This is in line with the many studies with English dyslexics reviewed by Rack et al. (1992).

The lower section of Figure 2.1 presents the mean reading times per item. The pattern of results for reading speed largely complements the error results, even though only reading times for correctly read items were included. Overall, the English dyslexic children showed longer reading times than the German dyslexic children and a larger word–nonword difference, particularly for the one-syllable items. The increase in reading time with increasing item length was similar for both groups. Both dyslexic groups showed a specific reading speed impairment, especially for nonwords, in relation to their reading-level controls, although this impairment was only reliable for the English children and was rather small for the German children.

Thus, as was expected, orthographic consistency does have an important influence on dyslexic children's reading performance. German dyslexic children show surprisingly high reading accuracy for both words and nonwords. This is the case even for items of three-syllable length that pose enormous difficulties to English dyslexic readers. German dyslexics also show considerably quicker reading speed than their English counterparts. However, it is important to note that their reading speed is nevertheless remarkably slow and similar to that of the considerably younger reading-level controls. For German texts, words of three- and four-syllable length are not atypical and a mean reading time of 2 to 3 seconds, as was achieved by the participants of the present study for three-syllable words and nonwords, is a considerable restriction of their reading fluency. German dyslexic children's reading speed was not even normal for short, high-frequency words. For a subset of one- and two-syllable high-frequency words, the German dyslexic children showed a mean reading time of 0.7s while a group of normally developing readers of the same age needed only 0.5s to recognize these items. This difference was reliable.

In another reading task, English and German children were presented with words that were not only similar, but in fact identical in the two languages (Landerl, 1996). Most of the items were words of English origin that are widely used foreign words in German (e.g. *Computer*, *Jeans*, *Walkman*). Half the presented word spellings were not pronounced according to the consistent grapheme–phoneme correspondences of German orthography and were thus irregular in German. We could therefore get some information about how German dyslexic children deal with irregular words that are very atypical for the orthography they are acquiring. The other half of the items conformed to German grapheme–phoneme correspondences and were thus regular in German (e.g. *Film*, *Hotel*, *Professor*). For these regular word spellings, the percentage of errors was once again considerably lower for the German than for the English dyslexic children (5.3% versus 27.6% errors). However, for the irregular words, the mean percentage of errors was as high for German as for English dyslexics (28.4% versus 25.4% errors). Two-thirds of the German dyslexic children's errors were regularizations, that is the children pronounced the word spellings according to the grapheme–phoneme correspondences of German (e.g. /gentlemən/ for *Gentleman*, or /walkmən/ for *Walkman*). Thus, once again it became evident that these children were competent in decoding grapheme sequences, but that this strategy was not efficient for the irregular items. It seems remarkable that the German dyslexic children's performance on these irregular words was not worse than that of the English dyslexics, since the presented words were familiar to the English children both with respect to pronunciation and orthographic structure, while the German children had to read foreign words based on unfamiliar orthographic structure.

In summary, the direct comparison of the two language groups shows that the reading difficulties of German dyslexic children are less severe than those of English dyslexic children. In general, reading accuracy is high, showing that in contrast to English dyslexic children, the German children are self-reliant readers and can decode more or less every grapheme sequence, although this decoding process is slow and sometimes extremely laborious. This is the pattern of reading performance that we typically find in German samples of dyslexic readers (Wimmer, 1993; Wimmer et al., 1998). The most obvious reason for German dyslexic children's comparably competent decoding abilities is the high consistency of the orthography that they acquire.

Cognitive deficits

The findings reported so far show that German dyslexic children's phonological decoding abilities are comparably good. A specific deficit in nonword reading for which phonological decoding abilities are indispensable is a consistent finding among English dyslexic children and this has been interpreted as one of the main consequences of an underlying phonological deficit (Rack et al., 1992). Although German dyslexic children made significantly more errors and showed reliably higher reading times than reading-level controls, their nonword reading accuracy is high in absolute terms and their reading speed is clearly higher than that of the English dyslexic children with whom they were compared. The question then is whether the reading difficulties of German dyslexic children are in fact due to a deficit in phonological processing? Or do we have to look for other cognitive deficits that might underlie their impairment?

Wimmer (1993) carried out several phonological processing tasks with samples of 8- to 10-year old German dyslexic children. One of the tasks was vowel substitution, where all vowels of verbally presented words and short sentences had to be replaced by the vowel /i/. This task requires segmentation of the presented word into its phonemic constituents, an explicit manipulation on the vowel phonemes and blending of the phonemes into a coherent pronunciation. Such explicit phoneme awareness tasks have been shown to pose specific difficulties for English dyslexic children and even adults (see Snowling, 1995, for a review). The 10-year-old normally developed German readers tested by Wimmer (1993) substituted 28.6 of the 30 vowels correctly. The dyslexic children of this age group provided 25.8 correct substitutions. Thus, it is obvious that the dyslexics were also quite able to perform the required phonemic manipulations. Their performance was significantly worse than that of the age-level control group, but did not differ from the performance of a group of grade 2 children who showed the same reading level (25.9 correct substitutions).

German dyslexic children's good phoneme awareness skills are also evident from a nonword spelling task, which requires not only correct segmentation of the speech stream, but also identification and translation into an adequate grapheme for each phoneme. Here, the finding is that although German dyslexic children have some difficulty in acquiring the process of nonword spelling in the first months of formal schooling, their performance is typically very accurate from grade 2 onwards (Wimmer, 1993, 1996).

A plausible reason for German dyslexic children's comparably good performance on phonemic awareness tasks is that the combination of a consistent orthography and the straightforward phonics teaching approach they experience is an excellent and intense training in phonemic awareness. Perhaps German dyslexic children's cognitive deficits become more clearly evident in tasks that are not as closely related to their reading abilities. In our direct comparison of dyslexia in German and English (Landerl et al., 1997) we confronted our subjects with a more complex phonological awareness task (spoonerisms) for which the consonantal onsets of two verbally presented words had to be exchanged (e.g. *man-hat* ➔ [han]-[mat]; *brown-fox* ➔ [fown]-[brox]). The task proved to be quite difficult even for 12-year-old normally developed readers (31.7% and 39.5% errors for German and English children). Interestingly, both groups of dyslexic children had comparable difficulties with this task (63.3% and 72.9% errors for German and English children respectively) and the German dyslexic children's performance was actually significantly worse than that of the matched group of 8-year-old reading-level controls (42.9% errors).

This was an important finding as it shows that German as well as English dyslexic children do have difficulties in the phonological domain. However, the spoonerism task is a very complex task involving segmentation and blending skills as well as phonological working memory processes. In detail, two words must be adequately segmented into onsets and rimes and then the segmented linguistic units must be held in phonological working memory until the onset of the second word is correctly blended with the rime of the first word and the onset of the first word is correctly blended with the rime of the second word (or the other way round). We cannot determine from children's poor performance alone which of these cognitive processes poses the problem for dyslexic children.

A consistent finding is that German dyslexic children have difficulties with rapid automatized naming tasks (Wimmer, 1993; Landerl, 1996). These tasks require the child to name a sequence of object drawings or colours or numerals as quickly as possible. Slow automatized naming is also reported for English dyslexic children (Wolf, 1991). One interpretation of this deficit is that it is also an indicator of the underlying phonological deficit of dyslexia. If phonological representations (i.e. mental representations of word pronunciations) are less accessible in dyslexic than in normal readers, this would explain why it takes them longer to activate these representations in rapid automatized naming tasks, and it would also explain why dyslexic children have difficulties performing explicit phonemic manipulations on these representations. But interestingly, the correlation between phonological awareness tasks and rapid automatized naming tasks is surprisingly low (Bowers, 1989; Wimmer 1993), suggesting that the deficit in rapid automatized naming has a different origin.

Some researchers suggest that dyslexia is caused by a general deficit in automatization skills (Nicolson and Fawcett, 1990). Such a general automatization deficit would of course also explain dyslexic children's deficit in rapid automatized naming tasks. Although this automatization deficit theory of dyslexia was put forward for English readers, it is especially interesting for German, for two reasons. First, the evidence on phonological processing deficits among German dyslexic children is inconsistent. Second, as was demonstrated in the first part of this chapter, reading accuracy is usually quite high in German dyslexics; their main reading problem is extremely low reading speed. Such a speed deficit would, of course, be compatible with a general deficit in automatization skills. In a recent study, we compared the phonological deficit and the general automatization deficit account with each other (Wimmer et al., 1998). In the course of a longitudinal study, the aim of which was to examine reading development over the primary school years, groups of 27 dyslexic and 20 closely matched control children were selected at the end of grade 2. The first assessment was done at the beginning of grade 1.

Several tasks assessed children's phonological processing abilities. At the beginning of grade 1, a rather simple rhyme detection task (e.g. 'What rhymes with *Feld*: *Geld* or *Gold*?') and an alliteration detection task (e.g. '*Mutter–Nadel–Beeren*: which word starts with /m/?') were carried out. At the end of grade 2, speech perception was assessed in two conditions. In the dual-speaker condition, the child heard a male and a female voice speaking different sentences at the same time and had to repeat the voice that was specified by the experimenter. In the second condition, the sentence that had to be repeated was masked by different levels of party noise. Phonological short-term memory was assessed in both grades 1 and 2 with different pseudoword repetition tasks. Furthermore, we developed a pseudoname learning task, which was carried out in grade 2. Here, children were shown drawings of three fantasy animals one after the other and were told their pseudoword names. The test trials then followed. The child was presented with one of the three animals and had to say the name. If the pseudoname could not be given correctly, it was provided by the experimenter and the child had to repeat it. The number of trials it took for all three pseudonames to be given correctly was counted. Thus, in contrast to pseudo-word repetition tasks, in which the items are typically repeated immediately after presentation, this task requires somewhat longer storage of unknown phonological sequences in memory.

The relevant task with respect to general automatization skills was a dual task that was developed by the proponents of this theory, Nicolson and Fawcett (1990, 1995). A general cognitive deficit in automatization skills should not only be evident in language processing, but also in other cognitive domains like motor skills that require a high degree of automatization. According to Nicolson and Fawcett, balancing qualifies as such a motor skill task, especially when conscious effort to compensate is prevented. In the sighted condition, the child had to stand one-legged on a beam for 30s. Error points were given if the child moved his arms to keep his balance, tapped the floor with his free foot or stepped down from the beam. In the dual-task condition, a semantic categorization task had to be performed while balancing on the beam, i.e. a sequence of nouns was presented from an audio tape and the child had to decide by a verbal 'yes' or 'no' response whether the noun denoted an animal. Finally, in the third condition children had to balance blindfolded. This task was carried out in grade 2.

Two other tasks that were performed at the beginning of grade 1 also assessed non-verbal skills. In a peg-moving task modelled after Annett (1985), the child had to move ten pegs from one line of holes in a wooden frame into the holes of a second line as quickly as possible. And in a visual search task the child had to cross out as quickly as possible all the drawings of apples in an upright position and ignore all apples with different orientation on a working sheet with seven lines of 12 apples each. Finally, rapid automatized naming skills and articulation speed were assessed both in grades 1 and 2.

Interestingly, these rapid naming tasks differentiated best between the dyslexic and the control children. But remember that deficits in naming speed can basically be caused by a phonological deficit as well as by a deficit in general automatization skills. The only other tasks that differentiated reliably between dyslexic and control children were the phonological memory tasks (pseudoname learning and the two pseudoword repetition tasks). There was absolutely no evidence for a deficit in balancing skills. In fact, dyslexic children's performance was identical to that of the control group in all three balancing conditions. The differences for the two other non-verbal tasks, peg moving and visual search were also not reliable. The visual search task is also relevant with respect to the classic theory that dyslexic children have difficulties in coding the exact visuospatial orientation of letter patterns. As was found in many earlier studies (e.g. Vellutino, 1979), there is no evidence for such a visual deficit in our German dyslexic sample.

The dyslexic sample tended to show somewhat poorer performance on the grade 1 alliteration detection task (77% versus 86% correct responses), but performance on the rhyme detection task was as good as that of the control group (85% versus 89% correct responses). In grade 1, dyslexic children showed slightly lower articulation speed than the control group, but in grade 2, there was no difference at all between the two groups. And on the speech perception task, there was a minimal difference between dyslexic and control children in the party noise background condition (69% versus 73% correct), but no difference in the simultaneous speaker condition (62% correct for both groups).

In summary, we could not confirm findings suggesting that dyslexia is caused by a general deficit in automatization skills. This theoretical account seemed even more interesting for German than for English, because although German dyslexic children acquire competent decoding skills early in their reading development, these skills do not reach the same level of automatization and fluency as in normal readers. A follow-up study in our lab (Wimmer et al., 1999) suggests that balancing skills are more closely related to attention deficit/hyperactivity (ADHD) than to dyslexia. A comorbidity of the two syndromes is well established (Pennington, 1991). A plausible explanation for findings suggesting deficits in balancing skills in dyslexic children is that only those dyslexics who show ADHD symptoms in addition to their reading difficulties perform poorly in this task.

On the other hand, there was clear evidence for difficulties in the phonological domain. Thus, as found for English, specific reading difficulties are due to a phonological deficit in the consistent German orthographic system. Interestingly, the phonological deficits of our German dyslexic children were more or less limited to the memory tasks and not evident in the receptive language tasks of speech perception and phonological awareness (alliteration and rhyme detection). The serious difficulties of our German dyslexic sample with pseudoword repetition and pseudoname learning are consistent with findings on English children (Vellutino et al., 1975; Snowling et al., 1986; Brady et al., 1987, 1989; Gathercole and Baddeley, 1990; Aguiar and Brady, 1991). Wimmer (1993) found no reliable pseudoword repetition deficit for another sample of German dyslexic children. The difficulty level of the task seems to be crucial for detecting the dyslexic deficit.

The negative finding with respect to speech perception is surprising in comparison to other empirical research showing clear speech perception deficits in dyslexic children (e.g. Werker and Tees, 1987; Reed, 1989). However, it should be noted that our task is rather crude in comparison to the refined measures of categorical phoneme perception used in these studies. The negative finding with respect to alliteration and rhyme detection also stands in contrast to findings with English children (e.g. Bradley and Bryant, 1978). One factor that might explain these different findings is that memory load is considerably larger in the Bradley and Bryant task, where children have to identify the odd one out of three or four items (e.g. *nod-red-fed-bed*). A previous study with older German dyslexic children used Bradley and Bryant's rhyme detection task and found a small deficit compared to age-matched control children (Wimmer, 1993).

How can deficits in naming speed and phonological memory processes cause difficulties in learning to read? A possible developmental course could be as follows. As a first consequence of deficits in phonological memory, one could expect children who later develop dyslexia to show a considerable delay in vocabulary development because it takes them longer to store new phoneme sequences in memory. However, although there is a close connection between language impairments and dyslexia (Catts, 1993), many dyslexic children do not show early language impairments severe enough to be diagnosed. Perhaps these children are able to establish the same number of phonological representations as other children, but their representations are less distinct (Rack et al., 1994; Elbro, 1996). Thus, their communicative skills are largely normal; only their pronunciations of certain words might sometimes be corrected by adults. And perhaps their somewhat sloppy pronunciations and word-finding difficulties are quite often not even recognized. In fact, recent studies show that children who later develop dyslexia or are at genetic risk for dyslexia because they have a dyslexic parent, show a delay in vocabulary development in the pre-school years (Scarborough, 1990; Frith, 1997).

This subtle language deficit becomes a serious problem once the child learns to read. In reading acquisition, representations of the sound structure of word pronunciations have to be stored in memory as earlier in language development, but this time in the form of letter sequences. Thus, we propose that orthographic representations are very similar to phonological representations and, indeed, models by Ehri (1992) and Perfetti (1992) suggest that the two kinds of representation are closely connected with each other. But in contrast to the earlier phase of language acquisition, storage of underspecified orthographic representations is no longer sufficient, so that the deficit in phonological memory leads to severe reading and spelling difficulties.

An illustrative example from German is the spelling of voiced and unvoiced stop consonants, which typically poses a serious problem for dyslexic children (Klicpera and Gasteiger-Klicpera, 1998). The standard explanation of this problem is that dyslexic children cannot clearly perceive the phonological difference between voiced and unvoiced stops. However, in the Austrian version of German, the phonological distinction between voiced and unvoiced stops is quite often neutralized, which means that there is no perceptual difference that would tell the child which words are spelled with unvoiced and which ones with voiced stops. For example, the first sounds in the words *packen* (English: to pack) and *backen* (English: to bake) are pronounced identically. Thus, the phonological representations of young children probably do not specify the phonological feature of voicing. When confronted with word spellings, children must specify if they are spelled with *p* or *b*. Whether this specification is added to children's underlying phonological representations of the particular words, or if the *b/p* distinction is only represented in the newly established orthographic representation, is open to further research. But it is obvious that this additional specification is usually no major problem for young readers and, in fact, many adults are sure that the words *packen* and *backen* are *pronounced* differently, although only the spellings are different. Dyslexic children, however, have serious and consistent problems memorizing whether a word is spelled with *b* or with *p*. An analogous English example is that many people are convinced that the word 'pitch' includes one sound more than the word 'rich' only because the spelling consists of one more letter (Ehri and Wilce, 1980)

Empirical evidence for dyslexic children's difficulty in establishing fully specified orthographic representations comes from Reitsma (1983), Lemoine et al. (1993) and Ehri and Saltmarsh (1995). In English, full specification of an orthographic representation is probably even more difficult than in German. Studies by Ehri and Wilce (1985) and Rack et al. (1994) show that orthographic representations that are consistent with the word pronunciation are easier to store. This would be a further explanation for the more serious reading difficulties of English in comparison with German dyslexic children described in the first part of this chapter.

The deficit in naming speed could simply be a consequence of the under-specified phonological representations. Perhaps these representations are not as accessible as fully specified ones and perhaps it takes slightly longer to set up an articulatory programme if not all of the features necessary for the phonetic output are specified in the phonological representation. Another account put forward by Bowers (1995) suggests a direct causal contribution of naming speed deficits to the deficit in orthographic memory. The argument here is that the establishment of memory representations for letter sequences cannot proceed smoothly if activation of the phonemes corresponding to each grapheme is too slow, such that no associations between the graphemes of the sequence can be formed. This would mean that dyslexic children do not learn to perceive larger orthographic units like typical syllables or morphemes as wholes.

Summary

The findings on dyslexia in German-speaking children reviewed in this chapter show that, as expected, orthographic consistency does have an important influence on reading abilities. German dyslexic children read more accurately and also considerably faster than a matched sample of English dyslexics. Lexicality (word versus nonword) and item length had more detrimental effects on English than on German children's performance. Even on irregular word spellings, which are very rare in German orthography and can only occur for foreign words, the performance of German dyslexics was not poorer than that of the English dyslexic sample. Consistent with the findings in English children, German dyslexic children showed a specific deficit in nonword reading, that is they read nonwords less accurately and more slowly than reading-age control children who were four years younger. Although the difference in nonword reading abilities was comparatively small, this finding can be interpreted as the first evidence that German dyslexic children also have specific difficulties with the phonological component of reading. However, the combination of a consistent orthography and a straightforward phonics teaching approach that emphasizes blending and segmentation processes enables dyslexic children to develop quite competent decoding abilities. Their reading accuracy is typically high, but their reading speed is deficient both for words and nonwords, showing that the processes of word recognition and nonword decoding do not reach the same level or automatization as for normal readers.

Further evidence that the phonological deficit hypothesis holds for dyslexia in German as well as English comes from studies showing that cognitive deficits are limited to this domain. Our research did not find any deficits in detailed visual processing abilities or general automatization skills. On the other hand, we found consistent deficits in rapid automatized naming and phonological memory. The findings of deficits in phoneme awareness that are so impressively evident in English dyslexic children and even adults, are inconsistent for German dyslexics. Probably the intensive training in phoneme blending and segmentation that German children receive via phonics teaching helps to compensate for such deficits, so that difficulties only become apparent in more complex tasks like spoonerisms (*brown-fox* ➜ [fown]-[brox]), which place heavy demands on phonological working memory.

In summary, we can conclude that dyslexia in German is caused by a deficit in phonological processing, but due to the high consistency of German orthography, children with such a deficit are less handicapped in their reading development than English dyslexic children for whom the high complexity of English orthography obviously poses an additional problem. Finally, I would like to express the hope that our findings on dyslexia in German help to stimulate more research on dyslexia in orthographies other than English, which will tell us more about how this impairment is influenced by the properties of a particular language or orthography. This kind of cross-language research makes an important contribution to our knowledge of dyslexia.

Acknowledgements

The research reported in this chapter was supported by grants from the Austrian Ministry of Science to Karin Landerl and the Austrian Science Foundation to Heinz Wimmer.

References

Aguiar L, Brady S (1991) Vocabulary acquisition and reading ability. Reading and Writing 3: 413-425.

Annett M (1985) Left, right, hand and brain: the right shift theory. Hillsdale, NJ: Erlbaum.

Bowers PG (1989) Naming speed and phonological awareness: independent contributors to reading disabilities. In S McCormich, J Zutell (eds) Cognitive and social perspectives for literacy research and instruction: 38th yearbook of the National Reading Conference, pp 165-172. Chicago: National Reading Conference.

Bowers PG (1995) A speculative account of several factors affecting the development of orthographic skill. Paper presented at the symposium of the American Education Research Association, San Francisco, April.

Bradley L, Bryant P (1978) Difficulties in auditory organisation as a possible cause of reading backwardness. Nature 271: 746-747.

Brady S, Mann V, Schmidt R (1987) Errors in short-term memory for good and poor readers. Memory and Cognition 15: 444-453.

Brady S, Poggie E, Rapala MM (1989) Speech repetition abilities in children who differ in reading skill. Language and Speech 32: 109-122.

Catts H (1993) The relationship between speech-language impairments and reading disabilities. Journal of Speech and Hearing Research 36: 948-958.

Ehri LC (1992) Reconceptualizing the development of sight word reading and its relationship to recoding. In P Gough, LC Ehri, R Treiman (eds) Reading acquisition, pp 107-143. Hillsdale, NJ: Lawrence Erlbaum Associates.

Ehri LC, Saltmarsh J (1995) Beginning readers outperform older disabled readers in learning to read words by sight. Reading and Writing 7: 295-326.

Ehri LC, Wilce LS (1980) The influence of orthography on readers' reconceptualisation of the phonemic structure of words. Applied Psycholinguistics 1: 371-385.

Ehri LC, Wilce LS (1985) Movement into reading: is the first stage of printed word learning visual or phonetic? Reading Research Quarterly 20: 163-179.

Eibl L, Lampée-Baumgartner T, Borries W, Tauschek E (1996). Mimi die Lesemaus [Mimi the reading mouse], 6th edn. Linz: Veritas.

Elbro C (1996) Early linguistic abilities and reading development: a review and a hypothesis. Reading and Writing 8: 453-485.

Frith U (1997) Brain, mind and behaviour in dyslexia. In C Hulme, M Snowling (eds) Dyslexia: biology, cognition and intervention, pp 1-19. London: Whurr.

Gathercole SE, Baddeley AD (1990) The role of phonological memory in vocabulary acquisition: a study of young children learning new names. British Journal of Psychology 81: 439-454.

Gleitman LR, Rozin P (1977) The structure and acquisition of reading I: Relations between orthographies and the structure of language. In AS Reber, DL Scarborough (eds) Towards a psychology of reading, pp 1-53. Hillsdale, NJ: Erlbaum.

Klicpera C, Gasteiger-Klicpera B (1998) Differenzierung zwischen orthographischem Wissen und phonologischem Rekodieren im Rechtschreiben bei guten und schwachen Schülern der 2. bis 4. Klasse Grundschule [Differentiation between orthographic knowledge and phonological recoding in spelling for good and poor pupils from grade 2 to 4]. Paper presented at the 41st congress of the German Society of Psychology, Dresden, Germany, September.

Landerl K (1996) Legasthenie in Deutsch und Englisch [Dyslexia in German and English]. Frankfurt: Peter Lang.

Landerl K, Wimmer H, Frith U (1997) The impact of orthographic consistency on dyslexia: A German–English comparison. Cognition 63: 315–334.

Lemoine HE, Levy BA, Hutchinson A (1993) Increasing the naming speed of poor readers: representations formed across repetitions. Journal of Experimental Child Psychology 55: 297–328.

Liberman IY (1982) A language-oriented view of reading and its disabilities. In H Myklebust (ed) Progress in learning disabilities, vol 5, pp 91–101. New York: Grune and Stratton.

Liberman IY, Liberman AM, Mattingly IG, Shankweiler DL (1980) Orthography and the beginning reader. In JF Kavannagh, RL Venezky (eds) Orthography, reading and dyslexia, pp 137–153. Baltimore: University Park Press.

Nicolson RI, Fawcett AJ (1990) Automaticity: a new framework for dyslexia research. Cognition 35: 159–182.

Nicolson RI, Fawcett AJ (1995) Dyslexia is more than a phonological disability. Dyslexia 1: 19–36.

Pennington BF (1991) Diagnosing learning disorders: a neuropsychological framework. New York: Guilford Press.

Perfetti CA (1992) The representation problem in reading acquisition. In PB Gough, LC Ehri, R Treiman (eds) Reading acquisition, pp 145–174. Hillsdale, NJ: Erlbaum.

Rack JP, Hulme C, Snowling MJ, Wightman J (1994) The role of phonology in young children learning to read words: the direct mapping hypothesis. Journal of Experimental Child Psychology 57: 42–71.

Rack JP, Snowling MJ, Olson R (1992) The nonword reading deficit in developmental dyslexia: a review. Reading Research Quarterly 27: 29–53.

Reed MA (1989). Speech perception and the discrimination of brief auditory cues in reading disabled children. Journal of Experimental Child Psychology 48: 270–292.

Reitsma P (1983) Printed word learning in beginning readers. Journal of Experimental Child Psychology 36: 321–339.

Scarborough HS (1990) Very early language deficits in dyslexic children. Child Development 61: 1728–1743.

Snowling MJ (1995) Phonological processing and developmental dyslexia. Journal of Research in Reading 18: 132–138.

Snowling MJ, Goulandris N, Bowlby M, Howell P (1986) Segmentation and speech perception in relation to reading skill: a developmental analysis. Journal of Experimental Child Psychology 48: 270–292.

Vellutino FR (1979) Dyslexia: theory and research. Cambridge, MA: MIT Press.

Vellutino FR, Steger JA, Harding CJ, Phillips F (1975) Verbal vs non-verbal paired-associates learning in poor and normal readers. Neuropsychologia 13: 75–82.

Werker JF, Tees RC (1987) Speech perception in severely disabled and average reading children. Canadian Journal of Psychology 41: 48-61.

Wimmer H (1993) Characteristics of developmental dyslexia in a regular writing system. Applied Psycholinguistics 14: 1–33.

Wimmer H (1996) The early manifestation of developmental dyslexia: evidence from German children. Reading and Writing 8: 171–188.

Wimmer H, Mayringer H, Landerl K (1998) Poor reading: a deficit in skill-automatization or a phonological deficit? Scientific Studies of Reading 2: 321–340.

Wimmer H, Mayringer H, Raberger T (1999) Reading and balancing: evidence against the automatization deficit explanation of developmental dyslexia. Journal of Learning Disabilities 32: 473–478.

Wolf M (1991) Naming and reading: the contribution of the cognitive neurosciences. Reading Research Quarterly 26: 123–140.

CHAPTER 3

Problems in the acquisition of fluent word decoding in Dutch children

PETER F DE JONG

The acquisition of reading involves the gradual development of connections between the spoken and the written forms of words. In alphabetic writing systems (orthographies), children have to learn the systematic correspondences between letters or multi-letter units and the sounds in spoken words (Ehri, 1998). This knowledge can be used to decode most words and, accordingly, might serve as a self-teaching mechanism for the development of word specific orthographic knowledge (Share, 1995).

In this chapter, the major determinants of learning to read fluently in Dutch are discussed. In addition, the specific deficits of those children who have problems with the acquisition of fluent reading and some attempts aimed to remediate these problems are described. First, however, a brief description will be given of the linguistic and educational environment in which Dutch children learn to read (for a more extensive description see Reitsma and Verhoeven, 1990).

Learning to read in Dutch

Two aspects of the environment seem to affect the development of early reading acquisition. One is the consistency of the grapheme-to-phoneme mappings in the language in which a child learns to read (e.g. Wimmer and Goswami, 1994). The other aspect is the particular teaching method used to reveal the relations between the spoken and written form of words.

Orthography

In Dutch orthography, the mapping of graphemes to phonemes is far more consistent than in English, but there is no perfect one-to-one correspondence as, for example, in Finnish. The Dutch orthography has about the same level of consistency as the German orthography. As in many languages, the grapheme–phoneme relations, which are important for reading, are more consistent than the phoneme–grapheme relations, which are used for spelling (Bosman and Van Orden, 1997). Because reading acquisition is the major topic of this chapter, the brief description of Dutch orthography will focus on grapheme–phoneme correspondences.

The 26 letters of the Roman alphabet are used to represent about 35 to 40 phonemes. A number of phonemes, primarily vowels, are symbolized by digraphs. Most of the consonant–grapheme relationships are entirely consistent. Exceptions are the letters *b* and *d*, which are normally pronounced as a voiced stop, but which represent the voiceless stops /p/ and /t/, respectively at the end of the word. This is a consequence of one of the principles of Dutch orthography, the principle of congruence, which states that a word's spelling is consistent across all derivations and compounds of the word. For example, while the *d* in *hond* (English: dog) is pronounced as /t/, it is written with a *d* because in the plural form, *honden*, the *d* is pronounced as /d/. Other exceptions are the digraphs *nk* and *ng*, which correspond to a single phoneme when they appear at the end of a syllable, as for example in *wang* (cheek), but otherwise reflect two separate phonemes as in *wangedrag* (misbehaviour).

The majority of the vowels are represented by digraphs. With one exception, these digraphs represent only one vowel. A number of graphemes (*a*, *o*, *e* and *u*) can indicate either long or short vowels, depending on their place in a syllable. At the end of a syllable these graphemes reflect long vowels, as in *pa* (daddy) and *boten* (boats). But, whenever a syllable ends with a consonant, called closed syllable the vowel sound is short, as in *pas* (step) or *bot* (bone). To represent a long vowel within a closed syllable, the grapheme is doubled and accordingly turned into a digraph. Thus, the long vowel in *boten* (boats) is doubled in its singular form *boot* (boat), otherwise it would read as *bot* (bone). However, to preserve the short vowel of *bot* (bone) in its plural form, the final consonant is doubled and the plural becomes *botten* (bones) so that it can be distinguished from boten (boats).

The most inconsistent grapheme is the *e*, as it maps on to at least three vowels, including the schwa, and can also be part of a digraph. As a schwa, *e* is often part of an affix. To read polysyllabic words that include an *e*, it is often necessary to divide a written word into its constituent morphemic units (Reitsma and Verhoeven, 1990). For example, *paarden* (horses) consists of the morphemes *paard* (horse) and *en* (more than one) in which case the *e* is a schwa (see also van Bon, 1993).

Though Dutch orthography has several inconsistencies, many words can be read by the straightforward translation of letters into sounds. Moreover, many departures from a one-to-one correspondence of graphemes to phonemes are rule-based. The least systematic relations between graphemes and phonemes are found in words that have been adopted from other languages, especially English and French. Due to the adherence of the etymological principle, in Dutch orthography the written forms of these words, as for example the word *cake*, have usually not been altered.

Reading instruction

In the Dutch school system, children enter primary school at the age of 4. The first two years encompass kindergarten. In these years, the children are predominantly engaged in various play activities, more general language activities, for example to support vocabulary acquisition, and some activities to improve fine motor control. Reading and reading-related skills are generally not taught. Teachers in kindergarten do not introduce the letters and their sounds. Phonological skills, other than rhyming, are not systematically trained. During this period, the acquisition of letter knowledge and phonological skills depend on the child and its home literacy environment. However, Dutch parents are not inclined to teach letter knowledge either. Alphabet books are seldom used at this age. Consequently, by the end of kindergarten the majority of children have little letter knowledge and their development of phonological abilities has just begun.

Formal instruction in reading starts in grade 1. By then the mean age of the children is 6 years and 5 months. Early reading instruction involves a great amount of phonics (Reitsma and Verhoeven, 1990; Blok and Otter, 1997). Most methods focus right from the start on the correspondence between graphemes in written and phonemes in spoken words. Initially, children are presented with four to six words. This written form has to be memorized. Then, a letter-to-sound rule is taught by presenting the word(s) that contain the letter of interest. For example, in one method, the word *maan* (moon) is initially used to illustrate the connection between the letter *m* and the sound /m/. Later on it is used to relate *aa* to /a/. After the introduction of several letter-to-sound rules, exercises are given to teach discrimination of the letters in the written form. In addition, children are taught to reflect on the sound structure of spoken words by means of activities such as phoneme deletion or the detection of phonemes in various positions in a word. Importantly, in most teaching methods, instruction about the sound structure of spoken words is linked to a manipulation of their written forms. For example, to illustrate the deletion of the /m/ from *maan* the letter *m* is deleted from its written form. Children are also given spelling and writing exercises from an early stage of learning.

After about five months of reading instruction most children are able to decode simple and regularly spelled written words. Such words can be accurately decoded by straightforward letter-to-sound translation and the blending of these sounds into the spoken form of the word. This method of decoding is therefore encouraged in the first six months of reading instruc-tion. Accordingly, children have a self-teaching mechanism at their disposal for the acquisition of word-specific knowledge. In the second half of the first year, deviations from one-to-one letter sound relations are introduced. In addition, the sensitivity for high-frequency, multi-letter units is stimulated to enhance sight word reading.

Determinants of early reading acquisition

Current belief is that phonological processing abilities are a major determi-nant of learning to read. Three types of phonological abilities can be distin-guished: phonological awareness, phonological coding in short-term memory (verbal short-term memory) and the retrieval of phonological codes from long-term memory (rapid naming). Phonological awareness refers to the sensitivity for and the accessibility of speech sounds in spoken words. Verbal working memory entails the temporary storage of verbal information. Rapid naming relates to the speed of access to the pronunciations of letters, digits and words.

A continuum of levels of phonological awareness can be distinguished with awareness of phonemes at the highest level and awareness for larger sound units, as rhymes and syllables, reflecting lower levels of awareness. Phonological awareness at the level of phonemes (phonemic awareness) is considered especially important for early reading acquisition. However, a considerable body of evidence now suggests that, in turn, the development of phonemic awareness is dependent on the acquisition of reading or reading-related skills. This has led several researchers to suggest a bi-direc-tional (Wagner et al., 1994) or even interactive (Perfetti, 1992) relationship between the development of phonemic awareness and reading acquisition.

The interactive view of this relationship holds that phonological aware-ness and reading ability develop simultaneously. However, as argued by Perfetti (1992), which skill develops more rapidly is determined by the linguistic and educational environment in which a child learns to read. In the Dutch educational system, the development of reading and letter knowledge during kindergarten will be minimal, as these are not taught. From the start of reading instruction in grade 1, emphasis is on letter–sound relations and the manipulation of sounds in words. During the first months of reading instruc-tion an acceleration of the development of phonological awareness can be expected. Indeed, such a sharp increase was observed by Mommers (1990), who tested an at-risk and a no-risk group of children every two weeks from the start of kindergarten. At the beginning of grade 1 none of the at-risk children and just about half of the no-risk children were able to segment simple words consisting of two to four phonemes. However, after about four months of reading instruction all children from the no-risk group and about half of the children from the at-risk group could segment these words perfectly. Mommers (1990) concluded that such a rapid development of phonemic awareness is not due to the development of more general cognitive abilities but should be attributed to reading instruction.

More recently, Wesseling and Reitsma (1998) assessed phonemic awareness from the second year in kindergarten through January of grade 1. Phonemic awareness was minimal halfway through the second year of kindergarten. A small increase in phonemic awareness was observed towards the end of the second year of kindergarten, just before reading instruction started. However, a far greater improvement was found between the end of kindergarten and January in grade 1, that is after about four to five months of reading instruction. Like Mommers (1990), Wesseling and Reitsma (1998) stated that reading instruction was responsible for this sharp increase of phonemic awareness from the end of kindergarten. In addition, Wesseling and Reitsma (1998) found that individual differences in phonemic awareness were quite stable during kindergarten, but were substantially less stable from the end of kindergarten to halfway through grade 1. The lack of stability of individual differences in phonemic awareness during the first months of instruction is probably due to the fact that children with adequate phonemic awareness at the start of grade 1 will benefit little from instruction, while of the children who start with minimal phonemic awareness some will respond quickly to instruction, some will gain phonemic awareness at a much slower rate and others may not develop any phonemic awareness at all during this period.

Although in Dutch education instruction in phonological awareness and reading are intertwined, phonological awareness is probably the most rapidly developing ability. In the first months of formal instruction, the focus is on the correspondence of letters to sounds and the detection of letters and sounds in written and spoken words respectively. Consequently, an effect of phonological awareness on the development of reading acquisition is the likely effect to be observed. Longitudinal studies are most adequate to test this hypothesis.

In one of the first Dutch longitudinal studies on the relationship between phonological awareness and reading acquisition, Mommers (1987, 1990) administered measures of phoneme segmentation and blending to 461 children at the start of grade 1. In addition, measures of more general cognitive abilities, such as Raven's progressive matrices, were given. After four and eight months of reading instruction, measures of reading, including word decoding, were administered. Word decoding ability was measured by recording how many words a child could read from a list of words of increasing difficulty within one minute. This is the standard procedure in

Dutch primary education to assess word decoding. The results revealed the effects of general abilities at the start of grade 1 on reading acquisition after four and eight months. But after these general abilities were taken into account, specific effects of segmentation and blending at the start of grade 1 on subsequent word decoding were found.

In a more extensive study, Bast and Reitsma (1998) took measures of phonological awareness, segmentation and blending before the start of reading instruction, that is at the end of kindergarten, and in the autumn of grade 1 after about three months of reading instruction. In addition, Bast and Reitsma (1998) included a measure of letter knowledge at the end of kinder-garten. As expected, Dutch children hardly had any letter knowledge before the start of reading instruction and were, on average, able to identify about four of the 26 letters. As in the study by Mommers (1990), phonological awareness in most of the children was negligible at the end of kindergarten but had increased significantly after three months of reading instruction. However, it should be noted that the minimal amounts of letter knowledge and phonological awareness that Bast and Reitsma (1998) report might be partially due to the fact that they included only kindergarten children whom kindergarten teachers expected to become average readers. Accordingly, they excluded the 10% of children with the lowest reading readiness skills and the children who belonged to the upper 25% with respect to early reading skills.

Bast and Reitsma (1998) followed the development of word decoding in their sample from the autumn of grade 1 to the end of grade 3. As in the study by Mommers (1987), they found that phonological awareness at the start of reading instruction had an effect on subsequent reading acquisition. The effect remained even after the influence of letter knowledge was controlled for. However, unlike the results of Mommers (1987), general cognitive abili-ties, including vocabulary and non-verbal intelligence, did not appear to influence early reading development. This may be a result of their specific sampling procedure, mentioned above. In addition to the effect of kinder-garten phonological awareness on reading achievement in the autumn of grade 1, individual differences in phonological awareness in the autumn of grade 1 had an effect on further reading acquisition, even after reading achievement in the autumn of grade 1 had been taken into account. These results suggest that, at least during the first six months of reading instruction, individual differences in the development of phonological awareness continue to contribute to subsequent differences in the speed of reading acquisition.[1]

---

[1]Bast and Reitsma also report an effect of phonological awareness on reading achieve-ment. However, the particular model they adopted to describe their data is questionable, as another model without this effect seems to be equally valid.

As in the acquisition of many skills, the determinants of initial differences in progress may differ from determinants that influence later development. For reading acquisition this means that the influence of phonological awareness and other phonological skills may, for example, be limited to the early phases of learning to read. This possibility of a changing relationship between phonological abilities and reading achievement was a major subject of a recent longitudinal study from kindergarten to the end of grade 2 (de Jong and van der Leij, 1999). Measures of phonological awareness, verbal working memory and serial rapid naming were administered in the autumn of the second year in kindergarten, in the autumn of grade 1 and again at the end of grade 1. Phonological awareness was measured with an oddity task which consisted of items that required the detection of a non-rhyming word (e.g. p*op*, d*op*, *bus*), a word with a different first sound (e.g. *m*uis, *room*, *m*eel) and a word with a different last sound (e.g. *teen*, roo*s*, kaa*s*). Measures of verbal working memory included a memory span task and a nonword repetition test. Finally, serial rapid naming required naming a series of pictures representing common objects as quickly as possible. In addition to these phonological ability measures, tests reflecting general cognitive abilities and reading-related knowledge were administered.

As was found in other Dutch studies, kindergarten children appeared to have very little letter knowledge and their phonological awareness was minimal. In particular, their performance on items that required an awareness of phonemes (first and last sound) was near chance level. But one year later, in the autumn of grade 1, performance on these items had increased significantly.

The major interest was in the effects of phonological abilities on the development of word decoding in the autumn and at the end of grade 1, and at the end of grade 2. The results revealed that, with the exception of serial rapid naming, kindergarten phonological abilities did not contribute to subsequent reading acquisition after more general cognitive abilities and letter knowledge were controlled for. Kindergarten serial rapid naming had a small effect on later reading achievement. The absence of an effect of kindergarten phonological awareness is not in accordance with the results of Mommers (1987) and Bast and Reitsma (1998), but note that these researchers assessed phonological awareness just before the start of reading instruction, while de Jong and van der Leij (1999) took their measures about one year before reading instruction began. Furthermore, Mommers (1987, 1990) did not incorporate kindergarten letter knowledge, while, surprisingly, in the study by Bast and Reitsma (1998), more general cognitive abilities in kindergarten appeared to be unrelated to reading achievement in grade 1.

From the autumn of grade 1, after a few months of reading instruction, de Jong and van der Leij (1999) observed substantial effects of phonological awareness, verbal working memory and serial rapid naming on subsequent reading acquisition, even when reading achievement in the autumn of grade 1 was taken into account. The effects of phonological awareness and serial rapid naming appeared to be independent, while the effect of verbal working memory could be fully accounted for by phonological awareness. After the end of grade 1, however, the additional effects of individual differences in the development of phonological abilities on reading acquisition decreased substantially. De Jong and van der Leij (1999) concluded that for Dutch children, the importance of phonological abilities for learning to read seems to be limited to the first year of reading instruction.

Recently, de Jong and van der Leij (1999) assessed the reading achievement of about 140 of their sample of children at the end of grade 3 (see also de Jong and van der Leij, 2002). In Table 3.1 the correlations of phonological awareness and serial rapid naming with reading achievement over three approximately equal time periods are presented. Correlations are given for reading words and reading nonwords. The results clearly show that the relationship between individual differences in phonological abilities and reading achievement is dependent on the time at which the former abilities are assessed. The correlation of both phonological awareness and serial rapid naming with reading achievement is lower from kindergarten to the end of grade 1 than in the subsequent periods. Although it may be argued that in kindergarten individual differences in phonological awareness could not be completely reliably determined, this is certainly not the case for serial rapid naming. Nevertheless, the pattern

Table 3.1 Relationships of phonological awareness and serial rapid naming with word and nonword reading

Phonological ability	Reading	Kindergarten (autumn) to grade 1 (end)	Grade 1 (autumn) to grade 2 (end)	Grade 2 (end) to grade 3 (end)
		Correlations		
Phonological awareness	Words	0.21*	0.45**	0.37**
	Nonwords	0.16+	0.42**	0.32**
Serial rapid naming	Words	0.26**	0.41**	0.39**
	Nonwords	0.25**	0.40**	0.37**
		Additional variance		
Phonological awareness	Words	0.0	4.1**	0.0
	Nonwords	0.2	4.9**	0.2
Serial rapid naming	Words	2.2*	3.7**	2.0*
	Nonwords	2.4*	5.3**	1.1+

+$p < 0.10$, *$p < 0.05$, **$p < 0.01$.

of correlations of both phonological abilities is about the same. Note also that the correlations of these phonological abilities with reading are similar for words and for nonwords. This suggests that individual differences in the development of word and nonword reading are determined by similar abilities.

In the lower half of Table 3.1, the additional percentages of variance explained by phonological awareness and serial rapid naming in subsequent reading achievement are presented, after general abilities and reading or reading-related skills have been taken into account. For example, after general cognitive abilities and letter knowledge have been controlled, phonological awareness in kindergarten does not explain any additional variance (0.0) in word reading at the end of grade 1. Individual differences in phonological awareness in the autumn of grade 1, however, explain an additional 4.1% of the variance in word reading at the end of grade 2, after general cognitive abilities and word reading in the autumn of grade 1 have been taken into account. The results in the lower half of Table 3.1 clearly indicate that the additional effects of phonological awareness are time-limited. Kindergarten phonological awareness has no additional effects on reading at the end of grade 1. After a few months of reading instruction, in the autumn of grade 1, individual differences in phonological awareness contribute to subsequent reading acquisition. After grade 1, however, these extra effects disappear. The effects of serial rapid naming decrease substantially after the end of grade 1, but do not disappear completely.

This pattern of results is in accordance with an interactive relationship between phonological abilities and reading acquisition (de Jong and van der Leij, 1999). In Dutch kindergarten, the development of phonological abilities and of reading ability is minimal. From grade 1, both abilities are improving under the influence of reading instruction, but phonological abilities are probably developing more rapidly. As indicated by all the Dutch longitudinal studies, individual differences in phonological abilities at the beginning or in the autumn of grade 1 contribute to learning to read. However, the current results suggest that their extra contribution is limited to about the first year of reading instruction, although they continue to underlie reading ability (see top half of Table 3.1).

De Jong and van der Leij (1999) speculated that the limited influence of phonological abilities, especially of phonological awareness, could be due to the relative consistency of the grapheme–phoneme mappings in Dutch orthography. They argued that at first, accurate decoding is an arduous process and high accuracy levels are obtained at the expense of a low reading speed (remember that the number of words read correctly in one minute is the dependent variable in most Dutch longitudinal studies). In this phase, individual differences in phonological awareness will be relevant. However, when speed rather than accuracy becomes the dominant factor in reading, as is characteristic for learning to read in more consistent orthographies, phonological awareness ceases to have an additional effect on reading acquisition. In short, de Jong and van der Leij (1999) hypothesized that individual phonological abilities are important as long as reliable individual differences in the accuracy of word decoding exist. In learning to read Dutch, this seems to be only during the first year of instruction. Accordingly, de Jong and van der Leij (1999) concluded that those children who fail to acquire phonological abilities within the first months of reading instruction are likely to develop reading problems.

Problems in reading acquisition

Children with reading problems or dyslexia might be expected to manifest deficits in the same abilities that have been found to affect the development of reading ability. Indeed, a large body of evidence now suggests that a phonological deficit is the core problem underlying dyslexia. Most of these studies have been concerned with problems in learning to read in English (e.g. Siegel, 1998).

The phonological deficit of dyslexic children is assumed to be particularly manifest in pseudoword reading. A pseudoword consists of an unknown letter string which can be converted into a pronounceable, but non-existent, spoken word. Thus, unlike known words that have usually been read several times and can be mapped on to an existing phonological representation, pseudowords are completely unfamiliar. To read these words draws heavily on phonological decoding, that is the ability to successfully apply grapheme to phoneme conversion rules (Siegel, 1998) and the ability to blend the constituent phonemes into a (new) pronunciation.

Wimmer (1993, 1996) provided evidence that Austrian dyslexic children learning to read German, have relatively few problems with the accurate reading of pseudowords but show large deficits in pseudoword reading speed. Wimmer (1993, 1996) argued that the relative consistent grapheme–phoneme correspondences in German orthography, possibly in combination with a phonics-oriented reading instruction, enable even dyslexic children to acquire adequate knowledge of grapheme–phoneme relations. In a language with a relatively consistent orthography, this knowledge is sufficient to decode most words. What remains a problem for dyslexic children is the development of sufficient decoding speed.

A similar case can be made with respect to Dutch dyslexic children. As already mentioned, the consistency of the Dutch orthography is similar to the German orthography. Yap and van der Leij (1993) examined word and pseudoword reading of Dutch dyslexic children with a mean age of 10 years but whose reading ability was about two years below normal. These children were compared to a group of normal readers of the same age (the chronolog-ical age-control group) and a group of younger normal-reading children in grade 1 with the same reading age (the reading-age control group). In addition, Yap and van der Leij (1993) incorporated a group of younger poor readers of the same reading age as the dyslexic children (the poor reading-age control group). In one of their tasks, the children had to read consonant–vowel–consonant (CVC) words (and pseudowords) in a speeded and a non-speeded condition. In the latter condition, a word remained on a computer screen until it was named. In the speeded condition, the words were flashed, that is they disappeared after a period of 200 ms. In both condi-tions, the measure of interest was the proportion of words (or pseudowords) that were read correctly.

The results of this study were clear-cut. For all groups the performance for words was better than the performance for pseudowords and the percentage correct in the unspeeded condition was higher than in the speeded condi-tion. For the reading of words, both speeded and unspeeded, minimal differ-ences were found between the dyslexics and the various control groups. The dyslexic children accurately identified over 90% of the words. However, in contrast to all the control groups, including the group of poor readers, the dyslexic children had extreme difficulties with the speeded identification of pseudowords. While in the control groups the performance in pseudoword reading dropped from above 90% correct in the non-speeded condition to about 85% in the speeded condition, the performance of the dyslexic children decreased from above 80% to just above 50% in the speeded condi-tion. These results strongly suggest that Dutch dyslexic children are particu-larly impaired in rapid phonological decoding.

A study by Assink and Kattenberg (1995; see also Assink et al., 1998) provides some indirect support for such a speed deficit. Instead of a naming task, Assink and Kattenberg (1995) used a word-matching task. In their second experiment, a group of dyslexic children and a group of younger children matched for reading age were compared. The children were required to decide whether two letter strings reflected the same word. The two letter strings could be words or pseudowords. One of the letter strings consisted of lower-case letters while the other string had upper-case letters. Strings that reflected the same word or pseudoword could be visually congruent or incongruent. In the congruent condition, the shape of lower- and upper-case letter strings was identical, such as in the pair *PULL–pull*. In the incongruent condition, this was not the case, for example as in *BEAR–bear*. Assink and Kattenberg (1995) recorded both decision errors and latencies.

The results revealed a very small proportion of errors, which did not differ between the groups and among the various conditions. There were, however, large differences in latencies. Most importantly, the performance of the younger normal and the dyslexic children was about equal for the identification of incongruent words, while the dyslexic children were far slower at the identification of incongruent pseudowords. This interaction was less pronounced for the identification of congruent letter strings. However, with these letter strings, global visual similarities could have been used to decide whether the strings reflected the same word (or pseudoword). With incongruent letter strings this seems impossible. To decide whether incongruent letter strings refer to the same word requires phonological decoding, especially when the letter strings are pseudowords. As the results indicated, this was exactly the condition in which the dyslexic children's identification speed was most impaired.

More direct evidence of the dyslexic children's deficiencies in the speed of pseudoword reading can be found in the study of de Jong and van der Leij. They selected a group of dyslexic children from the sample who had taken part in their longitudinal study (de Jong and van der Leij, 2002). By the end of grade 3, the reading performance of the dyslexic group was at the level of the controls at the end of grade 1, that is about two years below the performance of their normal reading peers, as indicated by a standard Dutch test for reading achievement. The dyslexic group was matched to a group of normal reading peers (chronological-age match controls), who read at the same level at the end of grade 1 as the dyslexic children at the end of grade 3. In addition, the groups were matched on measures of non-verbal intelligence and vocabulary knowledge which had both been administered before the start of grade 1.

The results are displayed in Figure 3.1. In Figure 3.1a, the number of words read correctly in one minute on a standard Dutch word reading test are given for the dyslexic group (DYS) and the chronological age-matched control group (CA) from the middle of grade 1 to the end of grade 3. The results for pseudoword reading are displayed in Figure 3.1b. The pseudoword reading test required the speeded reading of a list of CVC, CCVC and CVCC pseudowords. The number of pseudowords read correctly in one minute was recorded. Thus, unlike the discrete trial reading task in the study by Yap and van der Leij (1993), in this study, continuous (pseudo) word lists were given for both word and pseudoword reading. Because the words on the pseudoword list were not matched to those on the standard word reading achievement test – in fact, the former words were much shorter – the score on both lists cannot be compared. However, this does not hamper the interpretation of the results.

Close examination of Figure 3.1 reveals, once more, that dyslexic children have deficits in the rapid decoding of pseudowords. By the end of grade 1 the word reading performance of the CA group was equal to the performance of

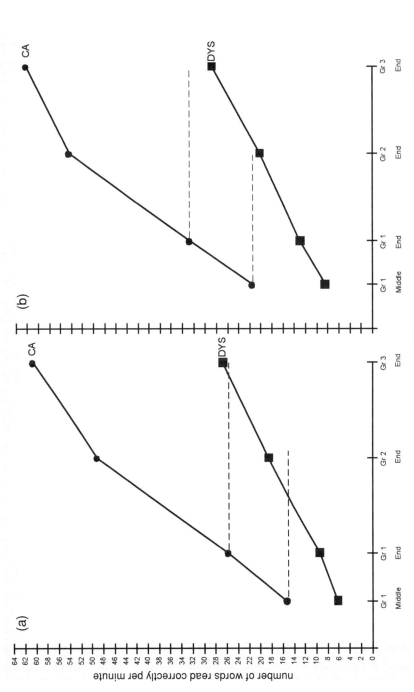

Figure 3.1 Development of the performance of dyslexic children (DYS) and their age-matched normal reading peers (CA) on a standardized word reading test (a) and on a pseudoword reading test (b) from the middle of grade 1 to the end of grade 3.

the DYS group at the end of grade 3. This is indicated by the higher dotted line in Figure 3.1a. Thus, at the end of grade 1, the CA group was in fact a reading-age control group; the group members are younger but read words at a similar speed to the dyslexic group at the end of grade 3. However, as Figure 3.1b reveals, at the end of grade 1 the pseudoword reading speed of the CA group was already higher than the speed of the DYS group at the end of grade 3 (see the higher dotted line). Interestingly, about halfway through grade 1 the pseudoword reading speed of the CA group appeared to be equal to the speed of the DYS group at the end of grade 2 (see bottom dotted line in Figure 3.1b). Turning to Figure 3.1a shows that by that time the word reading speed of the DYS group was higher than the word reading speed of the CA group halfway through grade 1 (see bottom dotted line in Figure 3.1a). This is, of course, exactly what one would expect given the hypothesis that dyslexic children are relatively more deficient in pseudoword reading than in word reading. One consequence of this hypothesis is that their pseudoword reading speed should be lower than the speed of a group of normal children with the same level of word reading. However, another consequence of this same hypothesis is that dyslexic children's speed of word reading is greater than the word reading speed of normal children matched for pseudoword reading ability. The latter consequence seems not to have been tested before.

The phonological deficit of dyslexic children is also assumed to result in poor phonological skills. These skills have been found to have a causal effect on reading acquisition, albeit time-limited in the Dutch situation. The importance of phonological skills for the development of dyslexia is particularly supported if dyslexic children manifest impairments on these skills in comparison to younger normal readers of the same reading age, that is a reading-age control group. In contrast to a comparison with their normal reading peers, it is difficult to interpret such a difference as a consequence of reading ability. The present discussion will be confined to Dutch studies that included a reading-age control group.

Dyslexic children's level of phonological awareness was examined by de Gelder and Vroomen (1991). Various levels of phonological awareness were assessed. Lower levels were measured with a rhyme judgement task. For higher levels of awareness an initial-consonant reproduction task and an initial-consonant deletion task were administered. The former task required the reproduction of the first consonant of a given pseudoword. In the latter task, the given pseudoword without the first consonant had to be produced.

In a first study, dyslexic children appeared to perform as well as chronological and reading-age controls on the rhyme judgement task. On the initial-consonant reproduction task the performance of the dyslexic children was high (80% correct). Their performance was somewhat lower than both control groups, but the difference was not significant. However, on the consonant-deletion task, the performance of the dyslexic children appeared to be substantially lower than the performance of the chronological-age control group and also lower than the performance of the reading-age control group. These results suggest that dyslexic children are able to perceive phonemes in words, as indicated by the initial-consonant reproduction task. But an impairment in phonological awareness is manifested when additional processing demands are made, as in the deletion task. Interestingly, such an impairment seems temporary. In another study reported by de Gelder and Vroomen (1991), dyslexic adults were compared to normal adult readers. No phonological awareness task differences were found between the groups. On the consonant-deletion task the mean score of the dyslexic adults was 92% correct.

Recently, Messbauer et al. (in press) included a phoneme-deletion task in a study on phonological deficits of Dutch dyslexic children. The task was similar to a task used by McDougall et al. (1994) and required the deletion of a verbally specified phoneme (always a consonant) from a single-syllable pseudoword. The specified phoneme could appear at any available position in the pseudoword.

A difference was observed between the performance of the dyslexic children and their normal reading peers. However, unlike the study of de Gelder and Vroomen (1991), the performance of the dyslexic children was similar to the performance of the reading-age control group. The difference between these results and those of de Gelder and Vroomen (1991) might be due to the fact that in the latter study, the dyslexic children attended regular schools, while the dyslexic children in the study by Messbauer et al. were in special education. Possibly, the children studied by Messbauer et al. had received more specialized training in phoneme deletion and segmentation, which might have advanced their phonological awareness.

Messbauer et al. also incorporated various measures of serial rapid naming ability. Children were required to name objects, letters and digits. The dyslexic children appeared to be substantially slower in naming than their normal-reading peers. For object and letter naming no differences were found between the dyslexic children and the reading-age matched group. For digit naming the mean speed of the dyslexic children was even higher than the mean speed of the reading-age control group. These results indicate that the letter- and object-naming speed of dyslexic children is in accordance with their level of reading, while their digit-naming speed is above this level.

Finally, verbal working memory deficits of dyslexic children have been considered in two recent studies. De Jong (1998) found that dyslexic children performed worse than their normal-reading peers on a digit-span and on a word-span task. No differences in verbal working memory were observed between the dyslexic children and a group of younger normal readers. Irausquin and de Gelder (1997) examined the performance of dyslexic children on a variety of word-span tasks, which differed in the phonological similarity (rhyming and non-rhyming words) and the length of the words (one or three syllables). The dyslexic children and the two control groups were matched on digit span. Nevertheless, Irausquin and de Gelder (1997) found that the overall performance of the dyslexic children on the word-span tasks was worse than the performance of their normal-reading peers, but better than the performance of the reading-age controls. Irausquin and de Gelder (1997) suggested that the impaired word-span performance of the dyslexic children compared to their normal reading peers, despite matching on digit span, might be due to a contribution from long-term memory to the word-span task. They argued that words are phonologically more complex than highly over-learned digits. Words might be activated more slowly and represented less precisely than familiar digits. Consequently, long-term memory would be more critical for the reconstruction of decaying words than for decaying digits.

In summary, evidence thus far is in accordance with a phonological deficit account of dyslexia. Dutch dyslexic children were found to have impoverished phonological abilities, as manifested by impairments in phonological awareness, verbal working memory and serial rapid naming. In most studies, their phonological abilities were similar to the abilities of younger normal readers. However, their pseudoword reading has been consistently found to be worse than the pseudoword reading of younger children of the same reading age. The deficiency of dyslexic children in pseudoword reading primarily concerns its speed and not its accuracy. Accordingly, the core deficit of Dutch dyslexic children concerns the rapid decoding of novel words.

Treatment of reading problems

Most treatments of impairments in reading speed have focused on reading practice under time constraints by limiting the exposure duration of words or pseudowords. Limited exposure duration is assumed to stimulate the use of multi-letter units because a letter-by-letter decoding strategy would be too slow (van den Bosch et al., 1995). The recognition of multi-letter units can be considered as an intermediate phase between letter-by-letter decoding and direct recognition, that is sight word reading. Multi-letter units can be any combination of letters from digraphs to morphemes. Of course, direct recognition of pseudowords is impossible, but the knowledge of correspondences between multi-letter units and sounds might greatly improve pseudoword reading speed.

In a number of studies, dyslexic children were trained in the rapid decoding of pseudowords. In these studies, the pseudowords were presented by a computer. Their exposure duration was dependent on reading accuracy, which was monitored on-line. Exposure duration decreased as long as accuracy was at a pre-set level. If accuracy dropped below this level, than exposure duration was increased again. In most studies, the dyslexic children were trained twice a week for 25 or 30 minutes for a period of about eight weeks.

In a first study, van den Bosch et al. (1995) obtained some support for the effectiveness of training rapid decoding. Their rapid decoding group read words and pseudowords faster than a group that was exposed to the same pseudowords but without time pressure. The accuracy of these groups was similar. In contrast, compared to a no-training group the children in the rapid decoding group read more accurately, but at a similar speed.

Wentink et al. (1997) also trained children in rapid decoding but to stimulate the processing of multi-letter units more directly, they emphasized the syllable structure of the pseudowords. All monosyllabic pseudowords and the first and third syllables of multisyllabic words were printed in bold face. The results indicated that the training group had improved more on a Dutch standardized measure of word-list reading speed than a no-training group. On a discrete word decoding measure the trained group read words and pseudowords more rapidly, but no differences in accuracy were observed with the untrained group. Unfortunately, in a similar study, Wentink et al. (1998) could not replicate these results. Wentink et al. (1998) suggested that the duration of this training was too short. These poor readers were trained for half as long as the poor readers in their previous study (Wentink et al., 1997).

Instead of enhancing the procressing of multi-letter units by training rapid decoding, Yap (1993) and Das-Smaal et al. (1996) trained dyslexic children directly in the speeded recognition of multi-letter units in words. In these studies, the child had to decide whether a word, presented by a computer, contained a given multi-letter unit. For example, the multi-letter unit was practised by presenting words like *ander* (other), *landen* (countries) and *brand* (fire). The exposure duration of a word was limited *and* adapted to the accuracy level of the child. The child had to decrease exposure duration while maintaining accuracy. Each unit was trained separately until a pre-set detection speed was reached.

Das-Smaal et al. (1996) trained dyslexic children in the recognition of multi-letter units in written words. Yap (1993) also incorporated a group of dyslexic children who were trained in the rapid recognition of spoken multi-phoneme units in *spoken* words and a group that was required to practise the rapid detection of spoken multi-phoneme units in *written* words. The children in the Das-Smaal et al. (1996) study were trained twice a week for 30 minutes for a period of eight weeks. The dyslexics in the studies by Yap (1993) received somewhat less training.

The main result of these studies was that each group trained in rapid unit detection outperformed a control group on the particular task the group was trained to do. For example, a group trained to detect a spoken multi-phoneme unit in a written word had a higher performance on this task than a control group. Mixed results were found for the transfer to word and pseudoword reading. Das-Smaal et al. (1996) did not observe any transfer. Yap (1993) found in the first study that right after the training, the rapid detection groups showed larger gains on a standard Dutch word-reading test than the control group. However, this difference had disappeared after three months. In addition, in the second study, no transfer to word reading was observed at all.

From this short review, it appears that, thus far, the effects of treatments aimed at enhancing word decoding speed are small. In most studies, treatment effects were restricted to tasks that were trained or to tasks that resembled the training task. In some studies, transfer effects to word or pseudoword reading were found, but often these effects could not be replicated or appeared to have vanished several months after the training had finished. In a previous review of such treatment studies, van der Leij (1994) concluded that 'possibly, one of the main characteristics of specific reading disability is the dependence on external structures in order to be able to perform adequately.... When deprived of such external guidelines the students may return to old habits' (page 266). This conclusion still seems to be valid.

Conclusion

Children learning to read in Dutch are faced with a fairly consistent orthography. Correspondences between spoken and written words are primarily taught by phonics-oriented teaching methods. By the end of grade 1, most children are able to use a grapheme-to-phoneme translation procedure to decode known and unknown words. Individual differences in normal reading acquisition are affected by individual differences in phonological awareness and serial rapid naming. However, the additional effects of these abilities seem to be limited to the first year of reading instruction. Children with problems in learning to read are found to have primarily phonological deficits. Their deficits include impairments in phonological awareness and serial rapid naming, although Dutch dyslexic children are most clearly deficient in the rapid decoding of pseudowords. Treatments of this deficiency have thus far concentrated on the use of time pressure to stimulate the encoding of multi-letter units during word reading. Improving on these treatments is an important challenge for future research.

References

Assink E, Kattenberg GAP (1995) The use of phonological and orthographic information by normal and poor readers of Dutch. Reading and Writing 7: 277–294.

Assink E, Lam M, Knuijt P (1998) Visual and phonological processes in poor readers' word recognition. Applied Psycholinguistics 19: 471–487.

Bast J, Reitsma P (1998) Analysing the development of individual differences in terms of Matthew effects in reading: results from a Dutch longitudinal study. Developmental Psychology 34: 1373–1399.

Blok H, Otter ME (1997) Vijf methoden voor aanvankelijk lezen onderzocht (Evaluation of five methods of early reading instruction). University of Amsterdam: SCO-Kohnstamm Instituut.

Bosman AMT, van Orden GC (1997) Why spelling is more difficult than reading. In CA Perfetti, L Riben (eds) Learning to spell: research, theory, and practice across languages, pp 173–194. Mahwah, NJ: Lawrence Erlbaum Associates.

Das-Smaal EA, Klapwijk MJG, van der Leij A (1996) Training of perceptual unit processing in children with reading disability. Cognition and Instruction 14: 221–250.

de Gelder B, Vroomen J (1991) Phonological deficits: beneath the surface of reading-acquisition problems. Psychological Research 53: 88–97.

de Jong PF (1998) Working memory deficits of reading disabled children. Journal of Experimental Child Psychology 70: 75–96.

de Jong PF, van der Leij A (1999) Specific contributions of phonological abilities to early reading acquisition: results from a Dutch latent variable longitudinal study. Journal of Educational Psychology 91: 450–476.

de Jong PF, van der Leij A (2002) Effects of phonological abilities and linguistic comprehension on the development of reading. Scientific Studies of Reading 6: 51–77.

Ehri LC (1998) Grapheme–phoneme knowledge is essential for learning to read words in English. In JL Metsala, LC Ehri (eds) Word recognition in beginning literacy, pp 3–40. Mahwah, NJ: Lawrence Erlbaum Associates.

Irausquin RS, de Gelder B (1997) Serial recall of poor readers in two presentation modalities: combined effects of phonological similarity and word length. Journal of Experimental Child Psychology 65: 342–369.

McDougall S, Hulme C, Ellis A, Monk A (1994) Learning to read: the role of short-term memory and phonological skills. Journal of Experimental Child Psychology 58: 112–133.

Messbauer VCS, de Jong,PF, van der Leij A (in press) Manifestations of phonological deficits in dyslexia: evidence from Dutch children. In L Verhoeven, C Elbro , P Reitsma (eds) Precursors of functional literacy. Dordrecht: Kluwer.

Mommers MJ (1987) An investigation into the relation between word recognition skills, reading comprehension and spelling skills in the first two years of primary school. Journal of Research in Reading 10: 122–143.

Mommers M (1990) Metalinguistic awareness and learning to read. In P Reitsma, L Verhoeven (eds) Acquisition of reading in Dutch, pp 29–42. Dordrecht, The Netherlands: Foris Publications.

Perfetti CA (1992) The representation problem in reading acquisition. In PB Gough, LC Ehri, R Treiman (eds) Reading acquisition, pp 145–174. Hillsdale, NJ: Lawrence Erlbaum Associates.

Reitsma P, Verhoeven L (1990) Acquisition of written Dutch: an introduction. In P Reitsma, L Verhoeven (eds) Acquisition of reading in Dutch, pp 1–13. Dordrecht, The Netherlands: Foris Publications.

Share DL (1995) Phonological recoding and self-teaching: sine qua non of reading acquisition. Cognition 55: 151–218.

Siegel LS (1998) Phonological processing deficits and reading disabilities. In JL Metsala, LC Ehri (eds) Word recognition in beginning literacy, pp 141–160. Mahwah, NJ: Lawrence Erlbaum Associates.

van Bon WHJ (1993) Spellingproblemen (Spelling problems). Rotterdam: Lemniscaat.

van den Bosch K, van Bon WHJ, Schreuder R (1995) Poor readers' decoding skills: effects of training with limited exposure duration. Reading Research Quarterly 30: 110–125.

van der Leij A (1994) Effects of computer-assisted instruction on word and pseudoword reading of reading-disabled students. In KP van den Bos, LS Siegel, DJ Bakker, DL Share (eds) Current directions in dyslexia research, pp 251–267. Lisse: Swets & Zeitlinger.

Wagner RK, Torgesen JK, Rashotte CA (1994) Development of reading-related phonological processing abilities: new evidence of bidirectional causality from a latent variable longitudinal study. Developmental Psychology 30: 73–87.

Wentink H, van Bon W, Schreuder R (1997) Training poor readers' phonological decoding skills: evidence for syllable-bound processing. Reading and Writing 9: 163–192.

Wentink H, Drent I, van Bon W, Schreuder R (1998) The effects of a flash card training program on normal and poor readers' phonological decoding skills. In P Reitsma, L Verhoeven (eds) Problems and interventions in literacy development, pp 257–276. Dordrecht: Kluwer Academic Publishers.

Wesseling R, Reitsma P (1998) Phonemically aware in a hop, skip, and a jump. In P Reitsma, L Verhoeven (eds) Problems and interventions in literacy development, pp 81–94. Dordrecht: Kluwer Academic Publishers.

Wimmer H (1993) Characteristics of developmental dyslexia in a regular writing system. Applied Psycholinguistics 14: 1–33.

Wimmer H (1996) The nonword reading deficit in developmental dyslexia: evidence from children learning to read German. Journal of Experimental Child Psychology 61: 80–90.

Wimmer H, Goswami U (1994) The influence of orthographic consistency on reading development: word recognition in English and German children. Cognition 51: 91–103.

Yap R (1993) Automatic word processing deficits in dyslexia: qualitative differences and specific remediation. Unpublished dissertation, Vrije Universiteit.

Yap RL, van der Leij A (1993) Word processing in dyslexics: an automatic decoding deficit? Reading and Writing 5: 261–279.

CHAPTER 4

Developmental dyslexia in Greek

DIMITRI NIKOLOPOULOS, NATA GOULANDRIS AND MARGARET J SNOWLING

The extent to which languages adhere to the alphabetic principle differs. Within the group of alphabetic scripts, Greek orthography presents an interesting contrast to English because of the significant differences in the phonology, morphology and syntax of the two languages. One of the basic features of Greek orthography is the high degree of orthographic transparency for reading. Two factors account for this: regularity, the reliable mapping between graphemes and phonemes, and the articulatory and structural simplicity of most Greek words. In most instances, each Greek grapheme is represented by one phoneme. Consequently there are few Greek words with arbitrary pronunciations (as in the English words *yacht*, *might* and *through*) and there are no words containing silent graphemes (as in *island*), silent syllables (as in *Gloucester*) or indistinct schwa vowels (as in the first and third syllables of *potato*). Since Greek readers pronounce every single grapheme, the need to memorize the pronunciation of words as a whole (e.g. *heal-health*) is significantly reduced.

In addition, the phonological structure of many Greek words is transparent due to the predominance of open consonant–vowel (CV) syllables, e.g. μητέρα /mi:'tɛra/ (mother) CV-CV-CV. In contrast, English contains many words comprising numerous consonant clusters such as *splash* and *strength*. As these clusters of consonants are co-articulated, it is difficult for a beginning reader to disentangle the component phonemes, rendering the phonological structure of English much more difficult to perceive than that of Greek.

However, although Greek sound–letter mappings are regular for reading, this is not the case for spelling, where many more ambiguities occur. The same vowel can be spelled using several alternative graphemes (see Table 4.1). This anomaly can be traced to the preservation of some Ancient Greek

Table 4.1 Spelling in Greek: vowel–phoneme correspondences

/a/	α	
/ɒ/	o, ω	
/ɛ/	ε, αι	
/iː/	ι, η, υ, ει, οι, υι	e.g. επιχείρηση =/ɛpiːˈhiːriːsiː/
/uː/	ου	

(4th century BC) vowel graphemes that denoted differences in pitch and duration. For example, the grapheme ω was used in Ancient Greek to denote the long vowel /əʊ/ (as in 'old') and the grapheme o the short sound /ɒ/ (as in 'hot'). Over the centuries, the long vowel pronunciation has been discarded, but the two alternative graphemes have been retained in Modern Greek despite the fact that their pronunciation is identical. Consequently, in numerous Modern Greek words, the same vowel phoneme is represented by several different graphemes (e.g. /iː/ *επιχείρηση* / ɛpiːˈhiːriːsi: / (company).

Another reason why spelling is more difficult than reading is the highly inflectional nature of the Greek language. In English, verbs are not usually inflected, although a final -*s* is used to denote the third person singular (*I write-s/he writes*) and the suffix -*ed* indicates a regular past tense. Nouns are also generally uninflected, although the suffix -*s* is tagged on to nouns to designate the plural. In Greek, spellers need to take tense (past, present, future, etc.), person (I, you, he), voice (active, passive) and mood (indicative, subjective) into account to determine the appropriate suffix and prefix required (see Table 4.2 for an example of verb conjugation). To spell Modern Greek correctly it is necessary to have extensive knowledge of the grammatical rules governing the inflection of nouns and adjectives and the conjugation of verbs in addition to orthographic information about the spelling of root morphemes.

Greece has a centralized educational system, so all schools across the

Table 4.2 Verb conjugation in English and Greek

	Singular		
I	play	εγώ	παίζω
you	play	εσύ	παίζεις
he/she	plays	αυτός/ή	παίζει
	Plural		
we	play	εμείς	παίζουμε
you	play	εσείς	παίζετε
they	play	αυτοί	παίζουν

country use the same books and reading materials. Traditionally phonics-based reading instruction has been adopted to draw the attention of Greek beginning readers to the constituent syllables and phonemes in words. From the first days in primary school, Greek children are systematically introduced to the letters of the Greek alphabet. Most children master the letters of the alphabet so rapidly that consonant clusters (e.g. $βδ$, $γδ$, $γμ$, $βγ$, $σπρ$, $στρ$, $ρμπ$) are introduced in the reading curriculum after a few weeks of schooling. Word segmentation also forms a basic component of daily reading instruction. Beginning readers are systematically taught to segment words into syllables and phonemes and to blend these smaller segments to form words (see Figure 4.1).

Learning to read and spell

There is an increasing amount of empirical evidence demonstrating that differences in the orthographic structure of languages exert a significant effect on the development of literacy and other metacognitive skills. Children learning to read more regular languages than English, readily learn to use letter–sound mappings and are able to apply alphabetic strategies shortly after the onset of reading instruction (e.g. Nikolopoulos, 1994; Wimmer and Goswami, 1994; Pinheiro, 1995; Goswami et al., 1998). They also develop phonological awareness skills at a much faster rate than English-speaking children (Caravolas and Bruck, 1993; Wimmer, 1993; Nikolopoulos and Goulandris, 2000).

Given this evidence and the interesting contrasts in the linguistic structure of the Greek and English languages, the aim of the study presented in this chapter was to investigate the effects of the orthographic transparency of the Greek language and the phonics-oriented reading instruction on a group of poor Greek readers. We predicted that the Greek-speaking poor readers would be significantly more accurate when reading words and nonwords than their English-speaking counterparts and that their phonological skills would also be more advanced.

To test these hypotheses we contrasted the cognitive profile of 28 dyslexic readers with that of average readers of either the same chronological-age or the same reading-age. These children were recruited from four primary schools in Athens, Greece. All were native speakers of the Greek language with regular school attendance. Two reading criteria were adopted for the assessment of reading competence: first, the number of reading errors on the single-word reading test, and second, the time taken to read aloud all the 131 items. Children whose reading speed and/or reading accuracy score lay between the 16th and 84th percentile ranks were characterized as average readers. Children were characterized as poor (dyslexic) readers if their reading speed was one standard deviation below the mean for their chronological age or their mean number of errors exceeded one standard deviation, equivalent to below the 16th percentile.

Sixteen grade 2 children and 12 grade 4 children were identified as dyslexic using these criteria. These 28 children were matched in terms of age and non-verbal IQ to 28 randomly selected average readers and to 28 younger children who were reading at the same level (see Table 4.3).

Table 4.3 Details of the children in the study. Means and standard deviations

	Grade 2		Grade 4		
	Dyslexic	CA-controls	Dyslexic	CA-controls	RA control
Age	7y 3m	7y 2m	9y 3m	9y 3m	7y 3m
(years, months)	(0.47)	(0.47)	(0.30)	(0.27)	(0.6)
IQ	91.5	91.1	93.3	93.8	99.0
(standard score)	(11.6)	(12.9)	(13.6)	(13.1)	(15.0)
Reading speed	586.2	387.6	404	198.1	401
(total time in s)	(145.2)	(82.6)	(82)	(42.3)	(79)

Standard deviations in parentheses.

All participants were seen twice, individually, in a quiet room near their classroom. They were given an extensive test battery of cognitive, linguistic and literacy tasks. This comprised tests of single-word reading, spelling and nonword reading tests of graded difficulty, a version of the British Abilities Scales Arithmetic subtest (Elliot et al., 1983), and a test of non-verbal reasoning (Standard Progressive Matrices; Ravens, 1987). Children's development of metalinguistic skills was assessed by a series of phonological awareness tasks, including phoneme and syllable counting and deletion, phoneme substitution, spoonerisms, consonant segmentation, verbal fluency tasks (alliteration and semantic fluency) and phonological processing tasks comprising speech rate, verbal short-term memory (STM), and rapid naming tasks for objects, colours, digits and letters (Denckla and Rudel, 1976; Pratt and Brady, 1988; McDougall et al., 1994; Frith et al., 1995).

Six measures were used in the assessment of syntactic awareness skills. Three of the tests, Recalling Sentences, Word Structure and Sentence Assembly, were adapted for the Greek language from the CELF–R test battery (Semel et al., 1987). The other three were constructed by the first author to assess children's sensitivity to the three genders of the Greek language, the agreement between subjects and verbs, and to the position of the stress in words.

The reading and spelling skills of Greek dyslexic children

Despite their comparatively poor reading ability for their age, Greek dyslexic readers read the majority of the words on the single-word reading test accurately. Both the second (aged 7) and the fourth graders (aged 9) were able to read 90% of the words correctly. Greek dyslexic readers also read nonwords with similar ease. The mean nonword reading accuracy score was 86% at age 7 and 90% at age 9. Furthermore, none of the children ever refused to read a word or nonword stimulus, no matter how difficult it was. In many instances the children were also able to self-correct any initially incorrect responses when reading.

A similar degree of competence in the use of alphabetic skills was also observed for spelling. Even though the poor readers' performance on the spelling test was significantly poorer than that of their chronological age peers, there was not a single instance of a non-phonetic error (an error in which the response did not sound like the target word). The majority of their spelling errors were orthographic, so that the spelling sounded like the target word but contained the wrong letter(s) (e.g. spelling the word '$βρύση$' (tap) as $βρίση$).

These findings demonstrate that, unlike English dyslexic readers, Greek poor readers develop a high degree of competence in the use of grapheme-to-phoneme correspondence rules for reading and of phoneme–grapheme rules for spelling. English dyslexic readers' difficulties with literacy are usually so severe that they are wont to produce many non-phonetic reading and spelling errors, e.g. spelling the word 'rough' as refet or the word 'believe' as beever (Bruck and Treiman, 1990). Moreover, a nonword reading deficit is considered a robust characteristic of developmental dyslexia in English (Rack et al., 1992). Even adults with childhood histories of dyslexia find nonword reading very difficult, attaining an accuracy score of about 65% (Bruck, 1990).

The present study confirms that the nonword reading accuracy deficit is not necessarily a characteristic of developmental dyslexia in the context of regular orthographies, as has been previously noted by other researchers (Wimmer, 1993). The orthographic transparency of the Greek writing system in conjunction with the 'phonics'-oriented reading instruction in Greek, enables normally developing children, as well as poor readers, to attain alphabetic competence early on. Mastery of alphabetic skills in turn permits Greek-speaking learners to attain high levels of reading accuracy at an early stage in their reading development.

Despite their proficient alphabetic skill, dyslexic readers read words and nonwords more slowly than average readers. In grade 2, dyslexic readers read words at a rate of 4.5 s per word compared to the 2.9 s per word of average readers. In grade 4, the dyslexic readers' mean rate was 3.2 s per word. There were also significant differences between the groups on the nonword reading task, with dyslexic readers taking 3.9 s per word in grade 2 and 3.1 s in grade 4 compared to the average readers' 2.6 s and 1.7 s respectively.

The importance of the reading speed criterion was also apparent when we examined individual differences in the development of reading skills. Of the 28 dyslexic readers, seven (25%) experienced problems with reading accuracy alone, ten with reading speed (36%) and the other 11 (39%) had problems with both reading accuracy and speed (see Figure 4.1). This means that the exclusive use of the traditional reading accuracy criterion in the Greek language would leave some children's problems undetected. Reading speed appears to be a more reliable and sensitive measure of individual differences in word recognition skills in regular orthographies, where the consistency of grapheme-to-phoneme correspondences facilitates the development of high levels of reading accuracy.

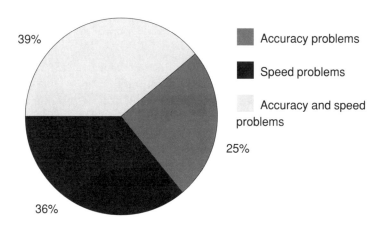

Figure 4.1 Individual differences in reading accuracy and reading speed: evidence from Greek dyslexic children.

Latent deficiencies in Greek dyslexic readers' word recognition systems were also revealed in a qualitative analysis of their reading and spelling errors. Despite the small percentage of reading errors, there were instances when the dyslexic readers were unable to read relatively easy high-frequency words correctly such as μαμά (mum) and τόπι (ball), as well as more difficult words such as ζωγραφίζω (to paint). The majority of errors were lexical substitutions, e.g. reading the word μαμά (mum) as μητέρα (mother), τόπι (ball) as σπίτι (home) or τηλεγράφημα (telegram) as τηλεφώνημα (telephone). The overall percentage of logographic errors indicating the adoption of a 'logographic' or partial visual reading strategy was 13% at age 7 (grade 2) and 15% at age 9 (grade 4). The remaining errors were unsuccessful sounding-out attempts in which children tried to sound out a word but were unable to produce the correct response either because they did not know the required grapheme–phoneme correspondence rule or because they failed to blend the phonemes correctly. This pattern of errors indicates that, despite the ortho-graphic transparency of their language, Greek dyslexic readers' reading strate-gies are by no means perfect and there are substantial individual differences among children of the same chronological age.

An item analysis revealed that over half (62%) of the 'non-phonetic' reading errors and letter omissions (56%) occurred on the low-frequency, multi-syllabic words containing difficult consonant clusters such as εκπυρσοκρότηση (detonation), εκτραχυλισμός (debauchery) or εγκάθειρκτος (imprisoned). The percentage of children making non-phonetic errors in shorter words with a simpler phonological structure did not exceed 4%. It appears that the combination of orthographic complexity, low word frequency and word length stresses the 'faulty' word recognition system, and it is only under these circumstances that Greek dyslexic readers' reading behaviour approximates English dyslexic readers' difficulty when asked to read unfamiliar words or nonwords.

In similar vein, although the spelling of Greek dyslexic readers was phonetically accurate, about 70% of them experienced difficulties with the orthographic accuracy of their spellings. The majority of their errors were the consequence of incorrectly selecting the wrong grapheme for phonemes with more than one spelling representation, e.g. writing the word μαχαίρι (knife) as μαχέρι or omitting one of the double letters (e.g. writing the word γραμματική as γραματική). Non-phonetic errors never occurred. An item analysis of spelling errors was performed to examine Greek readers' sensi-tivity to some of the inflectional morphemes of their language. Dyslexic and average readers' performance was contrasted on three major sets of inflec-tional morphemes. The first set comprised words containing common single-letter or two-letter inflectional morphemes used to mark differences in the gender of nouns. Two of them (i.e. -ος and -ης) are used in masculine nouns (e.g. ο φίλος (friend), ο ναύτης (sailor); one (i.e. -η) in feminine nouns (e.g. βρύση = /'vri:si:/ (tap); and the remaining two (-ο, -ι) in neuter nouns (e.g. δάχτυλο, παραμύθι). There were no significant differences in the perfor-mance of the dyslexic and average readers on the single-letter morphemes, possibly because these are the focus of explicit instruction from the first months in primary schools.

The second set of words contained two of the most frequently used verb endings (i.e -αίνω and -ώνω and eight less common bound morphemes. These multi-letter inflectional morphemes occur frequently in nouns (e.g.

-είο as in the nouns σχολείο, γραφείο, φαρμακείο) and verbs (e.g. -αίνω as in the verbs μαθαίνω, πηγαίνω, κατεβαίνω). Dyslexic children experienced considerable difficulty spelling both the high- and low-frequency morphemes in this set. For instance, only 25% of the dyslexic readers spelled the morpheme -αίνω correctly, while average readers attained an accuracy score of 64% – a highly significant difference. Similar differences in magnitude were also observed in the spelling of the other high-frequency morpheme -ώνω: (54% vs 80%) and the less-common bound morphemes (e.g. -ικό: 35% vs 65%; -αίνς: 4% vs 50%). These errors suggest that Greek dyslexic readers find it diffi-cult to learn common high-frequency spelling patterns that are underpinned by morphology. This may be because they are unaware of the morphemic structure of spellings. More generally, they may be insensitive to the statistical regularities in the orthography (cf. Treiman et al., 1995). Speculatively, this may be because of an over-reliance on single grapheme–phoneme correspon-dences, reinforced by their reading experience in a highly regular language (see Goswami et al., 1998, for a similar argument).

Phonological awareness skills in Greek dyslexic readers

Much existing research indicates that the written language deficits of dyslexic children stem primarily from a core deficit in the phonological domain (Vellutino, 1979; Stanovich, 1988). English dyslexic readers have consistently been reported to have deficits on various phonological aware-ness (Pratt & Brady, 1988; Bruck, 1990) and phonological processing tasks (e.g. Snowling, 1995, 2000). There is also evidence that the development of phonological awareness skills is at least partially a product of literacy skills (Morais et al., 1987). It has also been demonstrated that differences in the orthographic structure of languages can significantly affect the degree of saliency of different linguistic units (see Harris and Hatano, 1999, for reviews).

   The aim of the present set of analyses was to examine the development of phonological awareness skills in Greek dyslexic readers. Drawing on evidence that phonological awareness skills develop quickly in transparent orthographies (Wimmer,1993; Cossu, 1999), we predicted that Greek dyslexic readers would perform better than English-speaking dyslexic readers on many of the standard phonological awareness tasks. Moreover, if dyslexia can be traced to a universal and specific phonological deficit (Morton and Frith, 1995), then we should expect to find evidence of phonological impair-ment, either in the speed of processing phonological information or on tasks that tap phonological representations implicitly, such as short-term verbal memory tasks (Snowling and Hulme, 1994).

Our hypothesis that Greek-speaking dyslexic readers would have fewer problems with phonological awareness tasks that are difficult for English-speaking dyslexic readers was supported. The majority attained high scores on the phoneme and syllable counting and deletion tasks, scores ranging between 84 and 96% correct. Tasks requiring phoneme substitution or manipulation (e.g. spoonerisms and consonant segmentation) were more difficult, with mean scores ranging from 29 to 77% for dyslexic readers (see Table 4.4 for a summary of these data).

The high degree of competence attained on phonological awareness tasks that English dyslexic readers find difficult (e.g. Bruck, 1990) is in line with the view that the orthographic transparency of the Greek language enables learners to detect and manipulate phonemes at an early stage in reading development. Arguably, however, their superior performance may be an effect of intensive phonics instruction (Thompson and Johnston, 2000). It is not possible to distinguish between these possibilities here. Suffice it to say that the combination of a highly regular and consistent orthography and of a phonics-based reading instruction enables Greek dyslexic readers to develop conscious awareness of the phonemic structure of words earlier than most English dyslexic readers.

The absence of any significant differences in the performance of Greek dyslexic and average readers on some of the most commonly used tests of phonological awareness in English also highlights the issue of their diagnostic sensitivity for the identification of dyslexia in languages with a regular orthography. The orthographic transparency of the Greek language evidently creates such favourable conditions for the development of sublexical and phonological awareness skills that even poor readers attain high levels of competence at an early age. It is therefore only the more cognitive

Table 4.4 Performance of dyslexic and average readers on phonological awareness tasks: percentage correct

| | Grade 2 | | Grade 4 | |
	Dyslexic	Average	Dyslexic	Average
Syllable counting	96 (8.5)	97 (7.6)	94 (16.1)	99 (1.8)
Syllable deletion	82 (14.4)	96 (8.5)	87 (18.0)	97 (6.5)
Phoneme counting	85 (16.7)	87 (14.1)	81 (16.9)	93 (9.6)
Phoneme deletion	84 (10.9)	99 (2.5)	88 (9.9)	99 (1.7)
Phoneme substitution	59 (21.3)	80 (10.0)	65 (22.4)	91 (7.7)
Spoonerisms	31 (22.2)	48 (11.5)	29 (14.2)	62 (8.3)
Consonant segment	54 (10.8)	65 (13.7)	67 (20.2)	80 (4.1)

Standard deviations in parentheses.

demanding tasks such as spoonerisms,[1] that can discriminate poor from average readers.

Notwithstanding this evidence, there were significant differences between dyslexic and average readers in the time it took for them to complete phonological awareness tasks. In fact, it took the dyslexic readers almost twice as long as the controls to complete the phoneme substitution and spoonerisms tasks (Figure 4.2). This finding suggests an underlying deficiency, perhaps in the quality of underlying phonological representations, in so far as rate of access to them is impaired. In addition, the dyslexic group showed deficits in comparison to their peers on more common timed tests of phonological processing, notably speech rate, rapid naming and alliteration fluency.

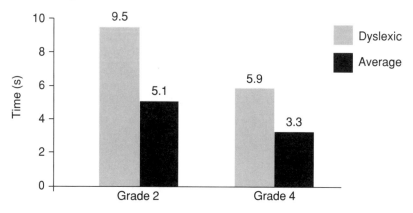

Figure 4.2 Mean reaction times of dyslexic children on the phoneme substitution and spoonerisms tests.

Cognitive deficits and dyslexia in Greek

We have argued that if it is true that Greek dyslexic children have poorly specified phonological representations, they should do less well on phonological tasks than their peers. Thus far, our data are somewhat equivocal. While Greek dyslexic children performed accurately on phonological tasks, they completed these tasks slowly. This pattern of performance raises the possibility that the children were responding by reference to orthographic representations that they created from the phonological input they received. Since rate of translation between orthographic and phonological codes was, by

---

[1]It should be noted that these more complex tasks may tap other cognitive resources, such as executive function, as well as phonological representations.

definition, slow in this group, it could be argued that the increased latencies they showed on the phonological tasks were an inevitable consequence of the way in which they were selected. To get around this problem of interpretation, it was important to compare the performance of the dyslexic children with that of the younger readers who were selected as reading at the same rate as they did (Table 4.3 for details). If the dyslexic children show deficits in relation to younger reading-level matched controls, then it is reasonable to infer that their difficulty stems from a deficit in phonological representation, not just in the rate at which they can evoke an orthographic representation.

When compared to younger reading-level matched controls, the dyslexic readers gained poorer scores on tests of nonword reading, phoneme deletion, spoonerisms and speech rate. The trend was in the same direction on the verbal STM, rapid naming and syntactic awareness tasks but failed to reach conventional levels of significance. There were no group differences on the simpler tests of phonological awareness. The dyslexic readers had no difficulty generating words from the same semantic category but had substantial difficulties with the phoneme fluency task in which they were asked to produce words beginning with a particular phoneme (e.g. /p/ → πατάτά, πολεμος, πεινάω, ποτέ).

To summarize, a similar pattern of results was obtained in the reading age comparison as in the age-matched comparison of Greek dyslexic and average readers. These data point to a specific phonological deficit in Greek dyslexic children that is evident even when they are compared with younger children who can decode words as efficiently as they can. In contrast, the dyslexic children did not show a deficit extending into the syntactic domain of processing.

To conclude, the similarity in the cognitive profile of Greek and English dyslexic readers is considerable and lends support to theories that view dyslexia as a universal phenomenon, the presenting characteristics of which may be influenced by culture, language and orthography (Frith, 1997; Snowling, 2000). The orthographic transparency of the Greek language moderates the severity of dyslexic readers' written language deficits and problems of phonological awareness. However, when more sensitive tests are used to probe the integrity of their phonological representations, for instance by measuring rate of access to them, then the characteristic markers of dyslexia can be seen.

Theoretical, educational and clinical implications

For many years, most of the evidence on the aetiology, manifestation and identification of developmental dyslexia has come from research into the 'deep' English orthography. According to a highly influential theory of literacy acquisition (Frith, 1985), the profound reading and spelling difficulties of English dyslexic readers are explained in terms of a developmental 'arrest' at the logographic stage of literacy acquisition, where word recognition is performed on the basis of partial cues. Frith (1985) postulates that most developmental dyslexic readers fail to make the transition to the alphabetic stage, during which most children gradually break the alphabetic code and establish a sound knowledge of grapheme-to-phoneme correspondence rules. Arrest at this essential stage of literacy acquisition results in severe problems with reading and spelling accuracy, and numerous non-phonetic errors (Bruck, 1990).

The findings of the present study, like others reported in this book, suggest that the actual stage at which development of literacy skills is arrested may depend, to some extent, on the degree of the orthographic complexity of the language being learned. Not all dyslexic children experience the same degree of difficulty with mastery of alphabetic skills. The orthographic transparency of the Greek language and the early introduction of Greek readers to phonics-oriented instruction facilitates the development of alphabetic skills more than the highly inconsistent English orthography. Greek dyslexic readers attain high levels of accuracy on reading and spelling single words and nonword reading from the age of 7, and make only a small percentage of logographic errors. The pattern of reading and spelling errors seen in this group resembles that of a group of English poor spellers, described by Frith (1985) as type-B spellers, rather than that of the more classic developmental dyslexics. Such children read well but spell phonetically. The same behavioural profile is replicated here in readers of Greek, where reading is easy for most children to master but spelling is not. Thus, it is imperative to reformulate some of the available theoretical accounts of literacy acquisition to account for the observed variation in the way in which literacy skills develop in different orthographic systems.

Professionals dealing with children who are learning to read a regular orthography should not expect dyslexic readers to exhibit the same pattern of reading and spelling difficulties as English dyslexic readers. The present research indicates that at least some of the typical signs of dyslexia in the English language (e.g. inaccurate word reading; letter or syllable omissions; reversals, substitutions or insertions in spelling; non-phonetic reading and spelling errors) are generally not characteristic of Greek dyslexic readers.

From an educational point of view, teachers and parents should be alerted to the fact that for Greek-speaking children, dyslexia does not present as a reading accuracy impairment but as slow, non-fluent reading alongside spelling difficulties. Other behavioural signs of underlying cognitive deficits include:

- sounding out the individual phonemes or syllables in words when other children of the same age decode words quickly and efficiently
- hesitating before long or difficult low-frequency words
- repeating the first syllable or article before deriving the pronunciation for the rest of the word
- occasional lexical substitution errors (especially under pressure of time).

Inaccurate spellings that sound like the target but contain incorrect vowels should also alert educationalists to the possibility of an underlying phonological impairment.

The results of the present study also have some important clinical implications for the identification of dyslexia. Significant differences in the diagnostic sensitivity of many cognitive measures that are commonly used in the identification of dyslexia in the English language warn against the uncritical adoption and use of these criteria across different orthographies. The results of the present study indicate that not all tasks or assessment criteria are sufficiently sensitive to detect the existence of underlying cognitive deficits. This appears to be particularly true for many common phonological awareness tasks. Greek-speaking children acquire alphabetic skills and high levels of syllable and phonemic awareness skills in the early years of schooling. Many phonological awareness tasks, such as phoneme and syllable counting, are too easy even for dyslexic children and thus inappropriate for diagnostic purposes. Only the more difficult and cognitive demanding tasks of phoneme deletion, substitution and spoonerisms are sensitive measures of individual variability in the development of phonological awareness skills. The significant differences in the time required to provide the correct answer also suggest the usefulness of a latency criterion, not only for the assessment of reading skills but also in the assessment of phonological skills. Phonological processing measures such as speech rate are also extremely useful tools for assessing the quality of underlying phonological representations in dyslexic as well as normal readers (Nikolopoulos and Goulandris, 2000). The poorer performance of dyslexic children on the consonant segmentation task and its significant and independent contribution to the prediction of reading ability (Nikolopoulos, 1999) also suggest the validity of devising new tests for the assessment of metaphonological skills.

Acknowledgement

This research was supported by a grant from the A.G. Leventis Foundation in Paris.

References

Bruck M (1990) Word recognition skills of adults with childhood diagnoses of dyslexia. Developmental Psychology 26: 439–454.

Bruck M, Treiman R (1990) Phonological awareness and spelling in normal children and dyslexics: the case of initial consonant clusters. Journal of Experimental Child Psychology 50: 156–178.

Caravolas M, Bruck M (1993) The effect of oral and written language input on children's phonological awareness: a cross-linguistic study. Journal of Experimental Child Psychology 55: 1–30.

Cossu G (1999) Biological constraints on literacy acquisition. Reading and Writing 11: 213–237.

Denckla M, Rudel RG (1976) Rapid automatized naming (RAN): dyslexia differentiated from other learning disabilities. Neuropsychologia 14: 471–479.

Elliot CD, Murray DJ, Pearson LS (1983) British Abilities Scales. Windsor: NFER-Nelson.

Frith U (1985) Beneath the surface of developmental dyslexia. In KE Patterson, JC Marshall, M Coltheart (eds) Surface dyslexia pp 301–330. Hillsdale, NJ: Lawrence Erlbaum Associates.

Frith U (1997) Brain, mind and behaviour in dyslexia. In C Hulme, M Snowling (eds) Dyslexia: biology, cognition and intervention. London: Whurr.

Frith U, Landerl K, Frith C (1995) Dyslexia and verbal fluency: more evidence for a phonological deficit. Dyslexia 1: 2–11.

Goswami U, Porpodas C, Wheelwright S (1997) Children's orthographic representations in English and Greek. European Journal of Psychology of Education 12: 273–292.

Harris M, Hatano G (eds) (1999) Learning to read and write: A cross-linguistic perspective. Cambridge, UK: Cambridge University Press.

McDougall S, Hulme C, Ellis A, Monk A (1994) Learning to read: the role of short-term memory and phonological skills. Journal of Experimental Child Psychology 58: 112–133.

Morais J, Alegria J, Content A (1987) The relationship between segmental analysis and alphabetic literacy: an interactive view. Cahiers de Psychologie Cognitive 7: 415–438.

Morton J, Frith U (1995) Causal modelling: a structural approach to developmental psychopathology. In D Cicchetti, DJ Cohen (eds) Manual of developmental psychopathology. New York: Wiley.

Nikolopoulos D (1994) The use of visual-orthographic and phonological strategies in English and Greek. Unpublished Masters dissertation, University of London, Institute of Education.

Nikolopoulos D (1999) Cognitive and linguistic predictors of literacy skills in the Greek language. The manifestation of reading and spelling difficulties in a regular orthography. Unpublished PhD thesis, University College London.

Nikolopoulos D, Goulandris N (2000) The cognitive determinants of literacy skills in a regular orthography. In M Perkins, S Howard (eds) New directions in language development and disorders. New York: Plenum Publishers.

Pinheiro AMV (1995) Reading and spelling development in Brazilian Portuguese. Reading and Writing 7: 111–138.

Pratt AC, Brady S (1988) Relation of phonological awareness to reading disability in children and adults. Journal of Educational Psychology 80: 319–323.

Rack JP, Snowling MJ, Olson RK (1992) The nonword reading deficit in developmental dyslexia: a review. Reading Research Quarterly 27: 29–53.

Raven JC (1987) Manual for Raven's progressive matrices and vocabulary scales, Section 3. Standard progressive matrices. London: HK Lewis & Co.

Semel E, Wiig EH, Secord W (1987) Clinical evaluation of language fundamentals, revised. Examiners manual. The Psychological Corporation, London: Harcourt Brace & Co.

Snowling MJ (1995) Phonological processing and developmental dyslexia. Journal of Research in Reading 18: 132–138.

Snowling MJ (2000) Dyslexia, 2nd edition. Oxford: Blackwell.

Snowling M, Hulme C (1994) The development of phonological skills. Transactions of the Royal Society B 346: 24–28.

Stanovich KE (1988) Explaining the differences between the dyslexic and the garden-variety poor reader: the phonological-core variable-difference model. Journal of Learning Disabilities 21: 590–604.

Thompson GB, Johnston RS (2000) Are nonword and other phonological deficits indicative of a failed reading process? Reading and Writing 12: 63–97.

Treiman R, Mullenix J, Bijeljac-Babic R, Richmond-Welty D (1995) The special role of rimes in the description, use and acquisition of English orthography. Journal of Experimental Psychology: General 124: 107–136.

Vellutino FR (1979) Dyslexia: theory and research. Cambridge, MA: MIT Press.

Wimmer H (1993) Characteristics of developmental dyslexia in a regular writing system. Applied Psycholinguistics 14: 1–33.

Wimmer H, Goswami U (1994) The influence of orthographic consistency on reading development: word recognition in English and German children. Cognition 51: 91–103.

CHAPTER 5
Dyslexia in Polish

MARCIN SZCZERBIŃSKI

Contributing a chapter to a book on dyslexia in different languages, I find myself faced with two tasks. The first is informative: providing the reader with an overview of Polish research into written language difficulties – information otherwise unavailable to him due to the language barrier. The second – and probably more important – is comparative: discovering what is *common* and what is *specific* about dyslexia in Polish, as compared to other languages.

I assume that the basic causes of dyslexia are the same in all languages – at least those written with an alphabetic script. Dyslexia stems from subtle cognitive deficits, mainly within the language-processing domain. Yet I will also argue that the specific mechanisms, manifestations and the course of dyslexic difficulties are influenced by the following linguistic and educational factors:

- the characteristics of the spoken language
- the characteristics of the orthography
- the methods of teaching literacy.

The problem is also embedded in the social context. Cultures, countries and educational systems differ in the value assigned to proficient literacy skills, the expectations of the learner, commonsense attributions of difficulties and the provision of remedial help (Figure 5.1). All these characteristics also shape the course and ultimate outcome of dyslexic difficulties.

The chapter begins with a description of the background factors. I will briefly characterize the basic features of spoken Polish, the orthography, and the ways of teaching reading and spelling. This will allow me to formulate some hypotheses about the specific features of dyslexia in Polish: its mechanisms, symptoms and developmental course from childhood into adulthood.

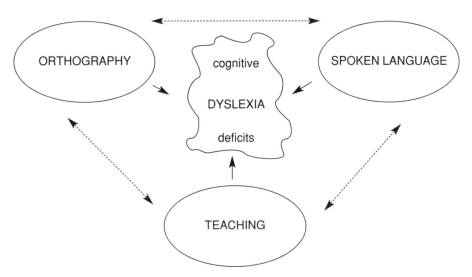

Figure 5.1 A simple diagram illustrating the relationship between linguistic and educational factors and dyslexia.

The second part of the chapter scrutinizes these hypotheses against the existing empirical data, thus addressing the central question: 'What is common and what is specific about dyslexia in different languages?'

The language

Together with Czech and Slovak, Polish belongs to the group of Western Slavic languages. It is more distantly related to Eastern Slavic (Russian, Ukrainian) and Southern Slavic (Bulgarian, Serbo-Croatian) tongues. With around 38 million speakers in the country, and possibly another 5 million worldwide, it is ranked among the 30 most widely spoken languages of the world (Webster, 1981; Ethnologue, 1996).

A detailed description of the language is beyond the scope of this chapter. Interested readers may refer to comprehensive English and Polish sources (Zagórska-Brooks, 1975; Fisiak et al., 1978; Strutyński, 1997). Listed below are some key features, which may also be critical for the task of reading and spelling.

• Syntax and morphology. Polish is an inflectional language, which expresses the relations between words in a sentence mainly by changing the words themselves – most typically by adding a suffix. Those inflectional changes occur in nouns, pronouns, adjectives and numerals (so-called declensions), and verbs (conjugations), e.g.:

Cztery małe dziewczynki pojechały na wycieczkę.

Four   little   girls   went   for a trip.

Czterej mali chłopcy pojadą na wycieczkę.

Four   little   boys   will go   for a trip.

Opiekowałem się małymi chłopcami i dziewczynkami w trakcie wycieczki.

I was looking after   little   boys   and girls   during   the trip.

Characteristically, some inflected words not only take on a suffix, but also undergo some alterations of their stem, e.g.:

pies/pjes/ – psy/psɨ/   wieźć/vjeɕtɕ/   –   wiózł/vjusw/

dog   dogs   to carry   (he) carried

Derivation (forming new words) is done by adding prefixes or suffixes. Again, the word stem is often altered in the process, e.g.:

rzucić – wyrzucić   chodzić – odchodzić   książka – księga   szkoła – szkolny

to throw   to throw away   to walk   to go away   a book   a big book   a school   school
                                          to walk away   a tome   [noun]   [adjective]

As a consequence of those morphological processes, a reader has to deal with constantly changing phonological and visual word forms (e.g. compare English *cat, cats, cat's* with Polish *kot, kota, kotu, kotem, kocie, koty, kotów, kotom, kotami, kotach*).

• **Segmental phonology.** Foreign listeners often perceive Polish as being spoken with 'almost no vowels'. Indeed, all formal descriptions of the Polish phonology (e.g. Rocławski, 1981; Strutyński, 1997) list relatively few vowels (no more than eight: six short oral and two nasal; the latter often described as diphthongs) but many consonants (at least 28). With 3.5 times more consonants than vowels, Polish indeed looks like a very consonantal language – the analogous figure for English is 1.2.[1] However, when we compare the frequency of usage, rather than the number of segments, we find nearly identical figures for English (39% vowels), Polish

---

[1]Following Longman Dictionary of Contemporary English (1995), which specifies 20 vowels (including eight diphthongs) and 24 consonants.

(40%) and French (41%). These three languages may be contrasted, with more consonantal German (vowel frequency only 36%) on one hand, and with Italian and Finnish on the other (48% and 51% frequency of vowels, respectively) (Fry, 1947 in Crystal, 1991; Rocławski, 1976; Kyostio, 1980). What gives Polish its specific consonantal quality is probably not the high proportion of consonants, but the numerous consonant clusters.

- **Consonant clusters** (up to four consonants long) occur frequently in various positions within the word, e.g.:

    pstra /pstra/   *państw* /paŋstf/   *odstrzał* /ɔtʃtʃaw/

Syllable-initial (onset) clusters are most frequent, as open syllables prevail (Bethin, 1992). Adjacent consonants tend to adjust their place and manner of articulation, which may lead to the reduction of a consonant cluster. Orthographically, this results in silent letters corresponding to 'potential' phonemes that occur only in slow, careful speech.

- **Word length.** Compared to English, Polish words tend to be slightly longer (Szczerbiński and Coleman, 1999) and more often polysyllabic. As a consequence there are relatively few rhyming monosyllables, so characteristic of English (e.g. *pat-bat-mat*). In contrast, multi-syllabic rhyming words (e.g. *krówka-główka-sówka-pocztówka...*) are very frequent. They are often grammatically related, sharing the same suffix (e.g. they are plural nouns, diminutives or verbs in the same number, gender and tense form).
- **Stress.** Polish is a syllable-timed language with fixed-word stress, falling on the penultimate syllable. Thus, stress never serves a lexical function of differentiating words (cf. English ób*ject* [noun] vs ob*jèct* [verb]) Unstressed vowels generally do not change their phonological quality – nothing like 'half vowel', analogous to the English 'schwa' /ə/ sound, exists.

The orthography

Polish is written with the Roman script, adapted to the phonological system of the language by using diacritics and combining letters into digraphs. Thus, the contemporary Polish alphabet incorporates 23 Roman letters (excluding *q*, *v* and *x*) and supplements them with nine diacritized letters: *ą*, *ę*, *ć*, *ń*, *ś*, *ź*, *ó*, *ż*, *ł*. Most diacritics represent a single distinctive phonemic feature: nasality (nasal vowels, written *ą*, *ę*, as opposed to their oral counterparts *o*, *e*) and place of articulation ('soft', palatal *ć*, *ń*, *ś*, *ź* as opposed to 'hard', dental *c*, *n*, *s*, *z*; alveolar *ż*, distinct from dental *z* and palatal *ź*). An additional seven digraphs (*ch*, *cz*, *dz*, *dź*, *dż*, *rz*, *sz*) are taught to the first grade children in the same way as single letters. They represent fricatives and affricates. Letter names always incorporate a respective letter sound (unlike English *w* and *y*, for example) and in the case of vowels, letter names and sounds are identical.

All orthographies represent some linguistic units by means of conventional visual symbols (graphemes). They differ, however, in terms of *what linguistic units* they choose to represent, and *how systematic the mappings are* between those units and the graphemes. Those differences are described in terms of orthographic *depth* and *consistency*, respectively. In 'shallow' orthographies, word spellings are 'phonetic': they represent surface phonology. 'Deep' orthography spellings directly represent morphemes – an example being the English regular past tense and plural suffixes, generally spelled as *-ed* and *-s*, regardless of their alternative pronunciations. In a fully consistent orthographic system, there is only one way to pronounce every string of graphemes or to spell any spoken word; the inconsistent orthographic system contains alternative sound-symbol mappings and exceptions.

Polish orthography is characterized by a very *high consistency for reading* (letter-to-sound mappings) but rather low consistency for spelling (sound-to-letter mappings). Practically every letter string – word or made-up nonword – can be read in only one, predictable way. Although letters may represent two or more phonemes when considered alone (e.g. *w* = /v/ or /f/), their pronunciation is always disambiguated by the context (preceding or following letters). There are practically no exceptional spellings (such as *have*, *pint* or *yacht* in English) nor homographs (one spelling – several pronunciations corresponding to different meanings, e.g. *wind – to wind*). The situation is different with spelling, however: most words can be written down in more than one way so that the spellings are phonologically plausible, but the orthographically correct option has to be chosen from the alternatives. Homophones (one pronunciation – different spellings corresponding to different meanings, e.g. *their – there*) also occur, although they are relatively infrequent. Spellings reflect the 'deep' features of the Polish orthography. Morphemes (word roots, prefixes and suffixes) are often spelled the same, although their pronunciation changes following the phonological rules of assimilation, final devoicing or cluster reduction (see Figure 5.2)

As these examples illustrate, morphological knowledge about related words (derivations) or different forms of the same word (inflections) usually provides clues to the orthographically correct spelling. In some words, however, the spelling is a matter of a historically motivated convention, cannot be derived from a morphological rule and has to be memorized on an item-specific basis.

Highly consistent reading, inconsistent spelling and the partially 'deep' structure observed in Polish seem typical of the majority of the alphabetic orthographies, such as German (Wimmer, 1993) and Portuguese (Pinheiro,

/-ẓba/		/-as/		/-apka/	
↓↑ ↓↑		↓↑ ↓↑		↓↑ ↓↑	
GROŹBA	PROŚBA	LAS	GAZ	CZAPKA	JABŁKA
/groẓba/	/prɔẓba/	/las/	/gas/	/t͡ʃapka/	/japka/
threat	request	forest	gas	hat	apples (Nom.)
⇓⇑	⇓⇑	⇓⇑	⇓⇑	⇓⇑	⇓⇑
GROZIĆ	PROSIĆ	LASY	GAZY	CZAPEK	JABŁEK
/grɔʑit͡ɕ/	/prɔɕit͡ɕ/	/laṣi/	/gaẓi/	/t͡ʃapek/	/jabwek/
to threaten	to request	forests	gases	hats (Gen.)	apples (Gen.)

Figure 5.2 Examples of assimilation, final devoicing and cluster reduction processes and their effect on letter-sound correspondences.

1995). Those orthographic systems can be contrasted with Finnish or Serbo-Croatian (which are even more shallow and consistent) on one hand and English or French (which have a very deep structure and low degree of consistency for both reading and spelling) on the other.

Education, literacy and dyslexia

The school system

Polish children start compulsory primary education in the year of their 7th birthday. However, 95–99% of children start formal reading instruction at the age of six, attending non-compulsory preparatory classes (so-called 'zero grade'). Thus, formal schooling starts at approximately the same age as in the USA, later than in Britain, but slightly earlier than in Germany, Austria or the Scandinavian countries.

The first three grades of compulsory primary education are called the period of 'initial education', where the basic literacy and numeracy skills are the main focus of the curriculum. It is during this period that children are expected to acquire core reading and spelling skills. Later on, teaching devolves into specialized subject areas.

Teaching literacy

Teaching literacy starts in the 'zero' grade and is largely phonics based. Letter–sound correspondences are gradually introduced, and word analysis and blending skills are drilled using real word material. It is initially restricted to 'easy' letters, with Polish digraphs and diacritics being introduced somewhat later. Reading syllable-by-syllable is encouraged as an intermediate

step to whole-word recognition. Writing is not taught until the beginning of
1st grade – almost a year later than reading. Cursive script is used from the
start and letter-forming skills (shapes, direction of strokes, etc.) are taught
explicitly. Spontaneous, emergent spelling is not encouraged, and the importance of spelling accuracy is stressed from the beginning throughout the
entire school period. The explicit teaching of orthographic rules (accompanied by drill exercises) is a very important part of the curriculum from the 1st
until at least the 5th grade. Similarly, teaching of general grammar is emphasized. Since the orthographic rules of Polish are grammatically motivated, the
two areas partially overlap.

Phonological awareness exercises play a very important part in preparing
and facilitating literacy acquisition from kindergarten on. Syllable and
phoneme analysis and blending, as well as alliteration recognition exercises,
are employed most often.

This is the mainstream approach towards reading: it has its distinct
varieties and also outright opponents. Alternative teaching methods, based
on whole-word (Dobrowolska-Bogusławska, 1991) or language experience
approaches (e.g. Majchrzak, 1995) have become popular recently.

It should be added that, in terms of functional literacy (the ability to put
reading skills into practical use), the Polish population fares badly in comparison to other Western societies. Reading comprehension was found to be
relatively poor in children (Foshay et al., 1962) and adults (OECD, 1995). It is
unclear what cultural, socioeconomic or educational factors are responsible
for this unfavourable outcome.

Dyslexia in Polish: what may be common and what specific?

Given the linguistic and educational characteristics outlined above, I would
like to formulate some hypotheses regarding the symptoms, cause and
mechanisms of dyslexia in Polish.

1. Spelling disorder, rather than reading disorder, may be typical for Polish

Reading difficulties were observed in all languages studied so far (Stevenson
et. al., 1982; Tansley and Panckhurst, 1991). However, it is likely that consistent orthographies are easier to learn, hence they reduce the incidence and
severity of those problems (Downing, 1973). There is some evidence to
support this hypothesis from experiments using a simplified orthography
(the Initial Teaching Alphabet; Downing, 1967) and from cross-linguistic
studies (Lindgren et al., 1985). Given the structure of the Polish orthography
(high consistency for reading, low for spelling) we may expect that a specific
spelling disorder should be a dominant form of written language difficulty in
Polish; in contrast, specific reading disorder may be relatively rare.

2. The symptoms and the course of the difficulties may be language-specific

Poor decoding skills are considered to be a core characteristic of dyslexia (Rack et al., 1992). However, this conclusion is based mainly on English language studies, and its validity may be limited to inconsistent orthographies. *Consistent orthographies facilitate decoding*: their users are more accurate at reading all types of novel, unfamiliar words (Wimmer and Goswami, 1994; Goswami et al., 1998). This advantage extends to consistent orthography dyslexics: their decoding problems are mild and limited mainly to the first months of reading instruction. High reading accuracy does not mean that difficulties are completely eliminated: their reading remains stubbornly *slow* and they make numerous *spelling errors* (Wimmer, 1993, 1996; Landerl et al., 1997). Such a developmental course of symptoms is likely to occur in Polish dyslexics, too.

Not only overall accuracy, but also the types of *errors*, vary across languages and orthographies (Fowler et al., 1977; Ognejovic et al., 1983; Cossu et al., 1995). Errors generally tend to involve inconsistent letter–sound correspondences. Their likelihood is heightened even more when the inconsistency overlaps with graphemic or phonological similarity (two similar-looking or similar-sounding letters are inconsistently mapped on to phonemes). As different letter–sound correspondences are affected by such problems in each orthography, cross-linguistic differences in error patterns should emerge.

3. The predictors and mechanisms of the difficulties may be language-specific

It is widely accepted that most dyslexics' reading and spelling problems are caused by linguistic deficits – especially deficits in processing the sounds of words (phonology). What deficits are most critical and how they disrupt learning remains controversial, however. As different orthographies represent different linguistic elements (morphemes, syllables, onset-rhymes, phonemes), the demands for the learner may vary accordingly. The mastery of every alphabetic orthography should require *phonemic awareness* – the ability to identify, segment and blend phonemes (e.g. Byrne, 1998). Some alphabetic systems with very unpredictable letter–sound mappings (like English) are more consistent at the level of longer letter strings that map on to *rhymes* and *onsets*. Learning such orthographies may, then, additionally require sensitivity to those larger phonological units (see Goswami and Bryant, 1990; Goswami, 1999; Seymour et al., 1999 for a comprehensive discussion of this controversial hypothesis). Good *morphological awareness* – the ability to manipulate morphological units – may be required in deep orthographies, particularly at the later stages of development, in the context of learning morphologically motivated spellings (Bryant et al., 1998).

Apart from deficits in linguistic awareness, dyslexics were also found to be slow at naming familiar stimuli (objects, digits or letters; Wolf and Bowers, 1999). Rapid naming difficulties probably reflect problems in learning any arbitrary symbol–name associations, including letter–sound correspondences and the pronunciation of frequently encountered orthographic units (Manis et al., 1999). Whereas dyslexics learning inconsistent orthographies are deficient in both linguistic awareness and naming, their consistent orthography counterparts show mainly naming impairment; their problems with phonological awareness are mild and limited mainly to earliest phases of learning (De Gelder and Vroomen, 1991; Wimmer, 1993). It seems that dyslexia in a consistent orthography is mainly a problem with learning *orthographic skills*: making word recognition automatic and producing spellings that are orthographically 'legal' (not merely 'sound right'). Dyslexics learning an inconsistent orthography, on the other hand, may struggle with *alphabetic decoding* (letter–sound translation) as well as higher-order orthographic skills.

Dyslexia in Polish: the research findings

What are the forms of literacy difficulties?

In the previous section I hypothesized that, in Polish, spelling difficulties may be a more typical form of written language disability than reading difficulties. Even the common usage of the term 'dyslexia' seems to support this conjecture: listening to Poles using the word one may get the impression that dyslexia is primarily about 'bad spelling' rather than 'bad reading'.

Several incidence studies (e.g. Spionek, 1973; Szurmiak, 1974) gave 9–17% estimates of childhood written language difficulties. The largest epidemiological study (Jaklewicz, 1980; Bogdanowicz, 1985) distinguished specific reading and spelling disorder[2] from poor reading and spelling that was commensurate with low general ability. Specific written language disorders were diagnosed only when children met the exclusionary criteria (IQ more than 85, no gross sensory or neurological impairment), made a number of errors considered 'typical' (e.g. confusions based on phonological or graphemic similarity of letters) and showed some perceptual or motor deficits. Reading skills were operationalized as reading rate (number of words read *correctly* per minute); to diagnose reading disorder, at least a two-year delay in reading rate was also required. Among 4th grade (10–11 years old) students, 9.2–10.9% reading-disordered and 13.1–16.7% spelling-disordered children were identified; literacy difficulties of specific and non-

---

[2]The Polish literature usually labels them as 'dyslexia' and 'dysorthography', respectively.

specific nature were present in as many as 30% of the sample. Socioeconomic factors played some role: children who lived in the country were at slightly higher risk than city dwellers. All children with reading disorder were also spelling disordered. Children with 'reading + spelling' disorder profile exhibited more severe perceptual–motor deficits than the 'spelling-only' disorder group.

The incidence of early reading problems was assessed by Bogdanowicz (1991, 1997). At the end of the first year of tuition ('zero' grade) 4.7% of children were unable to read any words, while another 5.5% could achieve no more than two words per minute (wpm). In contrast, average children read between five and 13 wpm, and very good readers over 35 wpm. Such early discrepancies appeared remarkably stable, even over a 10-year period (Jaklewicz, 1980, 1982; Bogdanowicz, 1991, 1997), although their magnitude seemed to gradually diminish with age.

In adolescents, poor spelling seems the most apparent manifestation of written language difficulties, as it is the main reason concerned parents and teachers refer students for psychological assessment. However, systematic assessment reveals additional reading difficulties (especially slow reading speed) in at least 70% of adolescent poor spellers (Jaklewicz, 1980; Wszeborowska-Lipińska, 1995, 1996).

In general, the incidence estimates presented above correspond to those obtained in other countries (Tansley & Panckhurst, 1991) or are even higher. Specific problems with both reading and spelling are observed at different age levels, and largely overlap. There is, therefore, little support for the hypothesis that the consistency of the Polish orthography helps to reduce the incidence of reading problems. It is probably the severity of underlying cognitive deficit that is crucial: 'reading + spelling' disorder profile stems from more serious deficits than in the 'spelling-only' condition. There is, however, some (albeit circumstantial) evidence that the Polish orthography may enable dyslexics to overcome their decoding difficulties eventually. Teenage dyslexics make rather few reading errors, and reading rate differentiates them from normal controls better than simple accuracy (Wszeborowska-Lipińska, 1995, 1996). Low reading speed and orthographically inaccurate spelling seem, then, to constitute a persistent manifestation of written language disorder in Polish. Younger dyslexics, however, do exhibit considerable decoding difficulties: the author's small sample of 2nd and 3rd grade dyslexics (see below) decoded correctly 85–92% of the single words, but only 47–65% of the nonwords. This performance is clearly worse in comparison with German or Spanish dyslexics of a similar age (67–96% nonword reading accuracy; Wimmer, 1993; Wimmer et al., 1999; Rodrigo and Jimenez 1999), though still better than English dyslexics, who showed similar, or worse, accuracy reading shorter, one-syllable words (Rack et al., 1992).

What are the manifestations and the developmental course of literacy difficulties?

I hypothesized that the types of dyslexic errors may be language- and orthography-specific. The problems identified among Polish dyslexics include: semantic word substitutions and guessing; gross word distortions; word and letter reversals; letter substitutions; omission of diacritics; confusion of suffixes; poor punctuation – to name just a few (Bogdanowicz, 1994). Some of the problems are, therefore, language- and orthography-specific (e.g. diacritics), while others seem universal.

Spelling error corpuses collected with normal students (e.g. Kiken, 1935; Polański, 1973; Grzędowa, 1976) and poor spellers (Jaklewicz, 1980) show that the vast majority of errors are phonetic: misspellings 'sound right' but disregard higher-order orthographic rules (which are usually morphologically motivated). Errors thus tend to cluster in relatively few orthographic areas where sound-to-letter mappings are most complex, and word sound provides insufficient clues to correct spelling. There are no studies that would directly investigate whether dyslexic misspellings are qualitatively different from errors produced by normal students or merely more frequent. Clinical observations suggest that beginning readers with dyslexia/spelling disorder – unlike normal children – frequently distort words beyond recognition, which suggests poor awareness of phonological word structure and deficient recoding skills. As they grow older, however, their errors become more phonetic, similar to those made by normal students, yet still more frequent. It seems, therefore, that at least in the majority of dyslexic cases sufficient recoding skills are eventually learned.

Many authors also refer to the immature 'reading technique' of poor readers. Typically, young Polish readers overtly sound out and blend individual letters (Sochacka, 1998), but quickly move into an orthographic whole-word recognition phase. Dyslexics often seem to be arrested in the letter-by-letter decoding phase for much longer – while 91% of very good readers already recognize whole words directly at the end of 'zero' grade, only 43% of dyslexics do so in the 4th grade (Bogdanowicz, 1997).

Poor handwriting (labelled 'dysgraphia' in the Polish literature) also frequently co-occurs: among children with joint reading and spelling problems, 23% produce poor or illegible handwriting (Bogdanowicz, 1985). This relationship seems to diminish with age (Bogdanowicz, 1997), but others (Wszeborowska-Lipińska, 1996) found that even among adolescent dyslexics, half present with poor handwriting.

It seems plausible that those symptoms that are most directly related to core dyslexic deficits are also most resistant to treatment. The most 'stubborn' problems identified in various long-term intervention studies with younger primary school dyslexics (Markiewicz and Zakrzewska, 1978; Trzeciak, 1980;

Maurer, 1990) included: slow reading speed; misreading word endings (suffixes); and certain, orthography-specific types of spelling errors. Spelling seemed generally harder to improve than reading. However, the problems identified as most difficult to remediate varied from study to study. The general conclusions from the intervention studies were rather positive: it was possible to improve various aspects of reading and spelling and sometimes even to enable reading-impaired children to catch up with their peers.

The emotional, educational and social consequences of dyslexia are potentially serious. Spionek (1973), Jaklewicz (1980, 1982) and Wszeborowska-Lipińska (1995, 1996) showed that untreated dyslexic problems led to frequent neurotic and psychosomatic symptoms as well as disruptive behaviour. As they grew older, dyslexics often lagged more and more behind their peers in terms of knowledge and IQ. A large proportion of them left school earlier, with fewer formal qualifications, and performed less responsible jobs. The family environment appeared to be absolutely crucial in preventing such a negative train of events. Dyslexics who succeeded at school had parents who valued education, accepted their 'difficult' children and offered active support (helping with homework, arranging a tutor, etc.). Some personality traits of dyslexics also seemed to play a role in determining ultimate educational success or failure.

The Polish findings reviewed above are comparable with those obtained elsewhere, indicating general similarity of dyslexia symptoms, the course and long-term consequences across countries and languages. Both reading and spelling problems are observed; they are persistent (though remediable) and, if untreated, may seriously compromise educational and employment prospects. The actual reading and spelling errors, however, may be orthography-specific to some degree, being easily elicited by complex, multiple letter–sound mappings, which are different in each orthography. A prolonged letter sounding-out and blending reading phase may be characteristic of dyslexics taught to read with phonics methods.

What are the predictors and mechanisms of literacy difficulties?

Virtually all the research carried out in Poland started with an assumption that dyslexia is a cognitive and (ultimately) biologically-based disorder. Early research (until the 1970s) focused on perceptual and motor functions. It was proposed that dyslexia stems from cortical deficiencies in processing visual and auditory stimuli, as well as in acquiring and executing motor programmes (Spionek, 1963, 1970, 1973; Bogdanowicz, 1978). The atypical patterns of laterality (lack of clear dominance for an eye, hand and foot, or a crossed dominance) were also supposed to play a role through their link with the abnormal visual–spatial orientation. Numerous studies have indeed found some support for these hypotheses. Compared with normal readers of the same age, dyslexics are inferior on non-verbal auditory processing (e.g. reproducing sequences of beats or taps) and 'phonematic hearing' (often operationalized as phoneme discrimination ability; Kania, 1982), visual discrimination (Maurer and Oszustrowicz, 1984), visual memory and visual-motor co-ordination, and occasionally also motor-kinaesthetic skills (see Table 5.1). Data on laterality are less consistent, yet generally atypical laterality (especially lack of clear dominance) occurs slightly more often among poor readers. Auditory deficits (both non-verbal and phonological) were found most frequently.

The findings, however, are ambiguous. Only a few studies (e.g. Wszeborowska-Lipińska, 1995, 1996) matched dyslexics and controls on IQ, age and education level. None employed a reading age-matched design (comparing dyslexics with younger, normal readers matched on reading skills), which allows researchers to identify the causes of reading breakdown more clearly than chronological-age comparisons. Undoubtedly, perceptual–motor deficits accompany poor reading, but it is questionable whether they are its causes. It is more plausible that they reflect more general learning difficulties, are a consequence of school failure, or sometimes are spurious. The need for more conceptually and methodologically rigorous research in this area has been indicated (Kostrzewski, 1981; Grabowska, 1994).

Table 5.1 Percentages of poor readers with perceptual–motor deficits identified in various studies

Study	% of poor readers with					
	visual deficit	auditory deficit	motor–kinaesthetic deficit	only visual deficit	only auditory deficit	only motor–kinaesthetic deficit
Spionek (1963)*	70	91	68	ns	ns	ns
Bogdanowicz (1991, 1997)	26	80	41	3	35	0
Wszeborowska-Lipińska (1995, 1996)	93	92	ns	7	8	ns
Jaklewicz (1980)* (4th graders)	76	100	50	ns	ns	ns
Jaklewicz (1980)* (young adults)	46	83	37	ns	ns	ns

*Nonverbal measures of auditory processing only; ns = not specified.

Similar criticism applies to the studies that explored dyslexia as a deficit of cross-modal integration. They investigated the transfer of information within and across sensory modalities (Bogdanowicz, 1991, 1997) or the role of multisensory mental images (Fenczyn, 1981, 1987). The tests of inter-modal and cross-modal integration indeed discriminated poor and good readers better than the measures of isolated perceptual and motor functions (Bogdanowicz, 1991, 1997). However, this can be explained by more adequate levels of test difficulty. Also, the tasks that were best at predicting reading usually involved some verbal–phonological component.

Interpreting perceptual problems as a concomitant of poor reading, yet not its cause, is suggested by the author's own data (Szczerbiński, 1999). A battery of linguistic and visual tests was administered to an unselected group of 1st–3rd grade children, who were also assessed on accuracy and speed of single-word reading. As expected, nearly all the tests correlated with reading. However, the visual tests – memory for abstract shapes and copying complex figures – could not predict reading and spelling once differences of age, vocabulary knowledge and non-verbal intelligence were taken into account. Among seven indices of visual processing only speed of letter discrimination remained a significant (albeit weak) predictor of reading. In contrast, most tests of phonological processing retained their predictive power. The best predictors represented two underlying (largely separate) factors: phonological awareness (tests of phoneme analysis, blending and replacement, alliteration detection) and verbal fluency and speed (rapid naming of digits, alliteration fluency). Each category made its own independent contribution to reading success. The situation was somewhat different in the case of spelling, where visual skills (namely, accuracy of letter and symbol discrimination) played some role.

Overall, the results suggest that the main constraints on reading development are linguistic, not visual–perceptual. It does not, however, preclude some additional role of visual processes. In the first months of reading instruction, Polish children appear to use a mixed strategy: they decode words alphabetically but also rely on visual cues (Sochacka, 1998). It seems plausible that poor decoders compensate for their difficulties by relying excessively on global, visual word recognition and context-driven guessing. Errors attributable to such reading strategies have been documented (Spionek, 1970, 1973). Possibly, if visual problems accompany decoding difficulties, then no compensatory mechanisms are available and profound early reading impairment ensues. Visual difficulties also tend to co-occur with low intelligence, so children with poor visual skills may have more generalized learning difficulties. This may explain Spionek's (1973) finding that visual deficits were most frequent among children whose reading difficulties were noticed early, during the first year of formal tuition.

Linguistic factors

The high frequency of *spoken language problems* in dyslexia has been acknowledged since the research began. Sawa (1971) found 81% incidence of literacy difficulties among children with apparent speech problems. Conversely, 62% of children with literacy problems exhibited concurrent speech and language difficulties, while 72% of them had a history of such problems. Dyslexia was associated with late speech onset, more persistent childhood agrammatisms (until the age of 7) and, most often, articulatory deficits. Stuttering and stammering were also a frequent correlate of literacy problems, yet appeared to be a consequence of lasting school failure, associated with emotional disturbances.

A language-oriented approach to dyslexia research, which has become popular in Poland since the late 1980s (e.g. Kołtuska, 1988), adopted a broad view of the relationship between written language acquisition and literacy. Whereas much of Western research stemmed from the hypothesis of dyslexia as a specific deficit in processing phonological information, Polish authors usually suggested multiple linguistic problems, not only on the level of *phonology*, but also *semantics*, *syntax*, *morphology* and *discourse* (Borkowska, 1997).

An early example of such a 'broad language' approach was given by Borkowska and Tarkowski (1990), who compared the performance of 2nd-grade dyslexics and the chronological age controls on a battery of linguistic tasks. The dyslexics scored significantly worse on nearly all the subtests assessing syntax, morphology and communicative competence. Both linguistic processing and communicative competence tasks correlated with reading and spelling performance, yet the correlation was stronger for linguistic processing skills. The authors suggested that semantic deficits were present in some cases of developmental dyslexia.

The semantic, syntactic and communicative skills were further explored by Krasowicz (1994, 1997) and Borkowska (1998) with 2nd- and 3rd-grade dyslexics. The tasks involved describing pictures and telling the stories depicted by them. Compared to age-matched controls, dyslexics produced shorter, poorly structured and less informative narratives. Their sentences were syntactically simpler, with more frequent hesitations, abrupt endings and occasional syntactic errors. This last finding is particularly striking, since dyslexics made more syntactic errors than controls, even though they had less opportunity for making them as they generally spoke less (Krasowicz, 1997).

Oszwa (1999) investigated morphological and syntactic skills, specifically the use of prepositions by 2nd- and 3rd-grade dyslexics. Large and highly significant differences emerged in comparison with age-matched controls. The dyslexics' use of prepositions was limited in both range and frequency, and generally lacked precision. They produced spatial descriptions that were impoverished or erroneous, sometimes involving left–right confusions. Occasional mismatches occurred between inflectional forms and prepositions, resulting in syntactic errors. Forming derivations – a task often involving adding prepositions as prefixes – was also impaired.

Those interesting findings are, however, open to alternative interpretations. Fuzzy criteria of dyslexia were used in some of the studies mentioned above, making it possible that some generally poor learners were included in the dyslexic samples. The analyses performed also do not make it clear whether the semantic, syntactic, morphological and communication difficulties observed in the dyslexics were primary cognitive deficits (as the authors claim) or a secondary product of other, lower-level deficiencies, such as poor working memory, word-finding difficulties, or small vocabulary and poor story-telling skills resulting from their limited reading experience.

Data from my own study (Szczerbiński, 1999), which also explored morphological skills of early readers, support the latter interpretation. Morphological skills (forming derivative forms, diminutives, comparison of adjectives, adding and deleting prefixes) correlated with reading ability (accuracy and speed of single-word and nonword decoding). However, those correlations disappeared or became weak once differences in non-verbal intelligence and vocabulary knowledge were statistically controlled for in multiple regression analyses. In contrast, most measures of phonological awareness and rapid naming remained strong predictors of reading. This suggests that reading development is directly constrained by phonological, but not morphological skills – at least as far as basic alphabetic skills are concerned. Insufficient spelling data were collected to investigate the possibility that the awareness of morphological structures may be necessary for higher-order orthographic spelling skills. This hypothesis requires further investigation.

Arguably, the most comprehensive evaluation of language processing in the context of reading difficulties was carried out by Krasowicz and Bogdanowicz (1999). It constituted part of an 18-month longitudinal study that investigated the role of linguistic awareness in the acquisition of literacy (Krasowicz, 1999; Krasowicz et al., 1999; Krasowicz-Kupis et al., 2000). Linguistic awareness tasks were administered at the beginning of 'zero' grade, before formal reading instruction began. They examined phonology (e.g. phoneme and syllable analysis, blending and deletion; rhyme and alliteration detection and production; phoneme replacement) as well as syntax and morphology (e.g. judging whether sentences are grammatically acceptable, completion and correction of sentences). Those measures were readministered twice: at the end of '0' and the 1st grade, together with reading tests. An IQ test was also administered at the end of the study. Children were classified as poor, normal or very good readers, depending on a reading rate score at the end of the 1st grade; the cut-off point for the poor readers group was one standard deviation below the mean. When the three groups were compared on their pre-school awareness skills, the largest differences emerged on alliteration detection and production, phoneme analysis and blending, as well as phoneme and last-syllable deletion tasks. On these tests, future poor readers were usually worse than children who went on to develop both normal and very good reading skills. Smaller differences appeared on word-syllable analysis, nonword-syllable blending, rhyme production and first-syllable deletion tasks, as well as some syntactic tests (sentence correction and grammatical acceptability judgement), with significant differences emerging mainly between extreme (poor and very good) reading groups. Syllable blending, nonword syllable analysis, rhyme oddity and sentence completion tasks did not differentiate the groups. It was, therefore, mainly the phoneme-level awareness that was problematic for children with future reading difficulties; their problems with rhyme, syllable and syntax awareness were less pronounced.

The following pre-school language profile was identified as characteristic of later poor readers:

• very low scores in first phoneme deletion task (around 0)
• low scores in syllable deletion task (below 33 percentile)
• low scores in alliteration detection and production, as well as phoneme blending tasks (equal or below 40 percentile)
• average scores in other phoneme tasks and rhyme oddity task (around 50–60 percentile).

When the same comparisons were carried out on language tasks administered one year later, together with the reading test, many more significant differences were observed. All the tests were able to discriminate the groups. Syllable analysis of nonwords, phoneme analysis and alliteration production were the most powerful indicators of poor, good or very good reading group membership. Although the absolute level of performance grew for all children and for all measures, the discrepancies between the groups were usually retained.

The linguistic tasks, however, were far from perfect predictors of reading acquisition, leaving a considerable percentage of reading variability unaccounted for. IQ score appeared to be a good predictor of reading, correctly classifying some 60% of poor readers. Typically, poor readers were characterized by lower verbal than non-verbal IQ scores. The poor readers group membership could be predicted much better when IQ and linguistic tests were combined.

The results of Krasowicz et al.'s study imply the crucial importance of phonological awareness in successful word decoding, with grammatical awareness possibly playing some minor role. Various levels of phonological representation (syllables, rhymes, phonemes) all contribute to reading, yet the control over the phonemic level seems most critical. Interestingly, the development of single phoneme awareness skills (especially alliteration detection, phoneme analysis and blending) was quicker than the development of rhyming skills (especially rhyme production). Rhyming was also a rather weak predictor of reading acquisition. This suggests that different languages, orthographies and teaching methods may selectively enhance different aspects of phonological skills. In Polish, a child's attention is directed towards alliteration, analysis, blending and syllabification, but less towards rhyming. Consequently, sensitivity to rhymes is not well developed (even in good readers) and is less important for literacy.

An unselected sample of early readers I tested recently (Szczerbiński, 1999) allowed me to identify and analyse a small number of dyslexic subjects. I tried to extend the results of previous studies in two ways: by including both chronological age and reading age control groups, and by contrasting two different forms of difficulties: low accuracy and slow speed dyslexia. Dyslexics and chronological-age controls were selected among 2nd- and 3rd-grade children. Reading-level controls came from a 1st-grade sample and were matched on accuracy and speed of word reading, respectively.

Low accuracy criteria (word reading accuracy at least 1 standard deviation (SD) below grade mean + discrepancy between vocabulary knowledge and reading accuracy of at least 1 SD) identified seven boys (10% of the sample) as dyslexics. The group was characterized by a clear alphabetic decoding deficit: they could read only 47% of nonwords correctly, which was significantly worse in comparison with the same-age peers (78% accuracy) and younger 1st-grade controls matched on accuracy of word reading (70% accuracy). Low-accuracy dyslexics were also significantly worse than chronological age controls on two phonological awareness tasks (vowel and consonant replacement), speed of digit naming, and speed of reading words and nonwords.

A somewhat different picture emerged when low-speed dyslexia was investigated. Seven dyslexics were again identified, three of them girls. Selection criteria were word reading speed at least 1 SD below grade mean and at least 1 SD discrepancy between vocabulary score and reading speed. There was practically no overlap between speed and accuracy dyslexia: only one child met both conditions. Low-speed dyslexics did not differ significantly from younger 1st-grade children matched on word reading speed, but were worse than same-age peers on rapid letter and digit naming, rhyme oddity and nonword reading time. Both dyslexic groups showed few problems with visual tasks and performed very well on phoneme analysis and blending – in fact, somewhat better than chronological-age controls. Further analyses using composite scores showed that both dyslexic groups had double deficits: comprising both phonological awareness as well as rapid naming. However, whereas low-accuracy dyslexics were worse on phonological awareness tasks than naming, the reverse was true for the low-speed group.

Those results were largely consistent with those obtained by other authors, who also differentiated low-speed and low-accuracy subgroups of dyslexia in English (Lovett, 1987) or German (Wimmer et al., 1999). The two conditions turned out to be at least partially separable. Poor-accuracy dyslexia seems to reflect the 'classic' syndrome of phonological awareness deficit (coupled with some naming difficulties), which inhibits all aspects of reading development. Low-speed dyslexia, on the other hand, may stem from various causes: difficulty in forming and using name–symbol associations (evidenced by poor naming performance), minor problems with phonological awareness or limited reading experience. These compromise primarily the *automaticity* of word recognition.

Tasks that are most sensitive indicators of reading difficulties change with age. This is apparent with phoneme analysis and blending skills. Krasowicz and Bogdanowicz (1999), as well as my own data, show that they are strong predictors of reading during the initial period of learning. After 1st grade, however, they are fully mastered by nearly all children and no longer differentiate good and poor readers. Presumably, analysis and blending are constantly exercised in the classroom and thus overlearned, even by children with underlying phonological deficits. Tasks that are less affected by classroom practice, however (e.g. phoneme replacement), are also sensitive indicators of phonological deficits (and of reading problems) at a later age.

Conclusions

The findings reviewed above point towards *general similarity in the incidence and causes of dyslexia in Polish and elsewhere*. Specific reading and spelling disorders are present at rates comparable with those obtained in other countries. There is growing evidence that they are closely related to the history of speech and language impairment and stem from linguistic deficits. The little data currently available suggest that dyslexia in Polish also fits the double-deficit model proposed in the context of other languages (Wolf and Bowers, 1999). Poor phonological awareness and inefficient activation of name–symbol connections (evidenced by slow naming speed) are two major constraints of reading development. Deficits in other linguistic domains (semantic, syntax, morphology) also accompany dyslexia, yet the evidence of their causal role is somewhat weaker.

Perceptual–motor deficits also seem a frequent correlate of poor reading and spelling in Polish, as in many other languages – their exact role, however, is not yet understood. We may speculate that dyslexics have a general problem with automatization of any complex skills, or with tasks that require precise co-ordination of different subprocesses under tight time constraints. Such an underlying deficit could explain the frequent co-occurrence of various, seemingly unrelated problems, which are verbal–linguistic (slow reading and naming speed and fluency, articulation difficulties) but also non-linguistic (e.g. poor motor co-ordination).

There are also indicators of *language-specific influences*. Considerable word decoding difficulties experienced by Polish dyslexics over the first few years of learning may reflect the complexities of the writing system. Judging by the frequency of errors, we may conclude that the Polish orthography is, after all, rather inconsistent. It does possess 'areas of particular difficulty' (such as letters of similar sound and shape and ambiguous letter–sound correspondences), which elicit most of the errors and further exacerbate the problems of otherwise poor decoders. However, Polish orthography is more consistent than English: this is reflected in the somewhat better decoding skills of Polish dyslexics. Some degree of consistency and phonics-based teaching may help Polish dyslexics to eventually overcome gross decoding problems and achieve reasonable reading accuracy. Specific features of orthography and teaching may also explain why some phonological aware-ness skills are mastered very well (e.g. phoneme analysis and blending) and are very important for reading acquisition, whereas other are not (rhyming). However, the influence of orthography and teaching is probably minor: *the severity of underlying cognitive deficits seems the most important factor determining the symptoms and course of dyslexia.*

It is impossible to have an adequate picture of dyslexia without considering its *developmental course*. Although dyslexia is persistent, its *symptoms and predictors change with age and experience*. In Polish, dyslexics initially struggle with phonological skills, yet gradually they develop some (at least rudimentary) word decoding and phonological awareness. Later on, lack of automaticity of word recognition and dysorthographic spelling become dominant problems.

The developmental perspective also helps us to understand subtypes of dyslexia. I postulated the distinction between 'low-accuracy' and 'slow-speed' forms. The former conforms to the *developmental deviance* model (low-accuracy dyslexics read differently, unlike any normal children), whereas the latter may be described as *developmental lag* (slow-speed dyslexics read as if they were younger). 'Accuracy'–'speed' differentiation probably maps closely on to the other, more commonly used distinction between 'phonological' and 'surface' developmental dyslexia (Ellis, 1993; Wimmer et al., 1999). However, the subtypes may be relative to the developmental phase. Most dyslexics initially struggle with phonological skills, yet many eventually acquire them. This may correspond to conversion from the 'low-accuracy' (or phonological) to 'slow-speed' (or surface) form. *Consistent orthographies and phonic teaching may facilitate such conversion*, resulting in a smaller proportion of 'low-accuracy' problems, especially in the population of older dyslexics.

Acknowledgements

I would like to express my gratitude to Dr Nata Goulandris and Professor Ruth Campbell for very detailed and helpful comments on the earlier versions of this manuscript. Dr Grażyna Krasowicz-Kupis, Dr Bożena Wszeborowska-Lipińska, Dr Urszula Oszwa and Krystyna Sochacka MA provided me with their unpublished manuscripts and shared many stimulating thoughts. Particular thanks to Ms Natalia Fijak for invaluable help with literature search.

References

The publications marked (PL) are written in Polish.

Bethin CY (1992). Polish syllables: the role of prosody in phonology and morphology. Columbus, OH: Slavica Publishers.
Bogdanowicz M (1978) Psychological analysis of children's difficulties in writing. Zeszyty Naukowe Wydzialu Humanistycznego Uniwersytetu Gdańskiego – Psychologia 1: 89–100. (PL)
Bogdanowicz M (1985) Investigation into the incidence of dyslexia, dysorthography and dysgraphy among Polish children. Zeszyty Naukowe Wydzialu Humanistycznego Uniwersytetu Gdańskiego – Psychologia 7: 143–154. (PL)
Bogdanowicz M (1991) The development and school career of children with dyslexia and dysorthography – a follow-up study. Zeszyty Naukowe Uniwersytetu Gdańskiego – Psychologia 10: 63–78. (PL)
Bogdanowicz M (1994) About dyslexia or specific reading and writing difficulties – answers to parents' and teachers' questions. Lublin: Wydawnictwo Popularnonaukowe 'Linea'. (PL)
Bogdanowicz M (1997) Perceptual-motor integration. Warszawa: Centrum Metodyczne Pomocy Psychologiczno-Pedagogicznej MEN. (PL)
Borkowska A (1997) Language disorders of children with reading and writing difficulties. In A Herzyk, D Kądzielawa (eds) Brain-behaviour relationship: perspectives from clinical neuropsychology. (PL)
Borkowska A (1998) The analysis of narrative discourse of children with developmental dyslexia. Lublin: Wydawnictwo Uniwersytetu Marii Curie-Sklodowskiej. (PL)
Borkowska A, Tarkowski Z (1990) Linguistic and communicative competence of children with reading and writing difficulties. Logopedia 17: 35–42. (PL)
Bryant P, Nunez T, Bindman M (1998) Awareness of language in children who have reading difficulties: historical comparisons in a longitudinal study. Journal of Child Psychology and Psychiatry 39(4): 501–510.
Byrne B (1998) The foundation of literacy: the child's acquisition of the alphabetic principle. Hove: Psychology Press.
Cossu G, Shankweiler D, Liberman IY, Gugliotta M (1995) Visual and phonological determinants of misreading in transparent orthography. Reading and Writing 7: 237–256.

Crystal D (1991) The Cambridge encyclopaedia of language. Cambridge: Cambridge University Press.

de Gelder B, Vroomen J (1991) Phonological deficits: beneath the surface of reading-acquisition problems. Psychological Research 53: 88–97.

Dobrowolska-Bogusławska H (1991) The methods of teaching reading in English-speaking countries and their adaptation to the Polish language. Warszawa: WSiP. (PL)

Downing J (1967) Evaluating the Initial Teaching Alphabet. London: Cassell.

Downing J (1973) Linguistic environments II. In J Downing (ed) Comparative reading, pp 217–243. New York: Macmillan.

Ellis AW (1993) Reading, writing and dyslexia: a cognitive analysis. Hillsdale, NJ: Lawrence Erlbaum Associates.

Ethnologue – languages of the world (1996) Dallas: Summer Institute of Linguistics. Also available online at http://www.sil.org/ethnologue/

Fenczyn J (1981) Perceiving in children with partial deficits of visual perception. Psychologia Wychowawcza 3/1981: 368–381. (PL)

Fenczyn J (1987) Predicting reading and writing difficulties at pre-school age. Praca habilitacyjna. Krakow: Wydawnictwo UJ. (PL)

Fisiak J, Lipińska-Gregorek M, Zabrocki T (1978) An introductory English–Polish contrastive grammar. Warszawa: PWN.

Foshay EW et al. (eds) (1962) Educational achievements of thirteen year olds in twelve countries. Hamburg: Unesco Institute for Education.

Fowler CA, Liberman IY, Shankweiler D (1977) On interpreting the error pattern of the beginning reader. Language and Speech 20: 162–173.

Goswami U (1999) Causal connections in beginning reading: the importance of rhyme. Journal of Research in Reading 22(3): 217–240.

Goswami U, Bryant P (1990) Phonological skills and learning to read. Hillsdale NJ: Lawrence Erlbaum Associates.

Goswami U, Gombert JE, de Barrera LF (1998) Children's orthographic representations and linguistic transparency: nonsense word reading in English, French and Spanish. Applied Psycholinguistics 19: 19–52.

Grabowska A (1994) Diagnosing left-handedness in the light of contemporary research into brain assymmetry. Psychologia Wychowawcza 2/1994: 121–137. (PL)

Grzędowa S (1976) Orthographic skills in the secondary schools of Wroclaw province. In Nauczanie ortografii w szkole. Materialy sesji naukowej 24 VI 1976, Wrocław. (PL)

Jaklewicz H (1980) A follow-up study of dyslexia-dysorthography. Praca habilitacyjna. Gdańsk: Instytut Medycyny Morskiej i Tropikalnej. (PL)

Jaklewicz H (1982). Dyslexia: follow-up studies. Thalamus (International Academy for Research in Learning Disabilities) 2: 3–9.

Kania I (1982) Phonematic hearing. In Szkice logopedyczne. Warszawa: WSiP, pp 77–103. (PL)

Kiken I (1935) Experimental research into orthography. Warszawa: Nasza Ksiegarnia. (PL)

Kołtuska B (1988) The role of linguistic processes in dyslexia. Zagadnienia Wychowawcze a Zdrowie Psychiczne 3: 45–51. (PL)

Kostrzewski J (1981) Reliability and validity of the Phonematic Hearing Test. Zagadnienia Wychowawcze a Zdrowie Psychiczne 1: 56–85. (PL)

Krasowicz G (1994) Linguistic structure of narratives produced by children with the specific reading disorder. Kwartalnik Polskiej Psychologii Rozwojowej 2(3-4): 74–103. (PL)

Krasowicz G (1997) Language, reading and dyslexia. Lublin: Agencja Wydawniczo-Handlowa AD. (PL)

Krasowicz-Kupis G (1999) Metalinguistic development and reading achievement of 6-9 years old children. Lublin: Wydawnictwo UMCS. (PL)

Krasowicz G, Bogdanowicz M (submitted) Assessment of linguistic abilities as predictors of developmental dyslexia in Polish children. Dyslexia (submitted).

Krasowicz G, Bryant P, Bogdanowicz M (1999) The role of children's awareness of phonemes, syllables and rhymes in learning to read. International Journal of Behavioural Development (submitted).

Krasowicz-Kupis G, Kaczmarek B, Bryant P (2000) Linguistic, reading and spelling development in Polish 6-8 years old children. In W Schneider, C Stengard (eds) Inventory of European longitudinal studies of reading and spelling (EUR 19233), pp 202-204. European Communities 2000.

Kyostio OK (1980) Is learning to read easy in a language in which the grapheme-phoneme correspondences are regular? In JF Kavanagh, RL Venezky (eds) Orthography, reading and dyslexia. Baltimore: University Park Press.

Landerl K, Wimmer H, Frith U (1997) The impact of orthographic consistency on dyslexia: a German-English comparison. Cognition 63: 315-334.

Lindgren SD, De Renzi E, Richman LC (1985) Cross-national comparison of developmental dyslexia in Italy and the United States. Child Development 56: 1404-1417.

Longman Dictionary of Contemporary English. 3rd edn (1995) Harlow: Longman.

Lovett MW (1987) A developmental approach to reading disability: accuracy and speed criteria of normal and deficient reading skills. Child Development 58: 234-260.

Majchrzak I (1995) Introducing a child into the world of writing. Warszawa: WSiP. (PL)

Manis FR, Seidenberg MS, Doi LM (1999) See dick RAN: rapid naming and the longitudinal prediction of reading subskills in first and second graders. Scientific Studies in Reading 3(2): 129-157.

Markiewicz J, Zakrzewska B (1978) The results of therapy of children with reading and writing difficulties and hyperactivity. Zagadnienia Wychowawcze a Zdrowie Psychiczne 5: 76-84. (PL)

Maurer A, Oszustrowicz B (1984) The AW Enfeld Reverse Figures Test as a diagnostic method of visual perception disorders. Zagadnienia Wychowawcze a Zdrowie Psychiczne 1/1984: 31-39. (PL)

Maurer A (1990) Supporting the auditory-linguistic development of children with low school readiness. Logopedia 17: 95-107. (PL)

OECD (1995) Literacy, economy and society. Results of the first international adult literacy survey. Canada: OECD.

Ognejovic V, Lukatela G, Feldman LB, Turvey MT (1983) Misreadings by beginning readers of Serbo-Croatian. Quarterly Journal of Developmental Psychology 35A: 97-109.

Oszwa U (in press) The analysis of agrammatisms in children with developmental dyslexia. In A Borkowska, M Szepietowska (eds) Diagnoza neuropsychologiczna. Metodologia i metodyka. Lublin: Wydawnictwo UMCS. (PL)

Pinheiro AMV (1995) Reading and spelling development in Brazilian Portuguese. Reading and Writing 7: 111-138.

Polański E (1973) Investigation of pupils' orthography. Katowice: Wydawnictwo Uniwersytetu Śląskiego. (PL)

Rack JP, Snowling MJ, Olson RK (1992) The nonword reading deficit in developmental dyslexia: a review. Reading Research Quarterly 27: 29-53.

Rocławski B (1976) The outline of phonology, phonetics, phonotactics and phonostatistics of contemporary Polish. Gdańsk: Wydawnictwo Uniwersytetu Gdańskiego. (PL)

Rocławski B (1981) The Phonostatic system of contemporary Polish. Gdańsk: Wydawnictwo Uniwersytetu Gdańskiego. (PL)

Rodrigo M, Jimenez JE (1999) An analysis of the word naming errors of normal readers and reading disabled children in Spanish. Journal of Research in Reading 22: 180-197.

Sawa B (1971) Speech disorders and reading and writing difficulties of primary school pupils. Psychologia Wychowawcza 2/1971: 188-193. (PL)

Seymour PHK, Duncan LG, Bolik FM (1999) Rhymes and phonemes in the common unit task: replications and implications for beginning reading. Journal of Research in Reading 22(2): 113-130.

Sochacka K (1998) Reading development in the middle of '0' grade. Paper presented during the Annual Conference on Developmental Psychology in Pulawy, May 1998. (PL)

Spionek H (1963) Children's reading and writing difficulties and the functional efficiency of their analysers. Psychologia Wychowawcza VI(3): 197-209. (PL)

Spionek H (1970) Psychological analysis of school difficulties and failures. Warszawa: PZWS. (PL)

Spionek H (1973) Pupils' developmental disorders and school failures. Warszawa: PWN. (PL)

Stevenson HW, Stigler JW, Lucker WG, Lee S, Hsu C, Kitamura S (1982) Reading disabilities: the case of Chinese, Japanese, and English. Child Development 53: 1164-1181.

Strutyński J (1997) The Polish grammar. Kraków: Wydawnictwo Tomasz Strutyński. (PL)

Szczerbiński M (1999) Cognitive correlates of reading and spelling acquisition in Polish. Unpublished manuscript.

Szczerbiński M, Coleman M (1999) Who has to read more? Comparison of written word length and text length in Polish and English. Unpublished manuscript.

Szurmiak M (1974) Attempts at solving the problem of therapy of children with dyslexia in Krakow-Nowa Huta. Kwartalnik Pedagogiczny 4: 135-152. (PL)

Tansley P, Panckhurst J (1991) Children with specific learning difficulties. Windsor: NFER-Nelson.

Trzeciak G (1980) Ameliorating reading and writing difficulties. A research report. Zagadnienia Wychowawcze a Zdrowie Psychiczne 4-5: 134-145. (PL)

Webster's New Collegiate Dictionary (1981) Toronto: Thomas Allen and Sons.

Wimmer H (1993) Characteristics of developmental dyslexia in a regular writing system. Applied Psycholinguistics 14: 1-33.

Wimmer H (1996) The nonword reading deficit in developmental dyslexia: evidence from children learning to read German. Journal of Experimental Child Psychology 61: 80-90

Wimmer H, Goswami U (1994) The influence of orthographic consistency on reading development: word recognition in English and German children. Cognition 51: 91-103.

Wimmer H, Mayringer H, Landerl K (2000) The double-deficit hypothesis and difficulties in learning to read a regular orthography. Journal of Educational Psychology 92(4): 668-680.

Wolf M, Bowers PG (1999) The double-deficit hypothesis for the developmental dyslexias. Journal of Educational Psychology 91(3): 415-438.

Wszeborowska-Lipińska B (1995) Adolescents with specific reading and spelling difficulties. Psychologia Wychowawcza 3/1995: 223-234. (PL)

Wszeborowska-Lipińska B (1996) Specific reading and writing difficulties in adolescents. Unpublished PhD thesis, University of Gdańsk. (PL)

Zagórska-Brooks M (1975) Polish reference grammar. The Hague, Paris: Mouton.

CHAPTER 6

Матрёшка, Матрёжка или Мотрёшка
(Matryoshka, Matryozhka or Motryoshka):
The difficulty of mastering reading and spelling in Russian

ELENA L GRIGORENKO

This chapter examines the distribution of spelling skills and the relationship between reading and spelling skills in three distinct samples of Russian primary school children. I believe such a descriptive account is helpful in order to understand the mastery of reading and spelling in Russian. The samples presented here are drawn from a number of state-funded schools comparable to each other in most educational characteristics. To set up the context for my analyses, I first briefly describe the challenges imposed on a young learner by the linguistic peculiarities of the Russian language.

Russian: a brief linguistic excursion

The Russian language belongs to a group of languages called Slavic languages. There are three major subgroups of the Slavic languages:

- *East* Slavic (e.g. Russian, Ukrainian, Belorussian)
- *West* Slavic (e.g. Polish, Czech, Slovak)
- *South* Slavic (e.g. Serbo-Croatian, Slovene, Bulgarian).

Slavic languages began differentiating about 1000 years ago, as a result of geographic and cultural separation. (As a whole, the group of Slavic languages diverged from the Indo-European languages; Greek, Latin, Sanskrit and most modern European languages are considered descendants of this latter group.) Modern Russian belongs to the so-called '*consonant*' group of languages, that is, languages in which consonants play a dominant role.

To mentally 'place' Russian on the continuum of difficulty associated with letter–sound correspondences, consider the following two questions (Hamilton, 1980): (i) Would knowledge of the spelling of a Russian word guarantee knowledge of its pronunciation? (ii) Would knowledge of the pronunciation of a Russian word guarantee knowledge of its spelling?

According to Hamilton (1980), the answer to the first question is *usually*. Actually, the answer would be *always*, except for a rather limited assortment of exceptions. For example, some letters are not pronounced (e.g. *солнце* /sóntsə/ (sun) - the phoneme /l/ is not pronounced), the pronunciation of some letters in certain words differs from their usual pronunciation (e.g. *ч* /tʃ/ sounds like *ш* /ʃ/ in *булочная* /buloʃnaia/ (bakery)), and the pronunciation of many foreign words differs from what general pronunciation rules would suggest (e.g. some consonants are hard before /e/ *кафэ* /kafæ/ (café)).

According to Hamilton (1980), the answer to the second question is *occasionally*. There are some words in Russian (e.g. *луна* /luna/ (moon)) in which the sounds cannot be represented by alternative letters. A typical Russian word, however, can be represented graphically in more than one way (e.g. based on is phonemic content, the word *вправо* /vpravo/ (to the right) should (!) be written as *фправо* /fpravo/).

Thus, the major challenge to young readers of Russian trying to master the language is not how to read a word when seen, but, rather, how to spell a word once it has been heard.

Up to the challenge: teaching Russian in Russian schools

A traditional course in Russian language arts in mainstream public schools[1] includes teaching of the basics of phonetics, morphology, orthography, grammar and semantics. The traditional course is phonetically based, that is, Russian students from the first grade on investigate both practical and theoretical aspects of Russian phonetics, morphology and orthography (Moiseev, 1975). Phonetically based Russian textbooks cover the phonological aspects of the language through explanations of such concepts as sounds, speech organs, voice-voiceless (*д*/d/ versus *т* /t/) and hard-soft (*ж* /ʒ / versus *ш* /ʃ/) sounds, vowels and consonants, stress, position, letter-sound correspondence, phonetic transcription and so on.

To teach Russian morphology, the texts concentrate on parts of speech (nouns, adjectives, etc.), word parts, word–word linkages and grammar. To

---

[1]The majority of Russian public schools (referred to here as mainstream public schools) still use the standard unified programme of teaching reading developed by the former Soviet Ministry of Education. Today, however, there are various 'reformed' schools. In such schools, the approaches to teaching reading vary dramatically. Of the 67,200 schools in Russia, only 9,126 (or 13%) are of a new type; 540 (0.8%) are private; and the rest are mainstream.

teach orthography, the textbooks concentrate on major parts and principles of Russian orthography. These 'formal' rules are than supplemented by work with reading-level-appropriate excerpts, stories and larger units of literature (novels, plays, etc.). As a subject, the Russian language is taught for nine years (grades 1 through 9). Beginning with grade 1, this instruction is supplemented by reading, and, in grade 4 (the first middle-school grade), reading is replaced by literature and composition. In grades 10 and 11 (the college preparatory grades), only literature and composition are taught. Note that the majority of old-fashioned, traditional Russian schools (with the exception of a small number of innovative schools where there is much systematic and asystematic deviation from classic textbooks) still use teaching techniques and principles so that reading and spelling are delivered to children by direct instruction.

In this part of the chapter, I will give examples of the rules of the Russian language that Russian students in the primary- and middle-school grades are expected to master. These illustrations, of course, do not cover the full range of knowledge required for mastery of written Russian, but they provide a fair representation of the challenges faced by young Russians mastering reading.

The basics: a sketch of Russian phonemics

A phoneme is a representation of a speech sound, a set of sound types used in each specific language to differentiate words and their forms and serve the purpose of human communication (Shcherba, 1963). The Russian linguist Shcherba gives this example: an interrogative particle 'a?', when pronounced loudly or whispered, is represented by very different sounds, both physiologically and biologically; from a linguistic point of view, however, it is the same particle, the same phoneme. In other words, a phoneme is the common component in a set of specific sound types (often referred to as sound shades).

There are non-distinctive and distinctive phonemes. For example, in Russian, the stressed /a/ sounds different depending on the consonants surrounding it in a word. For example, when the phoneme /a/ is located between dental consonants (as in надо /nædo/, to need), a frontal /a/ appears; when the phoneme /a/ is located between two-focus consonants (as in шашка /ʃəʃka/, draught), a back /a/ appears; when the phoneme /a/ is located after soft consonants (as in мята /'mata/, mint, where the sound of я simply indicates a softened consonant preceding the /a/), an /a/ that is like и /i/ appears; and when the phoneme /a/ is located between soft consonants (as in мять /mɛt'/, to crumple), an /a/ that is like e /e/ appears; and so on. All these shades of *a*, however, are known as the Russian phoneme /a/; each of these sounds is a specific representation of the phoneme /a/, and each representation is determined by the specific surroundings of the phoneme.

These specific representations of one phoneme are not opposed to each other, even though they might differ articulationally and acoustically (e.g. different shades of /a/ in words *шаль* /ʃəl'/, shawl and *сядь* /sɛd'/, to sit down). In these examples, different pronunciations of the phoneme /a/ (resulting from different dialects or foreign accents) will, most likely, not hinder a listener's understanding of the meaning of the word.

As an example of distinctive phonemes, consider the Russian vowels *a, e, o* and *y*. For example, there are a number of Russian vowels pronounceable between the two Russian consonants, *ш* /ʃ/ and *p* /r/, specifically *a* (*шар* /ʃər/, ball), *e* (*шерсть* /ʃɛrst'/, wool), *o* (*шорох* /ʃɔrokh /, noise) and *y* (*шура* /ʃura/, a female and male nickname), but to maintain the meaning of these words, they should always be pronounced as distinctive phonemes. If, in the word *шар* /ʃər/, the first consonant *ш* /ʃ/ is replaced with a different consonant (e.g. *д* /d/, *б* /b/, or *n* /p/, as in *дар* /dær/ (gift), *бар* /bər/ (bar), *nap* /pʌr/ (steam)), different shades of the phoneme /a/ will appear, but the speaker and the listener will deliver and perceive these differences not as different phonemes, but as variations of the same phoneme.

If each phoneme can exist in a number of different variants (phonemic shades), than how can one determine the core phonemic structure of a language? In Russian, the phonemic content of the language is determined when a letter is present in a word in its 'absolutely strong position', that is, in its main phonemic variant. The 'absolutely strong position' for vowels is their stressed position at the beginning of a word before a hard consonant; the 'absolutely strong position' for consonants is their position in a word before any variant of the phoneme /a/.

Each of these phonemes, however, has a number of realizations depending on the placement of the corresponding letter in the word, the letter surroundings and so on. For example, /a/ has a number of different realizations – /æ/, /ə/, /a/, and /ɛ/ (as in the *надо - шашка - мята-мять* ; example above).

In Russian phonetics, consonants are masters and vowels are slaves (Hamilton, 1980). Russian vowels get twisted and torn; their qualities change, depending on whether the consonants on either side are soft or hard. For example, consider the words *мять* /mɛt'/ (crumple) and *мат* /mæt/ (checkmate) – if the consonants on either side are soft, we have /ɛ/, as in *мять* ; otherwise the vowel will be /æ/, as in *мат*.

In the Russian alphabet, however, the situation is just the opposite – the vowels are masters and the consonants are slaves (Hamilton, 1980). The

---

[2]Note the degree of difficulty associated with an attempt to pronounce the word *шалый* with the phoneme /a/ as pronounced in the word *сядь* ;. The surrounding phonemic context of /a/ is so powerful that it takes special effort and training to succeed.

series of soft-vowel letters – *я* /iɑ/, *e* /iɛ/, *ё* /iɔ/, and *ю* /iu/ – provide information about the softness of a preceding consonant (this is also true for
Russian spelling). This allows maximum efficiency – five vowels determine
12 additional consonant phonemes. Thus, the Russian alphabet is a rather
clever system. But notice that it is precisely this cleverness that creates a
problem by producing misconceptions that are difficult to correct and that
are characteristic of both beginning readers and writers who are native
Russian speakers and many foreigners trying to master Russian. Specifically,
many students have the misconception that the vowel pairs *a* /ɑ/ and *я* /iɑ/
or *y* /u/ and *ю* /iu/, for example, are the symbols for two different vowel
sounds. In contrast, some individual consonants, for example *б* /b/ and *п*
/p/, are mistakenly regarded as the symbols for only one sound apiece.
Thus, Russian spelling, although delightfully systematic, is far from being a
one-to-one system of symbols (Hamilton, 1980).

Spelling rules in Russian

Spelling rules are the most apparent source of difficulty for children learning
to read and write Russian. In this section, I briefly review some of the major
peculiarities of spelling in Russian.

Stressed and unstressed vowels

Russian vowels differ on a number of dimensions. However, the most distinguishing feature of Russian vowels is stress. Stress matters over and above
other differentiating features of Russian sounds and creates crucial differences between words (for example, *за́мок* /zæmak/ (castle) versus *замо́к*
/zamɔk/ (lock); *мука́* /mukæ/ (flour) versus *му́ка* /muka/ (torture)). Under
stress, vowels are louder and longer. Reduced vowels, then, are shorter,
softer and less distinguishable from each other.

For example, there are three 'o's in the word *городо́к* (town), but two of
them are reduced to /ə/ and /a/, giving /gəradɔk/. The question is, then, how
do we know to spell *gorodók* with three 'o's rather than with one *o* and two
*a*s. We do hear /gəradɔk/! The way to 'detect' the true identity of a vowel is to
find each of the vowels stressed in words that we are sure contain the same
parts. Thus, the word *го́род* /gɔrəd/ (city) verifies that the first vowel is *o*,
and the word *междугоро́дний* /medzugərɔdnii/ (intercity) demonstrates that
the second vowel is also *o*. This operation requires some skill in finding
related parts of the investigated word embedded in other words. But this
technique has a clear underlying logic: the system of Russian spelling usually
follows the tradition of representing sounds with letters that stand for their
basic values. In addition, Russian has some distinct rules of spelling that are
presented in children's textbooks and are expected to be memorized.

Vowels after consonants

'Normal' Russian consonants exist in two phonemic forms – soft and hard; in spelling, the difference between the hard and the soft /s/, for example, is represented by a particular choice of vowel letters or by the presence of the soft *ь* sign. A vowel letter from the 'hard series' (*a* /ɑ/, *э*/ɛ/, *ы* /ɨ/, *o* /ɔ/, *y* /u/) will indicate a preceding hard /s/, while a vowel from the 'soft series' (*я*/ia/, *e*/iɛ/, *и*/i/, *ё*/iɔ/, *ю* /iu/) indicates a preceding soft /s'/.[3] There are, however, exceptions to this rule. There are five letters (*ш*/ʃ/, *щ*/sʃ/, *ц*/ts/, *ч* /tʃ/, *ж*/ʒ/) in which the softness–hardness rule is not applicable. It would have made Russian a much easier language if those letters which represent hard sounds (*ш*/ʃ/, *ц*/ts/, *ж*/ʒ/) only combined with the hard series vowel letters, and the other two (*щ* /sʲ/, *ч* /tʃ/), which represent soft sounds, only combined with the soft series vowel letters. Instead the spelling of Russian words with these five letters is governed by a complex set of spelling rules, in which the spelling of these words depends on the placement of corresponding letters in the words and surrounding letters. Similarly, there are letter-combination-dependent rules for velar consonants (those formed with the back of the tongue), *к*/k/, *г*/g/ and *x*/x/ (e.g., the only vowel letters which can be spelled after *к*, *г*, and *x* are the soft series *e* and *и* and the hard series *a*, *o*, and *y*). One would think that this would be enough – yet, there are also rules relating to the spelling of the silent letters *ь* and *ъ*. Here, in addition to dependency on the surrounding words, the spelling is conditional on the morphology of the words (i.e. the gender of the nouns).

It would have been much easier if the irregularity of Russian spelling had been limited to the rules of vowel reduction. However, Russian spelling of consonants also offers a few complications. Let us consider only some of them.

Assimilation

Often, when two sounds are pronounced together, one after the other, at a reasonable speed, one of the sounds affects another. Consider as an example the Russian word *лодка* /lótkə/ (boat). What happens in this word is that the *к* in *лодка* affects the *д*, and causes it to be pronounced as /t/ as if it goes through transformations *лодка* → * /lódkə/ → /lótkə/. In this particular example, /k/ and /t/ are both voiceless consonants and, therefore, are more

---

[3]The hard–soft series vowels are usually viewed in correspondence to each other (*a* as in /sa/ corresponds to *я* as in /s'a/, *э* as in /sɛ/ corresponds to *e* as in /s'e/, *ы* as in /sɨ/ corresponds to *и* as in /s'i/, *o* as in /so/ corresponds to *ё* as in /s'o/, and *y* as in /su/ corresponds to *ю* as in /s'u/). These correspondences (or, rather, the inability to understand them) are a major source of spelling errors in Russian.

similar to each other than /k/ and /d/ (d is a voiced consonant). The *d-to-t* transformation in *лодка* is an example of assimilation – a linguistic phenomenon in which one sound becomes more like (or completely like) another. There are three types of assimilation: (i) from voice to voicelessness (e.g. *дуб* /dúp/, /b/ → /p/) and from voicelessness to voice (e.g. *просьба* /próz'bə/, /s'/ → /z'/)[4]; (ii) from hardness to softness (e.g. *зонтик* /zón't'ik/, /n/ → /n'/) and from softness to hardness (e.g. *конца* /kansá/, /ts'/ → /s/), and (iii) of place (manner) of articulation (e.g. *солнце* /sóntsə/, /ln/ → /n/).

Let us consider the impact of different types of assimilation on Russian spelling. First, the results of devoicing[5] are not usually spelled (with the exception of prefixes containing basic *z* such as *из-* /iz/, *исследование* /issledovanie/ (study); *раз-* /raz/, *рассказ* /raskaz/ (story); *без-* /bez/, *беспокоить*; /bespokoit'/ (bother)). The verification of the spelling of voiced/devoiced vowels requires locating modified forms of the words of interest, where the effect of assimilation becomes obvious. For example, having learned the word *порог* /parók/ (threshold), one would know that its genitive is *порога*. Thus, when we see *порог*, we know that it is pronounced /parók/ because *r* is devoiced, but when we hear /parók/ we spell it *порог*. Unfortunately, however, there are many pairs of words in Russian[6] that, due to assimilation, sound exactly the same but have different meanings (homophones). For example, there is another word in Russian which sounds exactly like /parók/ (just like the word for 'threshold'!) but means vice (*порок* in Russian). The genitive of *порок* is *порока*, but in order to figure out how to spell /parók/, one needs to know whether the word at issue is *порог* or *порок*. Thus, with such pairs of words, spelling verification must be preceded by the verification of meaning. In other words, when such words are heard out of context, their spelling is a guessing game.

Second, to appreciate the impact of softness–hardness assimilation on Russian spelling, consider the following typical soft-assimilation spelling error. Many children spell *песня* /pes'nia/ (song) as *песьня*; they insert the silent letter *ь* to show what they hear – that *с* /s/ in *песня* is soft /s'/. To understand a cluster of spelling errors arising as a result of hardness assimilation, consider the following two examples. The *н* /n/ in *конец* /kon'ets/

---

[4]Note that English does not have devoicing of the type found in Russian. There are some traces of it, as in 'hafta' for 'have to', but it is not a basic ingredient in English phonology as it is in Russian. Some of the European languages with devoicing similar to Russian's are German, Czech and Polish.

[5]Note that there are certain dialects in Russian which do not carry out devoicing.

[6]Here are some other examples of pairs of words that sound exactly the same but are spelled differently: *молот* (hammer) and *молод* (young) – both sound /mólət/; *грусть* (sadness) and *груздь*; (milk-agarik) – both sound /grust'/; *мок* (was getting wet) and *мог* (could) – both sound /mok/; *тушь* (India ink) and *туш* (musical greeting) – both sound /tuʃ/.

(end) and the *л* /l/ in *жилец* /ʒ il'ets/ (tenant) are soft consonants. *Конец* has a soft *н* /n'/ which becomes hard when it is moved next to the always-hard consonant *ц* /ts/: *конца* (*конца* is a genetive of *конец*). Thus, in the derivation of the genitive, a hardness assimilation has occurred. *Жилец* also has a soft sound (*л* /l'/), but in the derivation of the genitive, *л* proves to be resistant to hardness assimilation: *жилец* turns into *жильца* (/ʒ il'ets/ → /ʒ il'tsa/) preserving the softness with the sound letter *ь*. This inconsistency is confusing, and it is not uncommon to see *жильца* spelled as *жилца*, or *конца* spelled as *коньца*.

Finally, let us consider a few examples of assimilation in the place of articulation. The sounds /s/ and /z/ in such words as *сшить* (sew/ ʃʃi t'/) and *сжать* (squeeze /ʒʒat'/) become articulated in a different place, making it difficult for the listener to figure out how to spell these words. Correspondingly, beginning spellers write *шшить* and *жжать* . Another example is the omission of a consonant where several in a row are spelled, as in *счастливый* (happy /sʃaslivɨi/); in this case the typical spelling mistake is to replace the consonant combination with a single consonant (*счастливый* is sometimes mistakenly spelled as *щастливый*, substituting *щ* for *сч*, or even *щасливый*, substituting *щ* for *сч* and omitting *т*).

The morphological principle of Russian orthography

Russian spelling is largely morphophonemic in nature: this means that in addition to the phonemic rules we have been reviewing so far, Russian spelling is highly linked to the morphological aspect of the language. Russian words are spelled in a way that often gives extra information to a speaker (or, more precisely, a pronouncer) about what a vowel should be if stressed, or about the values that a consonant will have before a vowel. This section briefly reviews the main morphological rules of Russian spelling.

The principle

A morpheme is a linguistic abstraction reflecting the most basic and, therefore, the most informative and revealing structural components of a word.[7] There are four main types of morphemes: roots, prefixes, suffixes and endings.

The root is the most important kind of morpheme, because it identifies the word itself (the prefix, suffix and ending are modification morphemes, whereas the root is a definitional morpheme). Sometimes the entire word, apart from its grammatical ending, consists simply of a root: *нос* {nos|}, *жена*

---

[7]In this chapter, morphemes are marked by curly brackets ({}), a morpheme's position with respect to the rest of the word is indicated by hyphens (i.e. -morpheme; -morpheme-, morpheme-), and morpheme boundaries are represented by vertical cut lines (|).

{ʒɛ n|a} and so on. Linguists have developed volumes that group vocabulary items together according to the roots they share (e.g., Wolkonsky and Poltoratzky, 1961). Russian words normally have one root, but it is possible to find some with two or even three roots.

The classification of other kinds of morphemes is based on their relationship to the root. Prefixes come before the root, and suffixes and endings come after it. For example, the morpheme *пере-* {pere-} in the word *переход* /perekhod/ (crossing) is a prefix. Both in form and meaning, prefixes resemble English prepositions. In Russian words, the root can be preceded by one, two or three prefixes.

Suffixes come after the root. There are two types of suffixes: derivational and inflectional. Derivation signifies the creation of one word from another: *писатель* /pisat'el'/ (writer) from *писать* /pisat'/ (to write). Inflection signifies the alteration of existing words, so that they suit the relationships between words in a sentence. For example, to reflect the gender of the subject of the sentence, Russians would say *Она ушла* /Ona uʃla/ (She left) and *Он ушёл* /On uʃɔl/ (He left). These word modifications are carried out by inflectional suffixes. As in the case of roots and prefixes, several suffixes can occur in one word.

Endings change to show relationships in a sentence without altering the basic meaning of the word. Notice that not all Russian parts of speech have endings. Specifically, prepositions (*на* /na/, *в* /v/), conjunctions (*и* /i/, *a* /ɑ/, *но* /nɔ/, *или* /ili/), particles (*бы* /bɨ /, *не* /nɛ/), interjections (*ага!* /aha/, *вот!* /vɔt/), indeclinable nouns (*кино* /kinɔ/) and adverbs (*очень* /otʃen'/) do not have endings.

Sometimes, for convenience, researchers (e.g. Aronoff, 1976) determine two types of morphological transformations, inflections and derivations. Inflectional morphology primarily addresses changes in endings and roots, whereas derivational morphology addresses changes in the word construction.

Inflectional morphology (such as plural forms) preserves the word class of the base and has highly predictable semantic consequences (*invite* versus *invites* in English and *пригласила* /priglasila/ versus *пригласили* /priglasili/ in Russian). Inflectional morphology is linked to grammatical knowledge and is considered to be mastered along with the development of oral language (in pre-school years).

In contrast, derivational morphology (for example, agentive and diminutive) usually changes word class and has opaque semantic consequences (*invite* versus *invitation* in English and *приглашать* /priglaʃat'/ versus *приглашение* /priglaʃenie/ in Russian). Derivational morphology is linked to lexical knowledge and is assumed to be mastered during formal schooling.

The morphological principle of Russian orthography is usually summarized by two rules:

1   Sounds in unstressed positions that are components of a single morpheme
    and alternate with sounds in stressed positions are symbolized by the
    same letters as the latter. In other words, the symbol signification of
    sounds in unstressed positions (the orthography of writing) is equated to
    the symbol signification of stressed sounds, determined by the Russian
    graphics. Thus, the task of the speller here is to go through enough words
    containing the same morpheme in order to find the one in which the
    sound in question is stressed: for example гэра́ (mountain)-г[о́]ры
    (mountains), therefore *гора* as in *го́ры* , even though it sounds as /gəra/;
    cá[t] (garden)-*ca[d]ы́* (gardens), therefore *сад* – even though it does
    sound /sat/ – as in *сады* .
2   Sounds in unstressed positions that do not alternate (when components
    of a single morpheme) are signified according to orthographic traditions,
    based on phonemic rules. Such words cannot be verified; they need to be
    memorized (e.g. *сарай* /sərai/, *собака* /səbaka/, *зигзаг* /ʒikʒak/, *кто*
    /hto/).

The principle: exceptions

Even though the morphological principle of Russian orthography is its ruler,
there are a number of exceptions, covering a large spectrum of specific
spellings. In other words, the same morpheme is spelled differently under
different circumstances. Below are some examples of such situations.

1   Prefixes with *з* /z/ and *с* /s/ endings. In prefixes with *з/с* endings, *з* is used
    before voiced consonants and *с* is used before voiceless consonants. For
    example, *без/бес*: (i) *безрадостный* /besradostnɨi/(joyless, *р* /r/ is a
    voiced consonant), but (ii) *бесползный*/bespoleznɨi/(useless, *п* /p/ is a
    voiceless consonant).
2   Prefixes *раз/с* and *роз/с*.
    In prefixes *раз/с* and *роз/с* - *о* is used when the vowel is stressed (e.g.
    ро́спись /rospis'/ (mural)), but *a* is used when the vowel is unstressed
    (e.g. *ро́спиcáние* /rəspisanie/ (schedule)).
3   Endings in adjectives, participles, numerals, pronouns and so on.
    When the vowel is stressed, the ending is spelled -ой /oi/, when the vowel
    is unstressed, the ending is spelled -*ый* /ɨi/(- *ий* /ii/ after soft consonants).
    For example, *молодой*/mələdoi/ (young), but *новый* /novɨi/ (new) and
    синий /sinii/ (blue).

The principle: limitations

In addition to the exceptions exemplified above, the morphological principle
has a number of limitations. In particular, two major groups of rules capture

these limitations: (i) the rules linked to the graphical limitations – the so-called positional graphical principle (e.g. the same case endings are spelled differently depending on the characteristics of the preceding consonants), and (ii) the rules linked to the historical alternation of sounds (e.g. some morphemes change depending on which speech part – noun, verb, adjective and so on – they appear in).

So, Russian orthography is about uncovering a deep structure for words, and relationships between words, which otherwise might not be noticed. These deep word representations serve to show the logical, regular structure that underlies a word alteration that may seem irregular at the surface level.

In other words, learning to spell in Russian is about (i) being able to reveal hidden relationships between words (applying the morphological principle), and (ii) remembering how to spell (memorizing the exceptions and limitations of the morphological principle). There are a limited number of Russian morphemes. Operations with morphemes determine the so-called deep level of word structure, whereas operations with phonemes determine the so-called surface level of word structure. Knowledge of Russian morphemes is, in large part, what determines winners and losers in a Russian spelling bee.

Spelling and reading skills: distributions and links to other individual differences indicators

In the first section of this chapter, I summarized some major features of Russian phonetics, morphology and orthography, and outlined a number of rules a student of Russian must master throughout his or her school career. This shows that, due to a number of difficulties imposed by Russian phonemics and morphology, mastering reading and spelling in Russian cannot be expected to be a trivial task.

In this section, I review a number of studies attempting to describe and quantify reading and spelling deficits in four different student samples: (i) a large sample of Russian primary school students; (ii) a mixed sample of primary, middle and high school students; (iii) a small sample of primary school students; and (iv) a sample of high school students.

Characteristics of spelling skills in Russian primary school students

This section gives some descriptive information about the distribution of spelling skills in a sample of Russian primary school children. All children enrolled in the study were native Russian speakers.

The major objective of this descriptive investigation was to quantify inter-individual variability on spelling among children of a unified language and educational background. In other words, the study sought to answer the following questions.

- Is there any inter-individual variability in spelling in native Russian children of comparable educational background?
- Is this variability comparable for boys and girls?
- Is the variability on spelling tests comparable to that on arithmetic tests? Is there a correlation between performance on spelling and arithmetic tests?
- When the subjects are categorized into two groups of normally achieving children (90% of the sample) and underachieving children (10% of the sample), (a) what is the gender breakdown in the group of poor spellers and (b) is there an overlap between poor spelling and poor maths performance?

The sample included 1085 students aged 6–9. The children were enrolled in three public schools in the city of Voronezh, Russia. The economic and demographic profiles of Voronezh make it comparable to many other large urban cities of Russian regions. Voronezh was chosen as the study site for a number of reasons. First, it is a large industrial city in Central Russia and is quite representative (unlike Moscow) of many Russian cities. Second, despite significant economic differentiation, geographical differentiation by income is still quite scarce within the city – people of different incomes live right next to each other, so it is easier to obtain a heterogeneous sample than it would be in many other environments. Third, we had good access to samples from this city.

Among these pupils, 172 (15.9%) were first graders, 461 (42.5%) were second graders, 394 (36.3%) were third graders and 58 (5.3%) were fourth graders. Overall, there were 521 boys and 529 girls; the gender of 35 children was not registered.

The testing took place at the end of the school year (May of 1996). All children were given 40-minute grade-appropriate achievement tests in spelling and arithmetic. For all the tests, the outcome indicator was the number of errors. For comparison purposes, the data were standardized within grades.

The distribution of spelling skills in the sample is shown in Figure 6.1. As is obvious from the figure, the distribution is positively skewed (the majority of children made few spelling errors) and characterized by high kurtosis (the dispersion of the values is wide). The range of the values was rather large (8.7), testifying to the existence of individual differences in spelling in a sample of Russian children. In addition, there were 32 extreme cases of very poor spelling (defined as ≥ 2.5 standard deviations (SD) below the mean).

Boys made significantly more spelling errors than girls. The distribution of spelling skills among boys and girls was quite different: (i) the range was smaller among girls (8.72 in boys and 5.02 in girls); (ii) the dispersion of the values was also smaller in the sample of girls and a significant proportion of them spelled flawlessly; and (iii) there were only 12 extreme cases of very poor spelling (defined as ≥ 2.5 SD below the mean) among girls.

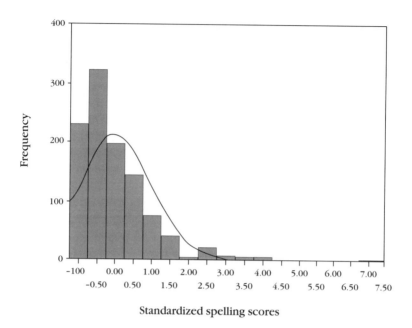

Figure 6.1 Distribution of spelling skills.

For the whole sample, there was a significant correlation between children's performance on spelling and arithmetic tests (p < 0.001). This was also the case for both subsamples of girls and boys.

When cross-classified, the clustering of poor versus normal-range spellers and poor versus normal-range performers on the arithmetic tests differed from the expected (p < 0.001 for the corresponding χ²-test). There were more children than expected who either did poorly on both tests or did well on both tests and fewer than expected children who did poorly on either of the tests. In addition, fewer than expected girls did poorly on either of the tests.

The DSM-IV-based (1994) definition of specific spelling/reading disabilities was used to select only those children whose performance on the arithmetic test was normal, but who underperformed on the spelling test. This group was comprised of 81 students (7.5% of the total sample evaluated), of whom 47 (58%) were boys, 31 (38%) were girls and three (4%) were children whose gender was not recorded. In this group, as expected, there was no correlation between students' performance on the test of spelling and the test of arithmetic. It is conceivable that this group of young children constitutes a group at-risk for developing specific reading disability in Russian.

Reading and spelling skills and intelligence

To extend the results presented above and to take a closer look at children whose reading/spelling performance suffers while their maths performance is at the average or above-average level, a second study was implemented. This study enrolled 506 children (276 girls and 230 boys), whose ages ranged from 8 to 17 (with a mean of 12.3 and a SD of 2.8). This sample was drawn from 16 schools of the city of Voronezh.

This study sought to answer the following questions.

- Do the children with specific reading and spelling difficulties differ from both children with non-specific reading and spelling difficulties and normally performing children on characteristics of general abilities (fluid and crystallized intelligence)?
- Do the children with combined reading/spelling difficulties differ from other children in the sample?

In this study, teachers of these children were asked to rate the children's performance in reading, spelling and maths using a 1–4 scale (1, poor; 2, mediocre; 3, average; 4, good), and children were asked to complete two brief tests of intelligence (for fluid and crystallized intelligence).

Children's and adolescents' fluid intelligence was measured with two subtests (Series and Matrices) of the Test of g: Culture Fair, Level II (Cattell and Cattell, 1973). To quantify crystallized intelligence, two parallel forms of the Test of Crystallized Intelligence (one for children of ages 8–12, and another for adolescents of ages 13–17) were utilized. Both forms consisted of two parts: (i) Analogies and (ii) Synonyms and Antonyms. The first part included 20 verbal analogies (KR20 = 0.83 for the children's form, and KR20 = 0.83 for the adolescents' form). Examples from the children's form are (i) pen - to write = knife - ? (a) to run, (b) to cut, (c) coat, (d) pocket; (ii) Russia - Moscow = Hungary - ? (a) Prague, (b) Budapest, (c) the Urals, (d) Yaroslavl'. The second part included 40 pairs of words, and the participants' task was to specify whether the words in the pair were synonyms or antonyms (KR20 = 0.91 for the children's form, and KR20 = 0.90 for the adolescents' form). Examples from the adolescents' form are: (i) beginning–end, and (ii) opinion–view. This test was developed specifically for this study and was based on items adapted and modelled from existing traditional tests of analogies and synonyms.

Based on teachers' evaluations, we divided students into groups of children reading and spelling adequately (i.e. children, whose teachers' ratings were 3 (average) or 4 (good)) and children experiencing some difficulty with reading and spelling and, therefore, making many mistakes (i.e. children, whose teachers' ratings were 1 (poor) or 2 (mediocre)).

Similar to the previous study, the variable of maths achievement was used as a control variable, permitting selection of those cases among poor readers and poor spellers who underachieve in language arts but not in maths. There were 25 poor spellers (5.3% of the sample) and 20 poor readers (4.1% of the sample) whose maths performance was average or above average.

The first question of interest was whether these groups of children with specific poor spelling and reading performance differ from the groups of: (i) poor achievers in spelling/reading and maths; (ii) average achievers in maths but poor achievers in spelling/reading; and (iii) average and above-average achievers (both in spelling/reading and maths) on indicators of fluid and crystallized abilities. These analyses were carried out controlling for gender and age.

All analyses showed the presence of a significant group effect. The mean differences are shown in Figure 6.2.

What is striking about these results is that the groups of poor spellers and readers do not show any other non-specific deficits. As a matter of fact, these groups are comparable to the groups of average and above-average achievers. The group demonstrating other non-specific deficits (i.e. lower levels of crystallized and fluid abilities) is that of poor performers on reading/spelling and maths tasks (the Spelling (Reading) '–' /Maths '–' group).

The second question of interest was whether those who are viewed by teachers as poor spellers tended also be viewed as poor readers. There were only 13 children who demonstrated poor performance in both spelling and reading (despite average or above-average performance in maths); 12 poor spellers were average (or above-average) readers and seven poor readers were average (or above-average) spellers. When this group of 13 children was contrasted to other children in the sample (once again, controlling for gender and age), they did not differ from other children on any of the screened indicators of intelligence.

Teachers' ratings and indicators of accuracy of reading

To validate the results of the previous study, a smaller-scale study where teachers' ratings were predicted by indicators of children's reading accuracy was conducted (for a detailed review of this study, see Grigorenko and Katz, 1999). In this study, there were 56 participants: 24 (12 girls and 12 boys) were third graders (mean age 10.1 years), and 32 (16 girl and 16 boys) were fourth graders (mean age 11.2 years).

To assess the accuracy of children's reading, two tasks were used – phonological awareness and single-word reading.

The phonological awareness test is a Russian modification of Rosner's Test of Auditory Analysis Skills. Children are required to make a new word by deleting a specified element (e.g. Say 'meat'. Now say it again, but don't

Cystallized ability

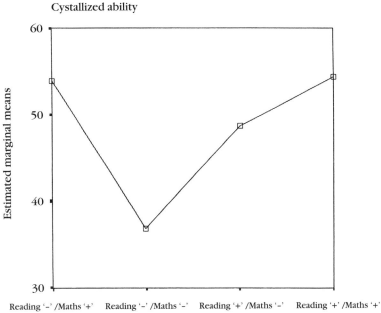

Fluid ability

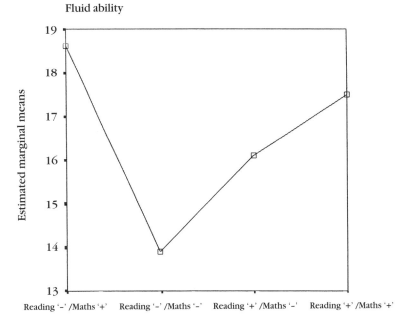

Figure 6.2 (a) Estimated marginal means (i.e. means adjusted for age and gender effects) in reading-by-maths performance groups.

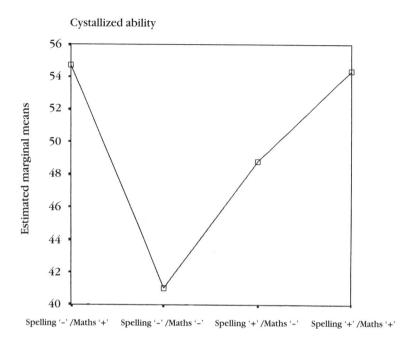

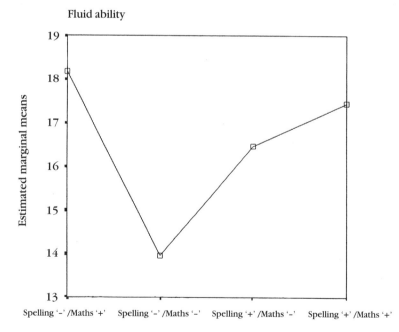

Figure 6.2 (b) Estimated marginal means (i.e. means adjusted for age and gender effects) in spelling-by-maths performance groups.

pronounce the t). The trial items and the first few test items involve deletion of a morpheme in a compound word or a syllable in a two-syllable word. The remaining items involve omitting a phoneme, first in the initial position, then at the end of the word and finally, from consonant blends at the start of the word. There are 40 items in this task.

In the single-word reading accuracy task, the child is presented with a list of 60 words, one at a time. Thirty words are four-syllable and 30 others are five-syllable words. Forty words are real words (20 regular and 20 inconsistent) and 20 words are nonwords. Each word is presented on a separate piece of paper so at any given time the child could see only one word.

Teachers' ratings of children's performance on reading tasks were predicted in a simple linear regression equation with indicators of phonological awareness and single-word reading tasks as independent variables, and gender and grade as control variables. The combination of variables explained 72% of the variance in teachers' ratings ($p < 0.000$). The contributions of both phonological awareness and single-word reading tasks were significant and substantial irrespective of grade and gender of the child.

A topology of spelling errors among high school children

In this study, we investigated spelling errors made by high school students. The study asked students to read five paragraphs. The paragraphs were followed by multiple-choice and free-response comprehension written questions. Free responses were recorded and studied for spelling errors. More than 600 high school students, both boys and girls, participated in this research. The age range of participants was 13–14 to 17–18 years. The data presented here are those generated in response to one question only. As discussed above, the spelling errors are classified as: (i) phonological errors (e.g. based on the principles of (a) stressed and unstressed vowels, (b) vowels after consonants, (c) assimilations (voicing–devoicing, hardness–softness and place of articulation); and (ii) morphological errors (e.g. based on a lack of understanding of both inflectional and derivational components). The outcome of this survey is presented in Table 6.1.

There are three observations of interest in this table. First, even in high school, students of Russian make spelling errors. Second, somewhat surprisingly, among these errors, there are phonology-based errors. (It is usually assumed that phonology of more regular languages such as Russian is mastered by the third or fourth grade; clearly, among Russian high school students there is a non-trivial number of those who have not mastered it). Finally, when percentages are compared, the highest number of errors is associated with morphology (30% of spelling errors were inflectional morphology errors and 23.3% were derivational morphology).

Table 6.1 Russian students' spelling errors

Source of complication	Examples	Percent observed
Stressed and unstressed vowels	виликанская correct spelling великанская	20
Vowels after consonants	синсацыонную correct spelling сенсационную	10
Assimilation	одиннокий, страный correct spelling одинокий, странный	16.7
Morphological mistakes (re: derivation and inflection)	добится correct spelling добиться	53.3

Conclusion

Different orthographies have different mapping rules from speech to spelling and vice versa, reflecting a huge variation in the degree of consistency with which alphabets around the world represent phonemes by graphemes. The continuum ranges from ideally transparent (i.e. having a one-to-one correspondence between phonemes and graphemes, like Turkish) to opaque (i.e. having a many-to-many correspondence between phonemes and graphemes, like English). Russian occupies the middle ground of the continuum, having elements of both transparency and opacity. It is possible that a universal reading-related deficiency presents different challenges in different orthographic systems and, consequently, manifests itself differently, both qualitatively and quantitatively. Therefore, models of reading deficiency developed in certain languages cannot simply be imposed on other languages and should be carefully verified on a broad, representative sample of readers.

A number of recent studies of normal reading development have provided some data suggesting that consistent (i.e. transparent) orthographies impose much less of a challenge compared to inconsistent orthographies. For example, children mastering reading in Spanish, Italian, Greek, Portuguese or German have been found to have significantly fewer decoding problems than English-reading children. Unlike the poor readers of English, who find it very difficult to read new words or pseudowords, poor readers in more transparent languages appear to master decoding by the second grade. Moreover, the English poor-reading children continue failing at phonological analysis (i.e. phonological awareness), while poor readers in less phonologically complex languages master this skill rather rapidly. However, poor readers in more consistent orthographies demonstrate impairments in reading speed and reading automaticity, and make many more spelling errors compared to their non-impaired peers (e.g. Harris and Hatano, 1999).

Russian orthography is largely simple and consistent, with most letters representing only one phoneme in the language and most phonemes represented by only one letter. Nevertheless, there are still some letters that are inconsistent: these letters have more than one phonemic expression. For this reason, Russian provides an excellent model for the study of cognitive operations involved in printed-word recognition and processing.

The studies presented above have demonstrated, in general, the presence of significant variations in reading and spelling skills among primary, middle and high school students all of whom were native speakers of Russian. The presented data have shown that Russian teachers using traditional methods of direct instruction are very sensitive in their evaluation of children's reading to their students' phonological awareness and single-word reading skills. Based on the information obtained from two independent large samples of children enrolled in Russian public schools, a hypothesis can be formulated that there are children mastering the written Russian language who experience specific difficulties while learning how to read and spell. These difficulties are not linked to general ability or behavioural deficits. Moreover, there is a significant but not complete overlap between poor reading skills and poor spelling skills.

References

American Psychiatric Association (1994) DSM-IV. Diagnostic and Statistical Manual of Mental Disorders. Washington DC: American Psychiatric Press.

Aronoff M (1976) Word formation in generative grammar. Cambridge, MA: MIT Press.

Cattell RB, Cattell HEP (1973) Measuring intelligence with the Culture Fair Tests. Champaign, IL: Institute for Personality and Ability Testing.

Grigorenko EL, Katz L (1999) Predictors of reading performance in Russian elementary school students: a teachers' prospective. Unpublished manuscript.

Hamilton WS (1980) Introduction to Russian phonology and word structure. Columbus, OH: Slavica Publishers.

Harris M, Hatano G (eds) (1999) Learning to read and write. A cross-linguistic perspective. New York: Cambridge University Press.

Moiseev AI (1975) Фонетика Морфология. Орфографиа [Phonetics. Morphology, Orthography]. Moskva: Prosveshchenie.

Shcherba LV (1963). Фонетика французского языка [Phonetics of the French language]. Moskva: Prosveshchenie.

Wolkonsky C, Poltoratzky M (1961) Handbook of Russian roots. New York: Cambridge University Press.

CHAPTER 7

Patterns of Developmental Dyslexia in Bilinguals

DENISE KLEIN AND ESTELLE ANN LEWIN DOCTOR

In this chapter we discuss several theoretical approaches to the study of reading, which have led to a better understanding of the normal reading process and of developmental disorders of reading. Three cases of bilingual developmental dyslexia are presented to show how models of monolingual reading may be extended to cover bilingual word recognition. We used tests from the bilingual version of the *Literacy Assessment Battery* to examine how these bilingual children's reading has been influenced by the orthographic structure, or relationship between letters and sounds, of their languages. We highlight the influence of orthographic structure on reading disorders and on the implementation of successful intervention programmes.

Investigations of word recognition using bilinguals offer an opportunity to differentiate universal from language-specific aspects of word processing. They also offer an opportunity to assess the wider application of current models of word recognition, which are based on data collected from monolingual readers. One such model of monolingual word recognition, the dual route model (Carr and Pollatsek, 1985; Coltheart, 1978; Humphreys and Evett, 1985), was developed to explain the two strategies that skilled readers of English use to read known and novel words. Dual route theories separate reading into a lexical (whole word) route for reading known words, and a sublexical (sound based) route for sounding out one-to-one letter–sound correspondences and rule-based words. Dual route theories are supported by patterns of reading observed in certain classic cases of developmental and acquired dyslexia, with some dyslexics and patients having difficulty with whole-word recognition, while at the same time being able to sound words out (Holmes, 1973; Coltheart et al., 1983; Bub et al., 1985), and others being able to recognize words by sight, but unable to sound out unknown words (Derouesné and Beauvois, 1979; Temple and Marshall, 1983).

This conception of the architecture of the reading system has been challenged. It was argued (Glushko, 1979; Marcel, 1980) that a single process can explain reading of previously seen as well as new words with novel items being read aloud by an analogy process that involves activating other familiar words. Therefore, the current debate centres on whether the two systems, lexical (whole word) and sublexical (partial word), operate independently. A separate challenge to dual route theory has come from computational models of single-word reading, such as the parallel distributed processing (PDP) model of Seidenberg and McClelland (1989), which at first proved unsuccessful in explaining reading of previously unseen nonsense words. However, the challenge was met by Coltheart et al.'s (1993) dual-route computational model, while Plaut and McClelland (1993) and Plaut et al. (1996) have developed a PDP model that performs well on reading made-up nonsense words. According to Plaut et al., (1996) regular words, exception words and previously unseen nonsense words may all be processed within a single system. Their theory thus stands in contradiction to dual route theory which postulates two systems, and for which the notion of phonological recoding of printed words to sound is an integral part of the reading process.

What evidence is there for phonological encoding? Several years ago it was demonstrated by the 'pseudohomophone' effect in lexical decision tasks (Rubenstein et al., 1971; Coltheart et al., 1977). In such tasks, a person is shown a string of letters and asked to decide if the string is a real word or a nonsense word. The 'pseudohomophone' effect occurs when pseudohomophones like *grane*, which both look and sound like real words, are rejected more slowly than non-pseudohomophones like *frane*, which look like real words but do not sound like them. One criticism of using this finding to support the notion of phonological encoding and the existence of a separate sublexical route is that the effect is based on reading nonsense words and has not been shown for real words in monolingual research (although such evidence has been found in bilinguals – see below). Phonological effects have also been observed in sentence verification tasks, such as, '*I know him*' versus '*I no him*' versus '*I noe him*' (Doctor and Coltheart, 1980),with young readers mistakenly accepting all three as being meaningful, and in semantic categorization tasks in which questions such as '*Is a rows a flower?*' (van Orden, 1987) are erroneously answered in the affirmative. Clear evidence of phonological recoding is also evident in bilingual lexical decision studies (Doctor and Klein, 1992). Bilingual adults took longer and were less accurate responding to interlingual homophones [*lake–lyk*], which sound the same in both their languages, than to interlingual homographs [*kind*]), which look the same but sound different in both languages, or language-specific words, which look and sound different.

To explain this bilingual effect Doctor and Klein (1992) developed a modification of the monolingual dual route model according to which there are separate, language-specific word recognition systems for print, termed 'orthographic input' and 'orthographic output' lexicons, one for each of the bilingual's languages, and also a language-independent letter-to-sound conversion system termed the 'grapheme–phoneme translator' (Figure 7.1).

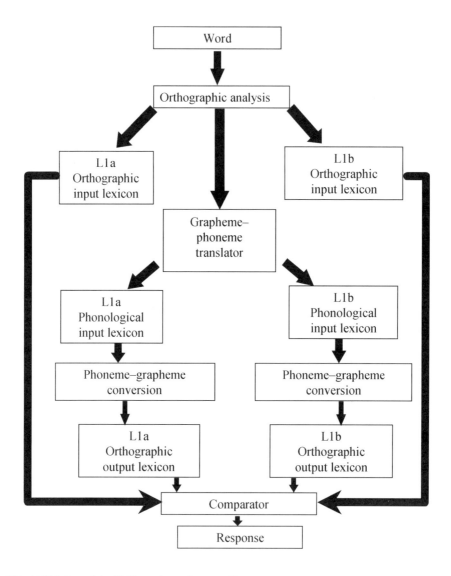

Figure 7.1 A model of bilingual word recognition.

According to this model, when any word is presented for recognition, each language-specific word recognition system or lexicon is searched, in parallel. If a match is not located in a lexicon, further processing in that lexicon ceases. At the same time, information about the word is sent in parallel to the grapheme–phoneme translator which translates letters into sounds. Being language-independent, this grapheme–phoneme translator may be accessed by words of either language.[1] The result of the letter–sound conversion process taking place in the grapheme–phoneme translator is a phonological representation of the word as it would be spoken, worked out according to rules stored in the translator. This phonological representation of the original printed word is then sent off to both language-specific phonological input lexicons, which are memory stores for heard words in both languages. If an entry is not found in the phonological input lexicon for one of the languages, further phonological processing in that lexicon ceases, but it continues if a match is found.

The next stage of processing is again language-specific. An 'orthographic' code is derived from the sound of the word. Thus, the sounds in the matched word are translated into letters, according to the rules of the language in which the match was found, in much the same way as it occurs for spelling to dictation. This information is fed into each of the language-specific orthographic output lexicons. These are separate memory stores for each language containing word spellings for that language. If no match is located in one of the output lexicons, processing ceases. If a match is found, a verification

---

[1]This claim is based on Doctor and Klein's findings in the study mentioned above, in which adult bilinguals were presented with mixed lists containing real words in both their languages as well as interlingual homophones and interlingual homographs. Because the stimuli were presented randomly, and there was an equal number of each word-type, it is unlikely that the readers could have predicted, before reading the word, to which language it belonged. Under these circumstances, and bearing in mind that phonological effects had not previously been demonstrated in monolingual research, one would not have expected any differences in responses to each of the four different word types. It was thus surprising that responses to interlingual homophones [*LAKE-LYK*] were significantly slower and less accurate than responses to the other word types. Furthermore, as the readers did not know in advance whether the stimulus was an interlingual homophone or not, it is unlikely that they could have adopted one processing strategy for interlingual homophones and a different reading strategy for other word types. To accommodate these findings we therefore postulated that the grapheme–phoneme translator operates simultaneously on all grapheme-phoneme correspondences associated with a particular grapheme, possibly because such a strategy would be accurate for all Afrikaans words as they are regular in their spelling-to-sound correspondences. While there is likely to be only one phoneme correspondence per grapheme for shallow orthographies, there may be several for deep orthographies.

procedure is implemented. The matched item located in the language-specific orthographic output lexicon is compared with the original word presented to the orthographic input lexicon. If the comparison is successful, a YES decision will be made, and the word will have been recognized. If a mismatch is detected (pseudohomophone, e.g. *grane*, or misspelling, e.g. *devellop*), rechecking will take place, resulting in longer latencies, or an error involving mistaken identification. This model has implications for dyslexia in bilinguals, which are discussed below.

Characteristics of Afrikaans and English

Writing systems or orthographies differ in the complexity of the rules linking the written language to speech (Rozin and Gleitman, 1977; Sasanuma, 1980; Hung and Tzeng, 1981). They have been categorized as either 'shallow' or 'deep', depending on the ease of predicting the pronunciation of a word from its spelling (Besner and Smith, 1992). In shallow orthographies, the letter–sound correspondence is transparent; in deep orthographies the reader must learn many arbitrary pairings. English and Afrikaans are both alphabetic scripts and, as Table 7.1 shows, they each have a similar number of phonemes (50 versus 57) They differ in the number of grapheme–phoneme correspondence patterns, with English sounds mapping on to many more symbols than Afrikaans sounds (104 versus 58) (Doctor et al., 1987). English therefore has a 'deeper' orthography than Afrikaans.

All Afrikaans words are pronounced consistently. For example, *hou*, *kou*, *vrou*, etc. would all be pronounced to rhyme with the English word 'toe' and the few ambiguities that occur in Afrikaans affect spelling more than reading. Consider, in contrast, *cough*, *rough*, *dough*, etc. A relationship has been suggested between the depth of the orthography and the type of processing strategy (whole word or phonological) preferred by readers of the language (Lukatela et al., 1980). The deeper English orthography may require a more

Table 7.1 Grapheme–phoneme correspondences in English and Afrikaans

	English (Wijk, 1966)	Afrikaans (Coetzee, 1985)
Vowel phonemes	25	30
Vowel graphemes	60	27
Consonant phonemes	25	27
Consonant graphemes	44	31
Total phonemes	50	57
Total symbols	104	58

whole-word approach and may act as a barrier to phonological involvement in fluent reading. In contrast, a whole-word reading strategy may be unnecessary for reading the shallow orthography of Afrikaans, and greater reliance on sounding out may be evident (Lukatela et al., 1980; Feldman and Turvey, 1983; Feldman et al., 1983).

The notion of two different reading strategies also underpins theories of reading development. Gough and Hillinger (1980), Marsh et al. (1981), Frith (1985), Seymour (1986) and Ehri (1992) have proposed stage theories of literacy development in which there is an early stage of logographic whole-word recognition based on partial cues, a later stage of alphabetic reading based on knowledge of letters and sounds, and finally, an orthographic stage based on understanding the complex orthography of English.

Certain predictions can be derived from the bilingual dual route model about processing at different stages of reading development in bilinguals. Bilingual readers at the early logographic stage should only be able to read words that constitute their sight vocabulary. According to Seymour and Elder's (1986) findings from monolingual beginner readers, frequency effects, which occur when familiar words are easier to recognize than unfamiliar words, are expected, as are lexicality effects, which occur when real words are easier to recognize than nonsense words. Regularity effects are not expected at this stage of development as regular and exception words are equally difficult to read. Bilingual beginners, using a purely logographic strategy, should also show frequency and lexicality effects and should produce reading errors that are visually similar to the target, or refusals, rather than regularizations or nonwords.

If an alphabetic strategy is available as well as access to a logographic vocabulary, then, in addition to known words being recognized by sight, new words can be sounded out. In bilinguals, this would involve accessing the language-independent grapheme–phoneme translator, which in turn would give rise to language-specific effects favouring the shallower orthography and would ensure similar performance for words and nonwords in Afrikaans. In the deeper English orthography, however, there will be regularity effects such that unfamiliar regular words will be recognized more accurately than unfamiliar irregular words, and reading of nonwords would be superior to reading of unfamiliar irregular words. Because two reading strategies are available (whole word and sounding out), errors will depend on the type of strategy that predominates, as well as on the orthographic structure of the language. A whole-word reading strategy may result in a refusal to respond to unrecognized words, or as one word being read as another, while a sounding-out strategy incorrectly applied to an irregular word will result in a regularization and possibly a nonsense word (*island* read as /ɪzland/). More visual errors may occur in reading Afrikaans words than English words, due to the greater visual similarity of words in Afrikaans because of the orthographic structure of the language. These 'neighbourhood' effects may lead to confusion that results in one word being read as another, the so-called 'lexicalization' error, for example *mooi* read as 'mooi'. Nonwords derived from the shallow orthography and presented to the reader for recognition may also give rise to visual errors, for the same reason.

It is only when the reader has reached the orthographic stage, and has available an orthographic framework that allows for both regular and irregular words to be identified and pronounced via a common process (Seymour and Evans, 1992), that equal performance is expected across both languages, irrespective of orthographic structure. If full acquisition has not taken place, there is a possibility that reading of words in the deeper English orthography reading will be impaired relative to reading of the shallower Afrikaans.

Many beginner readers have phonological processing difficulties that arise for different reasons and affect their reading. The child may have difficulty segmenting the word into letters, difficulty converting letters to sounds, or difficulty blending sounds to form a word. If the bilingual reader finds it difficult to convert letters into sounds, then performance will be equally restricted in both languages. On the other hand, if the reader can access only some grapheme–phoneme conversion rules, usually the most common correspondences, then orthographically shallow Afrikaans may show an advantage over English. The phonological dyslexic who, by definition, has difficulty converting print to sound, develops a compensatory strategy of guessing at words from partial clues and retrieving similar-looking words in the word recognition system for printed words (orthographic input lexicon). The effects may be more damaging for a language with a shallow orthography, such as Afrikaans, in which words resemble each other much more than in a deeper orthography. If the reader is able to segment the word, and knows some, but not all of the letter–sound correspondences, then the shallow orthography will again have an advantage.

Some children have reading difficulties because they cannot recognize words as wholes and so come to rely on grapheme–phoneme translation. The language with the shallow orthography (Afrikaans) is again likely to benefit from such a strategy by allowing the reader to decode more words in that language than in the other (English). Regularity effects should be evident in English, the deeper orthography, and nonword reading may be better than reading of unfamiliar irregular words.

Experimental investigation

Method

Participants

All the pupils in this study were classified as compound bilinguals (Ervin and Osgood, 1954) or primary language bilinguals because they had acquired English and Afrikaans simultaneously from their parents before the age of 5 years (Lamendella, 1977). Perfect dual competence is seldom maintained in South Africa because the child attends either an English-medium or an Afrikaans-medium class within a parallel-medium school. In such schools, half of each year is instructed predominantly in English and the remainder in Afrikaans. The result is that the child emerges with some degree of primary and secondary language competence instead of balanced bilingualism.

Control pupils. The 20 competent readers, five in each of four year groups, attended a parallel medium school. They were in grade 2 (7 years old), standard 1 (8 years old), standard 3 (10 years old) and standard 5 (12 years old). They had average to above-average IQs and age-appropriate reading and spelling skills.

Dyslexic pupils. The three pupils selected for the present study had normal birth and developmental histories. All had repeated a year at school and attended a special school for learning disabled pupils. Table 7.2 provides biographical and cognitive information. Their scores on the SSAIS (based on the WISC but standardized for South Africa) show that Karen and Shannon were of average intelligence; Barry was in the above-average range. Their competence in both languages was similar.

The dyslexic pupils were assessed twice, at an interval of two years. Barry was initially found to be dominant in Afrikaans but was later thought to be more proficient in English. Shannon was dominant first in English and later in Afrikaans. Karen remained English-dominant for both assessments.

Language Assessment

A full discussion of the language abilities of the dyslexic pupils is given by Klein (1993). In summary, they had difficulties acquiring language skills and with analysis, synthesis, sequencing and syllabification. They lacked phonological awareness, and this, as well as their other difficulties, put them at risk for reading and spelling (Bradley and Bryant, 1983; Content et al., 1986; Snowling et al., 1986; Goswami and Bryant, 1990).

Table 7.2 Bilingual pupils: biographical information

Subject	Sex	Age at 1st Assessment (years)	Age at 2nd Assessment (years)	VIQ²	PIQ³	Dominant Language FSIQ⁴	English	SSAIS¹ English	SSAIS¹ Afrikaans	HSRC Bilingual Competence
Karen	F	10:02	12:03	E	104	98	102	3*	3*	
Barry	M	11:07	13:06	A/E	124	134	135	2*	2*	
Shannon	M	12:05	14:09	E/A	107	117	113	6	5	

*= below average on Human Sciences Research Council's (HSRC) language competence test which compares competence in vocabulary, language usage, comprehension and spelling in English and Afrikaans and gives results in terms of stanine scores.

¹The SSAIS is the South African version of the WISC, used with children.

²Verbal intelligence quotient.

³Performance intelligence quotient.

⁴Full-scale intelligence quotient.

Materials

All pupils were assessed on a selection of tests from the bilingual version (English and Afrikaans) of the Literacy Assessment Battery (LAB). This battery provides a fine-grained analysis of children's reading and spelling difficulties, which serves as a basis for developing and evaluating teaching interventions designed to raise performance. The LAB is based on the dual route model of reading described above. Tests evaluate reading skills ranging from letter- to word-recognition. Tasks are designed to assess both lexical and sublexical processing, and beyond that to consider other aspects of reading that relate to the syntactic and semantic aspects of language. The words in the different language versions of the tests are matched as carefully as possible for frequency, length, imageability and number of syllables. The advantage of a bilingual version of the battery is that it permits direct comparison of the cognitive processes involved in reading and spelling in two different languages.

Tests

Experiment 1: Orthographic assessment

The purpose of the first assessment was to evaluate word recognition in both languages, using a Lexical Decision Task. The reader was asked to decide whether printed items were words or not, for example *GIRL* and *JIRL*. Comprehension of word meaning is not necessary to perform this task, although it facilitates correct responses to real words.

Materials. The test in each language consisted of 16 high-frequency and 16 low-frequency words. Word length ranged from four to seven letters, with four examples at each length. There were 32 derived nonwords. The lists were matched as carefully as possible across languages, and the stimuli in each language list were checked to ensure that no nonwords derived from English were real Afrikaans words and vice versa.

Results and discussion

Control pupils. The two age groups performed differently.[2] There was a gradual improvement in word-recognition skills with the younger group performing significantly worse than the older group.[3]

---

[2]$F_{(1,16)} = 6.50$, $p < 0.01$.
[3]Tukey hsd post-hoc multiple range test: 7- versus 12-year olds: $Q(16) = 6.24$, $p < 0.01$.

Table 7.3 Percentage correct responses given by Karen on the word-recognition task.

	English	Afrikaans
Total correct 10:02 yrs	66 (84)	50 (81)
Total correct 12:03 yrs	73 (92)	73 (91)

Scores of control children aged 10 years when Karen was 10, and 12 years when she was 12, are given in parentheses.

Table 7.3 shows that Karen's performance was well below that of the chronological-age matched controls.[4] At the time of the first assessment, when she was 10:02 years, her performance was at chance, and was similar to the 7-year-old control group. Two years later her performance was better than chance and similar to the 8-year-old controls. Her word-recognition skills were poor in both languages at both assessments. There were no frequency effects. At the time of the first assessment (T1) she showed lexicality effects for Afrikaans words and could reject only 16% of nonwords derived from Afrikaans words. At this time Karen was reading logographically, recognizing words by salient features. This conferred a spurious advantage on Afrikaans low-frequency words (88% correct recognition) and caused her to accept nonwords as real words, particularly in Afrikaans because of its orthographic structure. By the time of the second assessment (T2) her strategy had changed (see Table 7.3 above), and Afrikaans word-recognition had improved.

At the first assessment (T1), Barry, aged 11:07 years, displayed word-recognition skills that were at age level for Afrikaans. For English, his performance was at chance, indicating that he was guessing, and was significantly worse than the 10-year-old controls.[5] Table 7.4 shows that his English word recognition improved over time.[6] It was better than chance at T2, when he was 13:06 years, but it was still worse than the 12-year-old controls.[7] At T1, Barry was able to reject 88% of nonwords derived from Afrikaans, but only 63% of nonwords derived from English, and he could have been guessing. The phonological reading strategy which he had adopted made it easier for him to reject nonwords derived from orthographically shallow Afrikaans than

---

[4]T1 English: $z = -2.59$, $p < 0.01$; T2 English: $z = -7.41$, $p < 0.01$; T1 Afrikaans: $z = -2.28$, $p < 0.01$; T2 Afrikaans: $z = -3.09$, $p < 0.01$.
[5]BS versus 10-year-olds: $z = -3.74$, $p < 0.01$.
[6]$\chi^2 = 5.17$, df $= 1$, $p < 0.05$.
[7]BS vs. 12-year-olds: $z = -5.42$, $p < 0.01$.

Table 7.4 Percentage correct responses given by Barry on the word-recognition task.

	English	Afrikaans
Total correct 11:07 yrs	58 (84)	84 (81)
Total correct 13:06 yrs	78 (92)	84 (91)

Scores of control children aged 10 years when Barry was 11, and 12 years when he was 13, are given in parentheses.

from the deeper English orthography, possibly because half of these were derived from English words with irregular spelling patterns.

Shannon's word recognition was assessed once only, when he was 12:05 years. His performance was age-appropriate and approaching ceiling.

Summary

Karen appeared to be guessing at words on the basis of visual appearance. This conferred an advantage on Afrikaans low-frequency words, but penalised nonwords derived from Afrikaans. Barry also appeared to be guessing at words on their visual appearance, but he had access to sounding-out strategy as well, which allowed him to reject nonwords derived from Afrikaans and boosted his performance in that language. Because of their poor word-recognition skills, Karen and Barry were expected to display similar impairments in a range of reading tasks. Shannon was expected to display a different configuration of difficulties as his word-recognition skills, in both languages, appeared to have been consolidated.

Experiment 2: Phonological assessment

The aim of this assessment was to evaluate how the reading strategies these pupils had acquired would enable them to cope with a phonic system of different complexities. Those who were at a logographic stage were expected to show frequency and lexicality effects and make errors which were either refusals or visually similar to the target. Those who were at an alphabetic stage should show an advantage for Afrikaans, and frequency as well as regularity effects in English.

Materials

English and Afrikaans lists were devised, with 32 words and 32 nonwords per list. Half were high-frequency words and the remainder were low-frequency. They were matched to those in the lexical decision task for frequency and word length. Half the English words were regular and half were irregular, so that the pupils could use either lexical or sublexical strategies to perform the task. Comprehension was not assessed.

Results and discussion

Control pupils

The performance of the control readers on this task has been discussed by Klein (1996). She reported that the 7- and 8-year-old control pupils showed frequency effects in word recognition. Most errors were visually similar to the target, but some pupils were attempting to use letter–sound rules and produced nonword responses. Ten-year-olds with normally developing phonological skills were better at reading Afrikaans words and nonwords than English items. For English, they were better at reading words that were regular in their sound–spelling mappings, particularly if these words were also familiar to them. They found unfamiliar irregular words most difficult to pronounce. They were also good at reading nonwords derived from English. The 12-year-olds were able to read regular and irregular words equally well, supporting Seymour and Evans's (1992) finding for monolinguals. Orthographic depth affected performance, so that where full acquisition had taken place, words and nonwords derived from both languages were read efficiently.

Karen read high- and low-frequency words in both languages significantly worse than age-matched controls.[8] Her performance was more similar to the 7-year-old controls at the first assessment and to the 8-year-olds at the second assessment. Table 7.5 shows Karen's oral reading scores. At both assessments she read Afrikaans words more accurately than English words. At first, the difference between the two languages was not significant, but by T2, low-frequency Afrikaans words were read more accurately than low-frequency English words.[9] Frequency effects were observed at both assessments in English.[10]

Nonwords were read with less accuracy[11] than words, indicating difficulties with letter–sound conversion. At T1, she was better at reading Afrikaans

---

[8]T1 English high frequency: 10-year-old controls =100%; Karen = 68%; T1 English low frequency: $z = -7.55$, $p < 0.01$; T2 English high frequency: 10-year-old controls = 100%; Karen = 88%; T2 English low frequency: $z = -23.89$, $p < 0.01$; T1 Afrikaans high frequency: $z = -10.52$, $p < 0.01$; T1 Afrikaans low frequency: $z = -3.3$, $p < 0.01$; T2 Afrikaans high frequency: 12-year-old controls = 100%; Karen = 94%; T2 Afrikaans low frequency: $z = -8.88$, $p < 0.01$.

[9]$\chi^2 = 6.94$, df = 1, $p < 0.05$.

[10]T1: $\chi^2 = 6.22$, df = 1, $p < 0.05$; T2: $\chi2 = 8.29$, df = 1, $p < 0.05$.

[11]T1 English words: $z = -11.32$, $p < 0.01$; T1 English derived nonwords: $z = -9.5$, $p < 0.01$; T2 English words: $z = -24.27$, $p < 0.01$; T2 English derived nonwords: $z = -10.84$, $p < 0.01$; T1 Afrikaans words: $z = -5.42$, $p < 0.01$; T1 Afrikaans derived nonwords: $z = -11.43$, $p < 0.01$; T2 Afrikaans words: $z = -11.49$, $p < 0.01$; T2 Afrikaans derived nonwords: $z = -36.71$, $p < 0.01$.

Table 7.5 Karen: oral reading - percentage correct.

	English		Afrikaans	
	10:02 yrs	12:03 yrs	10:02 yrs	12:03 yrs
High frequency words	68 (100)	88 (100)	63 (98)	94 (100)
High frequency nonwords	38		13	
Low frequency words	19 (89)	31 (98)	44 (88)	75 (99)
Low frequency nonwords	31		0	
Total Words	44 (94)	59 (99)	53 (93)	84 (99)
Total Nonwords	34 (89)	31 (88)	6 (87)	38 (98)
Regular	64 (94)	85 (97)		
Irregular	53 (72)	62 (86)		

Scores of control children aged 10 years when she was 10, and 12 years when she was 12, are given in parentheses.

words than derived nonwords,[12] while English words and derived nonwords were read with similar low accuracy. Some improvement took place between the two assessments, as more words entered her lexicons and as she acquired some simple letter–sound correspondence rules. These benefited both languages but particularly low frequency Afrikaans words, by making it possible for her to sound them out. By T2, lexicality effects were evident in both languages and words were easier to read than nonwords.[13]

Karen's lexical decision data indicated a logographic reading strategy that encouraged her to guess at words from their salient features. Her oral reading errors showed that this strategy was coupled with knowledge of the simplest 1:1 letter-sound correspondences. The beginnings of words were most salient for her. Ninety-four percent of errors made on English derived nonwords shared the same initial letter as the target and only 25% the same final letter. Medial segments were guessed. The percentages for Afrikaans were 65% (initial) and 54% (final) respectively. Most of her errors were visual (English: 82%; Afrikaans: 98%), sharing 50% of the letters with the target, for example, *throng* → 'strong'; *bruid* → 'bruin'. At T1, 33% of errors on words in both languages and 50% of errors on nonwords were lexicalizations, for example: *thalk* → 'talked'. Errors were not phonologically plausible. By T2, although Karen's performance had improved quantitatively, she had not abandoned her logographic strategy, possibly because of her phonological processing limitations. Further evidence of this strategy and an inability to access meaning from sound was the absence, when she was 10 years old, of a

---

[12]$\chi^2 = 17.39$, df = 1, p < 0.01; Fisher p < 0.01.
[13]English: $\chi^2 = 4.04$, df = 1, p < 0.05; Afrikaans: $\chi^2 = 12.87$, df = 1, p < 0.01.

regularity effect in English. At that time there was no significant difference between her reading of regular and irregular words. Later, when she was 12 years old, and had developed knowledge of grapheme–phoneme correspondences, regularity effects appeared, in the expected direction, so that regular words were easier for her to read than irregular words.[14]

At T1, Barry (aged 11:07 years) could read aloud significantly fewer English and Afrikaans familiar and unfamiliar words than 12-year-old controls,[15] and was equivalent to 7-year-olds. As in word recognition, he demonstrated superior oral reading in Afrikaans,[16] for both familiar and unfamiliar words,[17] possibly because at that time he attended an Afrikaans-medium class and may have been exposed to more printed Afrikaans words. His reading strategy appeared to be logographic and as a result he was better at reading words than nonwords, thus showing a lexicality effect,[18] which had reduced two years later, at T2 (See Table 7.6). At the time of the first assessment, there was a trend for familiar words to be read aloud more accurately than unfamiliar words, but this was not statistically significant. The reading strategy which he had adopted conferred no real benefits.

Table 7.6 Barry: oral reading – percentage correct.

	English		Afrikaans	
	11:07 yrs	13:03 yrs	11:07 yrs	13:03 yrs
High frequency words	50 (100)	94 (100)	88 (98)	100 (100)
High frequency nonwords	38		56	
Low frequency words	38 (89)	63 (98)	75 (88)	88 (99)
Low frequency nonwords	25		38	
Total words	44 (94)	78 (99)	81 (93)	94 (99)
Total nonwords	31 (89)	63 (88)	50 (87)	91 (98)
Regular	64 (94)	85 (97)		
Irregular	53 (72)	62 (86)		

Scores of 10- and 12-year-old control children are given in parentheses.

[14] $\chi^2 = 4.17$, df = 1, p < 0.05.
[15] T1 English high frequency: z = -2.79, p < 0.01; T1 English low frequency: z = -2.03, p < 0.05; T1 Afrikaans high frequency: 12-year-old controls = 100%: BS = 88%; T1 Afrikaans low frequency: z = -8.88, p < 0.01.
[16] $\chi^2 = 8.066$, df = 1, p < 0.05.
[17] T1 high frequency: Fisher p < 0.05; low frequency: Fisher p < 0.05.
[18] $\chi^2 = 5.61$, df = 1, p < 0.05.

The most striking feature of the second assessment, when he was 13:06 years, and after he had transferred from an Afrikaans-medium class to an English-medium class, was the improvement in his English reading of words at both frequencies and the lack of improvement in Afrikaans. English oral reading had advanced from a 7- to an 8-year level and significant frequency effects emerged (Fisher p < 0.05). He still differed from the controls reading unfamiliar items in both languages.[19] Afrikaans word reading was comparable to 10-year-olds and significantly worse than 12-year-old controls,[20] particularly for unfamiliar words.[21] His reading of Afrikaans derived nonwords was also significantly worse than controls,[22] although the nonwords derived from Afrikaans were easier for him to read than the nonwords derived from English,[23] half of which were derived from English words with irregular spelling patterns.

Regular and irregular words were read significantly worse than controls at both assessments.[24] At the first assessment Barry's logographic reading strategy may have ensured that he did not show a regularity effect. By the time of the second assessment he had developed an elementary grapheme–phoneme correspondence system, which initially benefited the reading of Afrikaans words and later English regular words causing a regularity effect.[25]

Further evidence of the changes in his reading strategies appeared in his errors. At the time of the first assessment, 93% of his errors were visually similar to the target. Lexicalizations accounted for 42% of his errors on English words (*board* → 'borrowed'), 50% of his errors on Afrikaans words (*ryk* → 'kry') and 23% of his errors on nonwords. Although 58% of his errors on English words and 50% of his errors on Afrikaans words were nonwords, they were predominantly visual errors involving omissions, transpositions, additions, and derivations, for example, *steak* → 'streak', *thorough* → 'throg'. When he could not recognize a word directly he would try to pronounce it as a similar-looking word using visual features and simple

---

[19]T2 English low frequency: $z = 10.52$, $p < 0.01$; T2 Afrikaans low frequency: $z = -4.03$, $p < 0.01$.

[20]T1 words: $z = -11.37$, $p < 0.01$; nonwords: $z = -10.02$, $p < 0.01$; T2 words: $z = -12.68$, $p < 0.01$; nonwords: $z = -4.71$, $p < 0.01$.

[21]Words: $z = -4.03$, $p < 0.01$; nonwords: $z = -4.39$, $p < 0.01$.

[22]Nonwords: $z = -5.03$, $p < 0.01$.

[23]$\chi^2 = 5.52$, $df = 1$, $p < 0.05$.

[24]T1 regular words: $z = -19.28$, $p < 0.01$; T1 irregular words: $z = -10.67$, $p < 0.01$; T2 regular words: $z = -8.13$, $p < 0.01$; T2 irregular words: $z = -6.46$, $p < 0.01$.

[25]$\chi^2 = 4.51$, $df = 1$, $p < 0.05$.

letter–sound correspondences. This error pattern would be expected from a child who had difficulty with letter–sound conversion and relied on a reading strategy of recognizing words by visual features. By the second assessment, the quality of his errors changed as his knowledge of phonics increased, and there was an increase in the number of errors that were words misread as nonwords following an unsuccessful attempt to sound them out: *face →* 'fack'. Visual errors decreased to 69%, while lexicalization errors decreased for English words (29%) and derived nonwords, but not for Afrikaans.

When confronted with a word, Barry might look it up in either of his underdeveloped word-recognition systems, while simultaneously using a rudimentary letter-to-sound conversion process. The oddity judgement task (Bradley and Bryant, 1983) had shown that he found it difficult to attend to sounds in words. His letter-to-sound conversion system appeared to cope with single units of correspondence, and thus coped better with Afrikaans words than with English words. It also gave rise to a pseudohomophone effect in Afrikaans, so that he found it easier to read nonsense words that sounded like real words than those that did not, evidence that he was trying to use sound to access meaning. (An English example of a pseudohomophone would be 'seet'.)

The percentage of correct responses made by Shannon is shown in Table 7.7. At both assessments, he was as accurate as 12-year-old controls reading Afrikaans words and derived nonwords, and nonwords were read as well as real words. For English, word reading was significantly worse than controls at both assessments.[26] Further analysis of the data revealed that this was due to poor reading of low frequency words,[27] which did not improve between T1 and T2. Reading of nonwords, derived from English, did not differ from controls at T1 or T2.

Table 7.7 Percentage correct Oral Reading Scores obtained by Shannon.

	English		Afrikaans	
	12:05 yrs	14:09 yrs	12:05 yrs	14:09 yrs
Total words	88 (99)	88 (99)	97 (99)	100 (99)
Total nonwords	91 (88)	84 (88)	91 (98)	100 (98)
Regular words	92 (97)	97 (97)		
Irregular words	80 (86)	77 (86)		

Scores of 12-year-old control children are given in parentheses.

[26]T1: $z = -6.59$, $p < 0.01$; T2: $z = 6.59$.
[27]$z = -6.87$, $p < 0.01$.

Shannon, aged 12:05 years, was slightly but significantly weaker than the control group when reading regular words,[28] but did not differ from them in reading irregular words. Regularity effects were not expected and were not evident in the performance of the 12-year- old control group. At T1, Shannon did not show an advantage for reading regular words either, but 7/8 of his errors on irregular words were regularizations and this indicated a tendency towards using a phonic strategy when visual word recognition is unavailable, as it might be with unfamiliar words. Intrusion errors from one language to another constitute further evidence of his tendency to rely on letter-to-sound conversion rules, for example: Afrikaans *toe* → 'to'; English *folk* → 'volk'. (Shannon is the only experimental subject in this report to show substantial intrusion errors.) He also made stress errors, and they too may result from usage of a sublexical sounding-out strategy, since stress is assigned post-lexically, that is, you need to have heard an irregularly stressed word pronounced before you can pronounce it correctly yourself. Other errors reflected partial failures of grapheme–phoneme correspondence (e.g. *debt* → 'deb'). Because Shannon also had recourse to a visual reading strategy, some of his errors were lexicalizations (*strewn* → 'stew').

By the time of the second assessment, Shannon had transferred to an Afrikaans-medium school and reading of Afrikaans words and derived nonwords was superior to reading of English words. This may be explained by the additional exposure he was having to Afrikaans, but there is an indication from his performance on English words that he maintained a sublexical, sounding-out strategy. Regularity effects were evident,[29] and at this stage, all of his errors were regularizations. Shannon's results indicate that he was capable of deploying two different strategies when reading, and these affected performance in both languages differently. Further evidence of this is presented below in the discussion of imageability effects.

Experiment 3: Semantic assessment

To what extent is comprehension affected by the spelling structure or orthography of the language and by the strategies that bilinguals use to identify meaning? Readers who are at a logographic stage should be able to define only those words which they can recognize. They should perform similarly across languages, and show no differences between words that have a single sound and meaning, and homophones that share sound but have different meanings. Readers who are at the alphabetic stage, reliant on

---

[28]$z = -2.15, p < 0.05$.
[29]$z = -2.09, p < 0.05$.

grapheme–phoneme conversion, may find homophones more difficult to define than non-homophonic words because their reading strategy would generate two different meanings associated with the same sound. They may show a language effect caused by their reading strategy. If a shallow orthography encourages a phonological reading strategy, then it may be more difficult to define Afrikaans homophones.

Materials. There were 20 words and 20 homophones, matched for word frequency, for oral reading and definition in each language. Half the English set were regular, and half were exceptions.

Results and discussion.

The control pupils did not differ in their reading or defining of English or Afrikaans words, but all age groups found Afrikaans homophones more difficult to define than to read ($Q(16) = 8.45$, $p < 0.01$), and more difficult to read and define than English words (Pronunciation: $Q(16) = 8.13$, $p < 0.01$; Definition: $Q(16) = 15.42$, $p < 0.01$).

At T1, Karen, as expected, could only define those stimuli she could pronounce. By T2, when she had acquired some grapheme–phoneme correspondences, there were improvements in English pronunciation and definition. In Afrikaans, the improvements were restricted to words: homophones that require a lexical reading strategy were poorly defined.[30]

Barry's results go against the trend of Afrikaans homophones being more difficult to define. His definitions were more accurate in Afrikaans than in English, and because of his whole-word approach to reading, most of his errors in both languages were visual (English 70%; Afrikaans 90%). By T2, Barry had developed his phonics and his reading of English words had improved. Nevertheless, he still knew the meaning of more Afrikaans than English words (Fisher $p < 0.05$) and there was a non-significant trend, due to ceiling effects, in favour of Afrikaans homophones as well. This pattern of performance is likely to be due to his visual reading strategy benefiting homophone definition.

Shannon scored 100% for reading English homophones, and 90% for defining them. Afrikaans reading was 95% accurate, and definition 70%. He made a single homophone confusion error in English, but 3 (50%) in Afrikaans. Three non-confusion-type errors were made defining regular words and one defining an Afrikaans word. Shannon's performance on the oral reading task had demonstrated that he was capable of deploying two

---

[30]Afrikaans homophones versus words: Fisher $p < 0.05$; T2 English homophones versus Afrikaans homophones: Fisher $p < 0.05$.

[31]Homophones: Fisher $p < 0.05$; words: Fisher $p < 0.01$.

different strategies: a lexical strategy, which benefited reading of English words and which resulted in no difference between word and homophone reading and definition, and a phonological recoding strategy, which improved his oral reading but not his comprehension of Afrikaans words and resulted in a difference between them (Fisher p < 0.05). This strategy also resulted in a difference between word and homophone definition (Fisher p < 0.05) and in homophone confusions. Further evidence of his using two strategies was found in his oral reading of concrete and abstract words and in his performance on a synonym-matching task involving concrete and abstract words. He showed an imageability effect in English, but not in Afrikaans, in both tasks so that concrete words such as *skin* were easier to read than abstract words such as *fate*. This demonstrates again his usage of different strategies for processing print in different orthographies.

General discussion

The purpose of this study was to examine how reading strategy interacts with the structure of the written language to influence reading performance in normally developing bilingual readers and in bilingual developmental dyslexics. The normative data indicated that there are similar developmental trends in reading acquisition in both languages, regardless of orthographic differences in the writing systems. Seven-year-olds were at the early stages of processing, with few reading skills in either language. Eight- to 10-year-olds showed a greater tendency to read by translating letters into sounds. Normal readers in this study had reached ceiling on the tests by age 12 and even though Afrikaans biases readers towards a phonological strategy, most of the older readers realized that a whole-word, lexical processing strategy was necessary for complete success. Another similarity was that the same factors influenced word recognition in both languages: frequency, word length, part of speech, and imageability.

Many of the differences observed were due to the interaction of ortho-graphic depth with processing strategy. When the normally developing readers in the control group adopted an alphabetic reading strategy involving phonological recoding, their Afrikaans reading improved relative to English, and they found English regular words easier to read than irregular words. These readers were also capable of reading lexically and by the time they were 12 were able to read fluently by sight. Nevertheless, they made more use of this strategy for reading English than for reading Afrikaans as shown by their performance on the homophone definition task in which they made more errors on the Afrikaans version. They read English homophones via a lexical, whole-word recognition strategy, but adopted a phonological, sounding-out strategy for Afrikaans homophones.

Similar effects were evident in the dyslexics. Impairments in whole-word recognition and phonological processing were observed in both languages in each of the pupils. Karen and Barry displayed difficulty with phonological processing and consequently with letter–sound conversion. They relied on logographic strategies to access the words in the language-specific word-recognition systems. In this respect they performed similarly to monolingual beginner readers, and the difficulties they experienced are common in monolingual phonological dyslexics. Barry's reading strategy affected his two languages differently. He was developing letter–sound conversion strategies based on simple correspondences which favoured Afrikaans but not English. Consequently, he did not differ from control readers in his recognition and oral reading of Afrikaans words, but was significantly worse than they were in English. Initially, Karen had difficulty developing her word-recognition skills in both languages but her Afrikaans reading skills improved when she began to acquire alphabetic skills. Initially these skills had little immediate impact on English for Karen or for Barry because neither showed evidence of knowing rules, such as 'magic e', which are necessary for progress in English. Shannon's performance was qualitatively different from the others. He had developed whole-word recognition skills and was able to translate letters into sounds. His performance was similar to monolingual surface dyslexics, but in addition he made intrusion errors from one language to another. Observation of Karen and Barry over time showed that they did not abandon their logographic strategy while they were acquiring phonological procedures. In keeping with the predictions of the monolingual dual route model, as set out by Stuart and Coltheart (1988), they and Shannon showed dual use of both strategies for both languages, but the relative use of each strategy influenced performance differently in the two languages.

The current findings support the view that bilinguals do not develop special mechanisms for processing print that are different from those employed by monolingual readers and spellers (Caramazza and Brones, 1979; Masterson et al., 1985). What differs is the way in which they apply their skills to processing print in different orthographies or writing systems, and the effect which these processing strategies have on reading different types of orthographies. According to the bilingual dual route model described above, a printed word activates visual and phonological codes, sound-to-letter conversion, and a verification process before a single entry is accessed, which corresponds to the target letter string. In a shallow orthography, only a small subset of graphemes are interchangeable, the orthographic subunits are fewer and less distinctive than in a deeper orthography, and there are more lexical neighbours. Consequently verification is not as effective in Afrikaans as in English, resulting in the difficulties in homophone definition that were observed with normal readers and with Shannon. The verification process is costly in terms of time and accuracy. The monolingual debate about orthographic and phonological codes has centred on the time taken to activate these processes. Latencies are taken as evidence of processing. In this study, latency measures were unavailable but orthographic depth was found to exert an influence on processing strategies as reflected in errors. It is possible that the major factor that determines the origin of the phonetic codes in naming is not the speed of orthographic-code generation, but rather the ease of generating phonemic codes (Frost et al., 1987). It may be that the time course of the phonological code generation is affected mainly by the simplicity of the rules governing the spelling–sound correspondence, and that at the shallow end of the orthographic depth continuum, a sufficient portion of the phonological code can accumulate before the orthographic analysis can help word recognition. Reaction times may add power to the method used in this study for detecting effects which are apparent in latencies but not in error data (Seymour, 1990). Future studies should address this issue.

The cross-linguistic data presented here may be used to argue that the visual word-recognition system is more flexible than the orthographic depth hypothesis would allow. A shallow orthography is accessible using a visual strategy, but phonological recoding appeared to be sustained longer for readers of Afrikaans and existed as a viable strategy even in fairly skilled readers. In this respect, the present findings support others using lexical decision tasks, priming and naming in Persian (Besner and Smith, 1992), Afrikaans (Doctor and Klein, 1992), Spanish (Sebastian-Galles, 1991) and Dutch (Hudson and Bergman, 1985).

The bilingual version Literacy Assessment Battery, drawing on the dual route model of reading, allowed for the differentiation of lexical and sublexical processing strategies in deep and shallow orthographies and the discrimination of some language-specific from universal aspects of reading. Using the same methodology, further longitudinal studies are needed to investigate spelling as well as reading in normal and dyslexic children. Current models need to make explicit the underlying nature of developmental changes and must provide answers to questions about what causes bilingual children to acquire and develop their reading strategies.

References

Besner D, Smith M (1992) Basic processes in reading: is the orthographic depth hypothesis sinking? In R Frost, L Katz (eds) Orthography, Phonology, Morphology and Meaning. London: North Holland Press.

Bradley L, Bryant PE (1983) Categorising sounds and learning to read – a causal connection. Nature 301: 419–421.

Bub D, Cancelliere A, Kertesz A (1985) Whole-word and analytical translation of spelling to sound in a non-semantic reader. In KE Patterson, JC Marshall, M Coltheart (eds) Surface Dyslexia: neuropsychological and cognitive studies of phonological reading. London: Lawrence Erlbaum Associates Ltd.

Caramazza A, Brones I (1979) Lexical access in bilinguals. Bulletin of the Psychonomic Society 13: 212-214.

Carr TH, Pollatsek A (1985) Recognising printed words: a look at current models. In D Besner, TG Waller, GE MacKinnon (eds) Reading research: advances in theory and practice, vol 5, p 1082. Orlando, FL: Academic Press.

Coetzee AE (1985) Fonetiek. Pretoria: Academia.

Coltheart M (1978) Lexical access in simple reading tasks. In G Underwood (ed) Strategies of Information Processing, pp 151-216. London: Academic Press.

Coltheart M, Davelaar E, Jonasson JT, Besner D (1977) Access to the internal lexicon. In S Dornic (ed) Attention and Performance VI. Hillsdale, NJ: Erlbaum.

Coltheart M, Masterson J, Byng S, Prior M, Riddoch J (1983) Surface dyslexia. Quarterly Journal of Experimental Psychology 354: 469-495.

Coltheart M, Curtis B, Atkins P, Haller M (1993) Models of reading aloud: dual route and parallel distributed processing approaches. Psychological Review 100: 589-608.

Content A, Kolinsky R, Morais J, Bertelson P (1986) Phonetic segmentation in pre-readers: effect of corrective information. Journal of Experimental Child Psychology 42: 49-72.

Derouesne J, Beauvois MF (1979) Phonological processes in reading: data from alexia. Journal of Neurology, Neurosurgery and Psychiatry 42: 1125-1132.

Doctor EA, Coltheart M (1980) Children's use of phonological encoding when reading for meaning. Memory and Cognition 80: 195-209.

Doctor EA, Klein D (1992) Phonological processing in bilingual word recognition. In RJ Harris (ed) Cognitive Processing in Bilinguals, pp 237-252. Amsterdam: Elsevier.

Doctor EA, Ahmed R, Ainslee V, Cronje T, Klein D, Knight S (1987) Cognitive aspects of bilingualism. Part 1. External features. South African Journal of Psychology 17(2): 56-62.

Ehri L (1992) Reconceptualising the development of sight word reading and its relationship to recoding. In P Gough, L Ehri, R Treiman (eds) Literacy Acquisition, pp 107-144. Hillsdale, NJ: Lawrence Erlbaum Associates.

Ervin SM, Osgood CE (1954) Second language learning and bilingualism. Journal of Abnormal and Social Psychology 49: 55-72.

Feldman LB, Turvey MT (1983) Word recognition in Serbo-Croatian is phonologically analytic. Journal of Experimental Psychology: Human Perception and Performance 9: 288-298.

Feldman LB, Kostic A, Lukatela G, Turvey MT (1983) An evaluation of the 'basic orthographic syllabic structure' in a phonologically shallow orthography. Psychological Research 45; 55-72.

Frith U (1985) Beneath the surface of developmental dyslexia. In KE Patterson, JC Marshall, M Coltheart (eds) Surface Dyslexia: Cognitive and neuropsychological studies of phonological reading, pp 301-330. London: Lawrence Erlbaum Associates.

Frost R, Katz L, Bentin S (1987) Strategies for visual word recognition and orthographic depth: a multilingual comparison. Journal of Experimental Psychology: Human Perception and Performance 13(1): 104-115.

Funnell E (1983) Phonological processes in reading: new evidence from acquired dyslexia. British Journal of Psychology 74: 159-180.

Glushko RJ (1979) The organisation and activation of orthographic knowledge in reading aloud. Journal of Experimental Psychology: Human Perception and Performance 5: 674-691.

Goswami U, Bryant P (1990) Phonological Skills and Learning to Read. Hove: Lawrence Erlbaum Associates.

Gough PB, Hillinger ML (1980) Learning to read: an unnatural act. Bulletin of the Orton Society. 30: 179-185.

Holmes JM (1973) Dyslexia: A neurolinguistic study of traumatic and developmental disorders of reading. Unpublished Ph.D. thesis, University of Edinburgh.

Hudson PTW, Bergman MW (1985) Lexical knowledge in word recognition: word length in naming and lexical decision tasks. Journal of Memory and Language 24: 46-58.

Humphreys GW, Evett L (1985) Are there independent lexical and non-lexical routes in word processing? An evaluation of the dual-route theory of reading. Behavioral and Brain Sciences 8: 689-739.

Hung DL, Tzeng OJL (1981) Orthographic variations and visual information processing. Psychological Bulletin 90: 377-414.

Klein D (1993) Bilingualism and dyslexia: an investigation. Unpublished Ph.D. thesis, University of the Witwatersrand.

Klein D (1996) The effect of orthographic depth on dyslexia: an analysis with specific reference to the South African linguistic situation. In P Engelbrecht, SM Kriegler, MI Booysen (eds) Perspectives on Learning Difficulties. Pretoria: van Schaik Publishers.

Lamendella JT (1977) General principles of neurofunctional organisation and their manifestation in primary and non-primary language acquisition. Language Learning 27: 155-196.

Luketela G, Popadic D, Ognjenovic P, Turvey MT (1980) Lexical decision in a phonologically shallow orthography. Memory and Cognition 8: 124-132.

Marcel AJ (1980) Surface dyslexia and beginning reading: a revised hypothesis of the pronunciation of print and its impairments. In M Coltheart, KE Patterson, JC Marshall (eds) Deep Dyslexia, pp 227-258. London: Routledge & Kegan Paul.

Marsh G, Friedman M, Welch V, Desberg P (1981) A cognitive-developmental theory of reading acquisition. In GE MacKinnon, TG Waller (eds) Reading Research: advances in theory and practice, vol 3. New York: Academic Press.

Masterson J, Coltheart M, Meara P (1985) Surface dyslexia in a language without irregularly spelled words. In KE Patterson, JC Marshall, M Coltheart (eds) Surface Dyslexia pp 215-223. London: LEA.

Meyer DE, Gutschera KD (1975) Orthographic versus phonemic processing of printed words. Paper presented at the Meeting of the Psychonomic Society, Denver.

Meyer DE, Ruddy MG (1974) Bilingual word recognition: organization and retrieval of alternative lexical codes. Paper presented at the meeting of the Eastern Psychological Association.

Plaut DC, McClelland JL (1993) Generalization with componential attractors: word and nonword reading in an attractor network. In Proceedings of the 15th Annual Conference of the Cognitive Science Society, pp 824-829. Hillsdale, NJ: Erlbaum.

Plaut DC, McClelland JL, Seidenberg MS, Patterson K (1996) Understanding normal and impaired word reading: computational principles in quasi-regular domains. Psychological Review 103: 56-115.

Rozin P, Gleitman LR (1977) The structure and acquisition of reading II: the reading process and the acquisition of the alphabetic principle. In AS Reber, DL Scarborough (eds) Toward a Psychology of Reading. Hillsdale, NJ: Lawrence Erlbaum Associates.

Rubenstein H, Lewis SS, Rubenstein MA (1971) Evidence for phonemic recoding in visual word recognition. Journal of Verbal Learning and Verbal Behaviour 10: 645-657.

Sasanuma S (1980) Acquired dyslexia in Japanese: clinical features and underlying mechanisms. In M Coltheart, KE Patterson, JC Marshall (eds) Deep Dyslexia. London: Routledge & Kegan Paul.

Sebastian-Galles N (1991) Reading by analogy in a shallow orthography. Journal of Experimental Psychology: Human Perception and Performance 17(2): 471-477.

Seidenberg MS, McClelland JL (1989) A distributed, developmental model of word recognition and naming. Psychological Review 4: 523-568.

Seymour PHK (1986) Cognitive Analysis of Dyslexia. London: Routledge & Kegan Paul.

Seymour PHK (1990) Developmental dyslexia. In MW Eysenck (ed) Cognitive Psychology: An International Review, Chichester: Wiley.

Seymour PHK, Elder 1 (1986) Beginning reading without phonology. Cognitive Neuropsychology 3: 1-36.

Seymour PHK, Evans HM (1992) Beginning reading without semantics: a cognitive study of hyperlexia. Cognitive Neuropsychology 9(2): 89-122.

Snowling M, Stackhouse J, Rack J (1986) Phonological dyslexia and dysgraphia: a developmental analysis. Cognitive Neuropsychology 3: 309-339.

Stuart M, Coltheart M (1988) Does reading develop in a sequence of stages? Cognition 30: 139-181.

Temple CM, Marshall JC (1983) A case study of developmental phonological dyslexia. British Journal of Psychology 74: 517-534.

Van Orden GC (1984) A ROWS is a ROSE: spelling, sound and reading. Memory and Cognition 15: 181-198.

Wijk A (1966) Rules of Pronunciation for the English Language, Oxford: Oxford University Press.

CHAPTER 8

The dyslexic reader and the Swedish language

ÅKE OLOFSSON

This chapter begins with a brief description of various reading-related aspects of the Swedish language and the Swedish school system. Swedish orthography is then described in some detail and related to the development of word decoding ability. Finally, results of studies investigating normal reading development, children with reading problems and adults with a history of reading problems are reported.

Swedish is a Germanic language that resembles the English and German languages. Besides the common historical origin, the similarities have been augmented by the more recent uptake of loan words from German and English. The lexical similarity between modern written Swedish, English, French and German can be illustrated by examining their common morphemes. Ellegård (1982) has classified words in these languages according to whether they contain a common morpheme based on the 20,000 words listed in a typical school dictionary. A look at, for example, the Latin morphemes beginning with the letter *a* provides 81 words in French, 80 in English, 50 in Swedish and 48 German words. Thus, the overlap is considerable, although easily obscured by superficial differences in orthography and pronunciation.

The nearest 'linguistic' neighbour to Swedish is the Norwegian language, and both oral and written cross-linguistic communication is comparatively easy. Cross-linguistic communication is a bit more difficult with Danish and for the average Swede it is easier to understand written than spoken Danish. The Dutch language is one step further removed and it is not considered possible for Swedish and Dutch speakers to communicate, although the correspondence is close and the cross-linguistic comprehension impressive (see Strangert and Hedquist, 1989).

Reading instruction has a long and strong tradition in Sweden. Even before the introduction of compulsory schooling in 1842, the literacy rates were remarkably high. Prior to this, regular assessment of oral reading and reading comprehension was conducted by the parish priest and most of the historical documentation reporting this practice is still available (Johansson, 1987). Almost every Swedish child starts grade 1 at the age of 7 and there is a long and solid tradition of no formal reading instruction before school entry. Teaching is regulated by a master plan common to all public schools as well as to the rather small number of private schools. In recent years, many teachers have reported increasing levels of literacy among school entrants, a trend that is generally explained as a result of informal literacy exposure in kindergarten and at home (Lundberg, 1991). This development is probably furthered by a contemporary re-organization, which incorporated most of the kindergartens into the school system. It has also been suggested that the extensive Scandinavian research on phonological awareness has contributed to greater sensitivity to the needs of pre-schoolers among parents and educators (Olofsson and Lundberg, 1985; Lundberg et al., 1988; Olofsson and Niedersøe, 1999).

Methods of initial reading instruction are relatively uniform, including both writing and listening, and most teachers include phonics basics (e.g. sound blending, phonemic segmentation and explicit instruction in letter–sound correspondences) as well as meaning-oriented elements (emphasizing the understanding of connected text) in their teaching.

Description of Swedish vowels and consonants

The syllable structure of Swedish is typical of Germanic languages comprising many consonant combinations and closed syllables. A one-syllable root morpheme can have a maximum of three consonants (C) preceding the vowel (V) and three following it. Thus, the largest syllable has a CCCVCCC structure.[1]

Distribution of consonants

The Swedish consonants are presented in Table 8.1. The fricative system is complicated, as the phonetic similarity between the alveolar, palatal and velar fricatives is considerable. The situation is further complicated by the fact that the allophonic variation within the /ʃ/ and /ç/ is very broad. Elert (1995) reported seven or eight allophones of [ʃ]. (Swedish fricatives are further discussed in Sigurd, 1970.)

---

[1] In fact, there are a few rare words ending with more than three consonants, see Elert (1995).

Table 8.1 The phonemic inventory of Swedish: consonants

Manner of articulation	Place of articulation								
	bilabial	labio-dental	dental	dental-alveolar	alveolar	palatal	velar	glottal	labio-velar
plosive voiced	b			d			g		
voiceless	p			t			k		
fricative nonsib.vd.		v							
voiceless		f							
sibilant vl..					s [ʂ] ʃ	ç			
approx. central						j	[ɧ]	h	
lateral				l r					
nasal	m			n			ŋ		

Note: The fricatives [ʂ] and [ɧ] are two out of several allophones of the very complex phoneme /ʃ/ and attached here just to highlight the variability of this phoneme. The distinction sibilant/nonsibilant is typically not used in descriptions of the Swedish phonemes but is added here in order to facilitate comparisons with English. Also note that there is only one voiced fricative /v/ when /j/ is classified as approximant. (/j/ and /v/ may alternatively be treated as fricatives or approximants).

The Swedish system for initial consonants is typical of Germanic languages, allowing six different three-phoneme clusters, all starting with /s/ followed by the plosives /p/, /t/ or /k/. Like other Germanic languages, Swedish has numerous final consonant clusters. Many of these word endings are spelled in their fully articulated form, e.g. the word *hemskt* (frightening), but the reduced form /hɛmst/ is used in the spoken language.

As the Swedish language has many eligible consonant clusters it could be predicted that learning to read and spell might demand relatively high levels of phonemic awareness.

Distribution of vowels

The Swedish vowels are presented in Table 8.2. Each one of the nine vowels can occur in a stressed syllable and be represented by its long or short allophone. Thus, for practically all the regional dialects there are 18 contrastive vowels in stressed syllables. In unstressed syllables there are seven contrastive vowels in positions before the stressed syllable. In the subsequent positions following the stressed syllable, the number of contrastive vowels are seven, five and two. (The last one is typically a suffix.) The quantitative (length) distinction between the long and short versions of the Swedish vowels is also accompanied by qualitative differences, and the short allophones in general tend to be less phonetically distinct than the long ones. In some regional dialects there is no phonetic difference between the short allophones of /e/ and /ɛ/, which certainly can cause problems for the novice speller. True diphthongs are very rare in Swedish (except for some regional dialects), but vowel pairs occur when a suffix is added to a root morpheme with a final vowel, in some compound words and in a few loan words.

Consonant–vowel combinations

Swedish tends to avoid combinations of initial /sk/, /g/ and /k/ before front (palatal) vowels. (There are exceptions; mostly low-frequency words.) However, in Swedish spelling there are words with initial *sk-*, *g-* and *k-* followed by front vowels and the regular pronunciation is then respectively [ʃ], [j] and [ç].

Prosody

Stress, pitch and quantity are important in Swedish, but only the last is repre- sented in the orthography. Word stress is unfixed and the placement of stress is distinctive at the word level. There are two main types of word accent: words with one stressed syllable (acute accent) and words that have an

Table 8.2 The phonemic inventory of Swedish: vowels, long allophones

	Front	Back
High	i y	u
	ɪ	
	e	
Mid	ø	o
	ɛ	
Low	ɑ	

additional stress on the second syllable (grave accent). The grave accent is highly correlated with the pitch of the voice. Words with grave accent have two peaks on their pitch curve, a phenomenon which foreigners might perceive as a kind of 'singing' in spoken Swedish. The word accent is distinctive in Swedish because there are approximately 100 word pairs that have the same phoneme sequence and are differentiated solely by the position of the stress, e.g. the Swedish word *anden* pronounced with the first syllable stressed means 'duck', whereas *anden* with bisyllabic stress means 'spirit' or 'ghost'. For many of these word pairs the spelling is identical, but for some there is also an orthographic distinction.

Quantity (length) is also distinctive for stressed syllables. For Swedish vowels the duration of the short allophones is approximately 65% of the long ones, although the difference in duration varies between vowels (from 61% to 80%) (Elert, 1995). The difference in quantity is also accompanied by a difference in quality, e.g. *dit* (there, away there) and *ditt* (your, yours). In the first word, the vowel is long and sounds like the vowel in the English word 'see'. In the second word, the vowel is short, like in the English word 'hit'. Consonants also differ in quantity. Consonant length and vowel length in stressed syllables are complementary. A stressed short vowel is followed by a long consonant and a long vowel is followed by a short consonant (Garlén, 1988). Consonant length is often (but not always) reflected in the orthography as, for example, when the consonant is doubled after a short vowel.

Phoneme–grapheme relationships

In general, Swedish orthography maps on to phonemes very consistently. All but two vowels are represented by a single letter (with a few exceptions). /ɛ/ is spelled with *ä* or *e* and /o/ is spelled with *å* or *o*. For the learner the situation is, however, complicated by the fact that vowel length is often, but not always, marked by doubling the next consonant. Understanding when it is necessary to double a consonant or not, is a serious problem for young Swedish spellers.

Therefore all consonants except /h/ and /ŋ/ have at least two different orthographic counterparts representing quantity. For 12 of the consonants the alternatives are restricted to doubling or not (but 'double' /k/ is spelled *ck* and /j/ is never doubled). The orthographic alternatives for the remaining four (complicated) phonemes are presented in Table 8.3. Thus, the only prosodic feature systematically represented in print is vowel length. As vowel and consonant length are to a large extent complementary within a syllable, it is true that a double consonant is phonetically longer than a single one. However, in the educational context, the principle of consonant doubling is always formulated explicitly as reflecting vowel length. Learners are taught to double the consonant following a short vowel in a stressed syllable that precedes another vowel, a morpheme boundary or any of the 'sounds' /l/, /n/, /r/. In addition, they are instructed never to double *j* and very seldom *v* or *m*. There are however, also exceptions for prefixes, some high-frequency words (including many function words) and loan words.

Grapheme–phoneme relationships

To most foreigners there are some striking features of Swedish print, primarily the three 'non-ASCII' characters *å*, *ä* and *ö* (the three final letters in the Swedish alphabet). For the Swedish reader these letters are distinct, individual letters and they are not conceptualized as varieties of the letters *a* and *o* with diacritical markers. (For the very young learner, during the initial

Table 8.3 Phoneme–grapheme relationships for four Swedish consonant phonemes. (For the complete set of phonemes and graphemes, see Garlén, 1988)

Phoneme	Graphemes								
/s/	s	ss	c	z					
/ç/	tj	kj	ki	k	ch				
/ʃ/ [1]	sj	sk	skj	stj	sch	sh	ch	g	ge	ti
/j/	j	g	gj	hj	lj	dj			

Note 1. The most frequent graphemes are *sj* and *sk*. Garlén (1988) reports 22 different graphemes representing /ʃ/. Ekener (1982) uses a maximum of seven graphemes in her curriculum for poor spellers.

stage of letter-name learning, there is some confusion between these letters. But, in that early developmental phase many other visually similar letters also tend to be confused.) The non-trivial grapheme–phoneme relationships are presented in Table 8.4. It can be seen that most of the complex graphemes represent the phonemes [ʃ], [j] and [ç]. However, to a large extent these complex relationships are regular in the sense that the spelling is dependent on the local context.

Table 8.4 Phoneme–grapheme relationships in Swedish spelling

Phonemes	Graphemes																				
	c	cc	ch	dj	e	g	ge	gi	gj	hj	j	k	kj	l	lj	ng	o	ti	tj	y	z
ɑ					a																	
e					e																	
g						g																
j				j				j	j	j	j				j							
k		k										k										
l														l								
ŋ							ng									ng						
u																	o					
s	s																					s
ʃ			sj					sj	sj	sj	sj									sj		
ç			tj									tj	tj							tj		
y																					y	
o																	å					
ɛ				ä																		
ø																						ö
	ks	ks																				
	ts																					ts
	silent													*								

*In rl combinations l is usually silent).
Letters in the cells are the most frequently used graphemes for the actual phoneme. Single letter graphemes representing a single phoneme are (for simplicity reasons) not included in the table. These graphemes are: *a b d f h i m n p q r s t u v x å ä ö*. The less frequent graphemes *shi, si, sti, ssj, stg* (for the /ʃ/ phoneme) as well as *xi, xj* (for /kʃ/) and *ki* /ç/ are also excluded.

Swedish ABC books and readers

Methods of initial reading instruction have been quite uniform for many years and regulated by a national master plan. During the last century ABC books and readers have included a systematic introduction of letters combined with a phonics-based system for selecting the first words and sentences. Table 8.5 presents an outline of the order of introduction of the letters in three widely used readers over the last 60 years. Table 8.5 also includes letter groups based on their grapheme–phoneme relationship. There are great similarities between the letter order in the different readers and also, but to a lesser extent, between the readers and the grapheme–phoneme-based ordering. The readers do not include comprehensive explanations of the rationale behind the chosen pedagogical approach, so we do not know exactly on what criteria the authors have based the introduction of letter order. The grapheme–phoneme relationship seems to be one important aspect, but it is apparent that other factors are considered as well. One such factor is the ability to construct words and sentences based on the subset of letters learned so far. This may explain the early introduction of the letters *e* and *o*, which greatly enhance productivity with respect to Swedish CVC words. For example, *mor* in Swedish means 'mother'. Several high-frequency function words are easily constructed using this subset, for example *en* (the), *är* (is) and *i* (in). From Table 8.5 we can also conclude that the national Swedish letters, *å*, *ä* and *ö*, seem to be avoided initially. The reason for this is not clear, since all these letters occur in high-frequency words and all are productive in CVC settings. One plausible reason is that the letters may be spread out to avoid confusion based on the visual similarity between the letters with and without the 'marks above'. Table 8.5 also shows that in recent years there has been a tendency to move away from the traditional grapheme–phoneme relationship-based order of instruction. A closer look at Emilson-Benoit et al. (1985) reveals an emphasis on the construction of plausible and interesting phrases and more age-appropriate vocabulary compared to the slightly higher incidence of 'odd' sentence constructions in the earlier readers.

Reading acquisition

The International Association for the Evaluation of Educational Achievement (IEA) regularly conducts comparative evaluations of the general reading level in different countries (Elley, 1994). Swedish schoolchildren generally attain top scores (Lundberg and Linnakylä, 1992). This result is usually explained by educational factors, such as the structured teaching methods and a long tradition of teaching, in combination with socioeconomic and cultural factors, and is thus not primarily the consequence of the Swedish orthography (Lundberg, 1998).

Table 8.5 Order in which letters are introduced in three Swedish children's ABC-books and readers

Author (1)	Title	Year of publication	Letters in order of introduction			
Beskow and Siegwald	Vill du läsa	1935–62	m o r f a s ä i l	b n h e t å k v	d u p g j y ö x	c ck z qs
Borrman et al.	Nu ska vi läsa	1948–97	o s m r a f e k	n t i ä l	å b ö h u g j y	d v p c x zqw
Emilson-Benoit et al.	Läs med oss: Min egen bok	1985–	o l e s a r n i	v m t ä p u h k	j å y f b ö g	c d x z w q

Type of grapheme–phoneme relation	Letters		
Letters representing only one phoneme and never occurring in complex graphemes	a b f m p q r å ä ö		
Letters representing only one phoneme but may also occur in complex graphemes		d h i l n s t u v y	
Letters representing one of two phonemes		e o	
Letters representing more than one phoneme and often occurring in complex graphemes			c g j k
Low frequency letters representing one or two phonemes			w x z

Reading disabilities

From our description of spoken and written Swedish, a few predictions about reading acquisition can be made. As Swedish orthography has almost one-to-one mapping between letters and speech sounds (phonemes), learners who are sensitive to the phonological structure of the words have a distinct advantage. On the other hand, learners who do not have a clear representation of the phonological structure of words will have problems. Such learners may master the exact orthography of high-frequency words but will find it difficult to master the general principles of phoneme–grapheme relationships that will enable them to decode unfamiliar words. Furthermore, the prosodic features, vowel length and syllable stress, are reflected in the orthography. Native speakers do not generally have problems with these aspects of spoken language, but when a certain degree of explicit knowledge is needed, some pupils tend to find it hard deciding about vowel length. That is, they can hear the difference between the words, e.g. *dit* and *ditt*, but are unable to decide which word contains a short vowel and which a long vowel. Consequently children with impoverished phonological representations have problems acquiring the implicit 'rules' for consonant doubling.

Compound words can also pose major difficulties for learners. In Swedish, it is possible to construct compound words of theoretically unlimited length (e.g. the Swedish word for 'file conversion program' is *filkonverteringsprogrammet*). In compound words, the word stress for the component words is altered, as is in turn the pronunciation, but the spelling of the word remains unchanged. Readers who cannot rapidly access the component parts of a written string may have difficulty accessing compound words. In addition, spellers who are unaware of the structure of a compound word will find it difficult to derive its spelling, since the normal cues for syllable length in single words are often distorted by the altered stress pattern in the compound word. Consequently a reader may drop parts of long words and a writer may be uncertain about the need to double consonants.

Both good and poor readers have problems in the acquisition of the most complex phoneme–grapheme relationships, e.g. /ʃ/, /j/ and /ç/. The dyslexic reader may learn the exact orthography of high-frequency words but may fail to grasp the alphabetical principle and this will come to light especially when they spell and read low-frequency words.

Acquisition of word recognition and decoding

The past two decades of international reading research have resulted in a widespread acceptance of models of reading where word decoding and reading comprehension are seen as separate but related aspects of skilled reading (Hoover and Gough, 1990). It is also established that dyslexia is primarily a language-based problem affecting mainly word decoding ability (Vellutino, 1979; Share and Stanovich, 1995), although the definition problem is recognized (Tønnessen, 1997). Difficulties in word decoding may cause delayed or distorted reading development in a broader sense and may also affect reading comprehension to a more or less severe degree. Because of the primary role of word decoding in dyslexia and in reading acquisition, this chapter focuses on this component. Dyslexia from an international and Scandinavian perspective is covered in Høien and Lundberg (2000).

Research on word recognition has often used two different types of word decoding tasks to study the word recognition process. Originally these procedures were developed in the framework of dual route models, assuming that one route to lexical access is via grapheme–phoneme conversion (also referred to as the 'indirect' or 'phonological' route), and the other is via visual representations of familiar words or word-parts (also referred to as the direct or visual route). Within the more recent framework of connectionist models (see Plaut et al., 1996) and stage models of reading development (Høien and Lundberg, 1988), the second route is reconceptualized as an orthographic route building on sublexical information (that is, word parts like complex graphemes, spelling patterns and other less-specified regularities within words). (Discussion of word-recognition models is beyond the scope of this chapter and the interested reader is referred to Besner and Humphreys, 1991.)

In this chapter, word recognition will be considered in terms of phonological and orthographic skills, as Swedish tests of orthographic and phonological word processing have recently been developed (Olofsson, 1998). The developmentof word-recognition skills will be reported for three samples of Swedish readers. First, the normal development of skilled word recognition will be describedusing cross-sectional data. In the second study, adults with a documented history of reading problems are compared to age controls, and finally somecase studies of 14- to 15-year-old children with reading problems are reported.

Study 1

Swedish children start school at the age of 7 and by the end of first grade most children can read easy texts independently. By the end of grade 2 most children have acquired fast and accurate 'automatic' word-decoding skills. To investigate the normal development of word-decoding skills, children in randomly selected classrooms were given tests of phonological and orthographic coding.

Method

Participants

A total of 266 school children were randomly selected from four public schools in Umeå, Sweden, representing socioeconomic middle-class populations. A further 29 psychology students (mean age 24 years) from Umeå University volunteered to participate. The school children were 8–15 years old (in grades 1 to 9) with 59 children in grade 9 and 16, 34, 37, 39, 59 and 22 in grades 1 to 6 respectively. All children were native Swedish speakers and there were approximately equal numbers of boys and girls.

Materials and procedure

The testing, which took place in April and May, was undertaken by trained research assistants and administered as group tests in the children's regular classrooms.

Phonological coding in word recognition

This task was designed as a Swedish paper-and-pencil adaptation of the computerized phonological coding task used by Olson et al. (1994). The task was to select and underline one of two written pseudowords (nonwords) that sounded like a real word, as quickly as possible. For example, consider the two Swedish pseudowords *sox* and *seks*. The second one, *seks*, is pronounced exactly as the Swedish word *sex* (six) and is a pseudohomophone. Another example is *belk* and *bärj*, where the second pseudoword sounds exactly like the Swedish word *berg* (mountain). This task can only be solved using a basic grapheme–phoneme recoding strategy. The examples given illustrate that word-specific knowledge providing visual or orthographic information would not be helpful. A total of 80 pairs of nonword alternatives were presented on four pages with 20 pairs per page. The task was scored as the number of correctly chosen pseudohomophones selected in two minutes. The number of errors was very low. The maximum score was 80.

Orthographic coding in word recognition

This task was also a Swedish adaptation of the computerized orthographic coding task used by Olson et al. (1994). The participant had to identify and underline the word in word–pseudohomophone pairs presented in six lists of 20 pairs. As the phonological codes for the pairs are identical, both the word and its pseudohomophone are pronounced the same in Swedish. Examples of stimuli are *pizza/pitsa*, where the first word is correctly spelled in Swedish, or *tekst/text*, where the second word is correct (translation not needed). To make a correct response on this task the reader must use word-specific orthographic knowledge to select the correct spelling of the word. Both alternatives have the same pronunciation in Swedish, so pure phonological recoding would not differentiate the alternatives. The final score was computed as the number of words selected correctly in two minutes. Marginally more errors were produced in the orthographic coding task than in the phonological coding task although most normal readers make only one or two errors (Olofsson, 1998). The maximum score was 120.

Results

The typical normal development of word-decoding speed is illustrated in Figure 8.1. It can be seen that the beginning readers initially process both phonological and orthographic information at the same speed. Thereafter for about two years both skills develop almost in parallel, but after grade 4 the developmental curves show marked differences. Whereas phonological word-decoding speed seems to reach its asymptotic level by end of primary school (at age 12–14), orthographic coding speed continues to develop until adult-

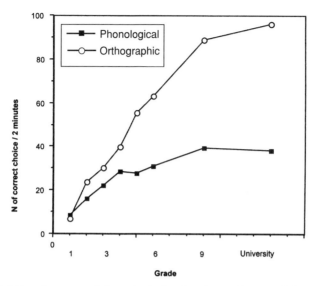

Figure 8.1 Development of phonological and orthographic word decoding skill in eight normal cohorts of Swedish readers.

hood. To illustrate the magnitude of the development after grade 4 (age 11), the change in the mean scores in Figure 8.1 can be expressed in terms of the standard deviation of each variable in grade 4. For the phonological word-decoding task, the difference in mean scores between grades 4 and 9 is equivalent to one standard deviation in grade 4. For the orthographic coding score the corresponding increase equals three standard deviations.

These findings suggest that Swedish children first become proficient at phonological word decoding in middle childhood, but then continue to extend their orthographic coding skills until adulthood. Similar results have also been found when comparing Swedish children at age 8 and 10 (Samuelsson et al., 1996).

Study 2

Olofsson (1999) investigated various aspects of phonological processing abilities and word decoding in a sample of adults with a history of reading problems. Twenty years ago the sample was identified on the basis of their reading problems in grade 2 (age 8). The selection criteria were based on the discrepancy between a non-verbal problem-solving task (Raven, 1960) and poor word recognition and/or spelling on two consecutive test occasions within a six-month interval (see Lundberg, 1985, for details). A control group of the same age but with normal reading and spelling performance was selected from the same classrooms. Now, at the age of 27, they were revisited and presented with a follow-up questionnaire. Some of them also agreed to take part in follow-up testing. Only the test data on word decoding and spelling will be reported in this chapter. (For the other variables, including digit naming, vocabulary, reading comprehension and meta-linguistic tasks, the reader is referred to Olofsson, 1999.)

Method

Participants

In the original study, the groups consisted of 46 and 44 children each. It was not possible to trace the whereabouts of about one quarter of the children in the original sample. About half the children were located and a questionnaire requesting information about their school history, educational background, social status, job, reading habits and future plans was sent to them. Twenty five (10 dyslexic and 15 control participants) volunteered to come to the university for a testing session. Thirty-seven participants filled in the questionnaire (15 dyslexic and 22 controls). All the participants except two in each group were boys. The missing cases did not differ from the participating ones on any of the primary school measures.

Materials and procedure

Testing was undertaken by a trained psychologist and took place at the university, except for one participant who was seen at his place of work.

Phonological coding in word recognition

This test was a modified version of the test used in Study 1. The task was to select and underline one of three or four pseudowords that sounded like a real word (i.e. a pseudohomophone) as quickly as possible. For example, among the three Swedish pseudowords, *belk*, *bärj*, *pulg*, the second one sounds similar to the Swedish word *berg* (mountain).

Orthographic coding in word recognition

The same task was used as in Study 1.

A spelling test was also constructed to provide a quick and inoffensive measure of spelling by focusing on the participants' knowledge of how to spell the Swedish /j/ sound. As already mentioned, the /j/ sound is one of the complexities in Swedish spelling. Eight low-frequency one- and two-syllable words with regular spelling of the /j/ sound were used. Swedish spelling generally represents /j/ by the letters *j* or *g* (see Table 8.4). For non-regular spellings the /j/ phoneme can be represented also by the letters *hj*, *dj* and *lj*. In Swedish, a strict rule-based spelling of the /j/ sound would give approximately 20% spelling errors. The following words were used: *sorg* (grief), *bälg* (bellows), (one-syllable words, final position *j* following a consonant); *gärs* (ruff (fish)), *gös* (pike, perch), *gyro* (gyro) (initial position *j* followed by a front vowel); *juvel* (jewel), *pjäs* (theatre, play), *miljö* (milieu) (otherwise spelled with *j*). The number of spelling errors was scored and the maximum score obtained was 6.

Results

The comparison of group means in Table 8.6 shows that the adults with a history of dyslexia scored significantly lower on both the phonological and the orthographic word-decoding tests. (The test scores are not directly comparable to the results in Figure 8.1, due to the use of slightly different versions of the tests and a different scoring procedure.) The dyslexics' spelling scores are also significantly lower. These results indicate that the young adults with a history of reading problems have not developed systematic understanding of the rules underlying the spelling of the Swedish /j/ sound. It is likely that this spelling problem would not have been revealed if we had used a spelling test consisting solely of high-frequency words.

The results of the questionnaire, which was answered by 15 adult dyslexics and 22 normal readers, clearly showed that the dyslexics had chosen a different path through the educational system, apparently avoiding reading and language studies, and eventually belonged to a group having no or only occasional access to university studies. There were 10 university students in the control group but none in the dyslexic group. A few of the dyslexics also stated that regardless of their interests, they selected studies that required minimal reading and spelling ability. However, awareness of the real basis for their decision did not arise until several years later. The dyslexics rated their spelling skill lower than controls and also reported having more problems with second language learning (English) than the controls. The frequency of using a dictionary or word book differed greatly between the groups. The adult dyslexics had a particular dislike for tasks requiring them to find anything according to alphabetical order.

Table 8.6 Mean scores, standard deviations (s.d.) and t-value for adults with and without a history of reading problems

Variable	Dyslexic[a] Mean (s.d.)	Normal[b] Mean (s.d.)	t
Phonological coding	11.0 (10.0)	23.1 (10.5)	2.88**
Orthographic coding	68.6 (20.5)	87.6 (19.6)	2.33*
Spelling (errors)	2 (1.33)	.73 (.88)	2.87*

Note: For all t-tests the df is 23. [a]N = 10. [b]N = 15. *p < 0.05; **p > 0.01.

Study 3

Olsson (1995) reported a study of children who were sent to a child guidance clinic or to the school psychologist. In addition to the standard battery of psychological tests used at the clinic, Olsson (1995) also used the two word decoding tests described above.

Method

Participants

The three oldest participants in Olsson's (1995) sample are reported here. The participants came from a small city (20,000 inhabitants) in the north of Sweden and included two 16-year-old boys in grade 9 and one 15-year-old boy in grade 8. The first (Case 1) was sent to the clinic for a dyslexia diagnosis, the second (Case 2) was sent to the clinic for making (and detonating) a bomb and the third (Case 3) for alcohol abuse. All three boys scored within the normal range on WISC (Wechsler Intelligence Scale for Children, Swedish translation 1977).

Materials and procedure

The testing was undertaken by a trained psychologist and took place at the child psychiatric clinic.

Phonological coding in word recognition

The same task as in Study 1 was used.

Orthographic coding in word recognition

The same task as in Study 1 and 2 was used.

Results and discussion

On the phonological coding test, their results were 20, 20 and 25 respectively. On the orthographic coding test, the scores were respectively, 20, 33 and 43. The word-decoding scores can be directly compared to Figure 8.1, yielding grade equivalents to grade 2 and 3 for the older boys and grades 3 to 5 for the grade 8 boy. Expressed as standard scores the phonological coding scores are -1.8, -1.8 and -1.4, and the scores on the orthographic coding test equals -3.4, -2.7 and -2.1 (Olofsson, 1998). It should be noted that the grade 8 boy also made an unusually large number of errors that are not accounted for in the reported scores. When using this kind of measure, it is not unusual to find that readers tend to increase their orthographic decoding speed at the expense of their error rate. The present three cases could be used to illustrate such a finding often reported by clinicians. That is, children with less severe phonological problems may compensate for their reading problem by increasing their orthographic coding speed at the expense of accuracy. Children with more profound phonological problems have greater problems in developing their orthographic coding speed. A difference between the first and the third case that might partly explain their differences in orthographic coding is that Case 1's reading problems were identified at primary school, whereas Cases 2 and 3 were unaware of any reading problems. Case 1 had a history of reading avoidance and was given extra support in several school subjects. Cases 2 and 3 reported that they did not do well in their studies, although they tried. Thus, an indication of some emerging orthographic coding skill in Case 3 may result from a limited amount of print exposure, unlike Case 1, whose long-term avoidance of reading resulted in inadequate levels of print exposure (cf Stanovich and West, 1989). For Cases 2 and 3, it remains to be seen if their new diagnosis and awareness will lead to better adjustment, which in turn could lead to more reading and to a subsequent increase of orthographic coding speed. Clearly, the inclusion of phonological and orthographic coding tests in the assessment of dyslexics adds valuable information to the diagnosis process.

General discussion

The results presented above lend support to the phonological processing deficit view of dyslexia, as well as to theories stating that dyslexia is mainly a word-decoding problem. The normal path of reading acquisition in Swedish commences with an initial phonological word-decoding stage. However, very soon, perhaps during the first year of instruction, orthographically based coding processes become increasingly more important for the development of word-recognition speed. Phonological processing ability is essential for skilled reading, but orthographic processing strategies predominate and phonological strategies are generally limited to instances when the skilled reader encounters an unfamiliar word. In short, a skilled reader has access to both phonological and lexical reading strategies and has the ability to adapt word recognition according to the demands of each specific reading task. In contrast, the Swedish dyslexic reader has impaired phonological word decoding, often accompanied by other phonological problems in, for example, rapid naming and phonemic awareness, as well as less-developed orthographic knowledge. Compensated dyslexics, persons with a history of reading problems who are able to perform quite well on many reading tasks, frequently still have specific problems when the reading task is demanding. They continue having deficits both in phonological processing and in orthographic knowledge (Felton et al., 1990; Bruck, 1992; Elbro et al., 1994; Olofsson, 1999; Gustafsson, 2000).

Explicit tests of the component processes used for word recognition seem to be an effective tool in the diagnosis of dyslexia. Swedish is a typical Germanic language and Swedish orthography has rule-based complexities at both the grapheme–phoneme and phoneme–grapheme levels. Thus, the present findings are relevant to other languages with similar types of orthographies. The early manifestation of developmental dyslexia in Swedish shows similarities to the pattern for German readers, that is, the children are accurate but slower readers (Wimmer, 1996). In less consistent orthographies like English, the use of simple grapheme–phoneme correspondences is less effective and this may encourage the child to rely on more visual or 'direct' coding strategies (Wimmer and Goswami, 1994). Wimmer and Goswami (1994) predicted that these initial decoding differences in reading strategy will diminish as the reader develops automatic and rapid decoding skill. However, the Swedish results show that when reading speed is taken into account, deficits in phonological processing ability continue to be a distinctive feature of developmental dyslexia, even for adult readers. But, as word recognition becomes more 'direct' and orthographically based, and reading speed increases, dyslexic readers still have residual orthographic impairments and fail to appreciate the complex regularities inherent in Swedish orthography.

Acknowledgements

The study was supported by grant F0395/96 from the Swedish Council for Research in the Humanities and Social Sciences (HSFR) and grant 12481/541 from the Joint Committee of the Nordic Social Science Research Councils (NOS-S). Correspondence concerning this chapter should be addressed to Åke Olofsson, Center for Reading Research, Postboks 2504 Ullandhaug, N-4091 Stavanger, Norway (ake.olofsson@slf.his.no).

References

Beskow E, Siegwald H (1935). Vill du läsa? Första skolåret (Do you want to read? The first year of schooling). Stockholm: Bonniers.

Besner D, Humphreys GW (eds) (1991) Basic processes in reading: visual word recognition. Hillsdale, NJ: Lawrence Erlbaum.

Borrman S, Salminen E, Wigforss F (1948) Nu ska vi läsa: första boken (Now we are going to read: the first book). Stockholm: Almqvist & Wiksell.

Bruck M (1992) Persistence of dyslexics' phonological awareness deficits. Developmental Psychology 28: 874–886.

Ekener H (1982) Rättskrivning (Orthography). Stockholm: Esselte.

Elbro C, Nielsen I, Petersen DK (1994) Dyslexia in adults: evidence for deficits in non-word reading and in the phonological representation of lexical items. Annals of Dyslexia 44: 205–226.

Elert C-C (1995) Allmän och svensk fonetik (General and Swedish phonetics, 7th edn). Stockholm: Norstedts.

Ellegård A (1982) Internationellt morfemlexikon (International morpheme dictionary). Stockholm: Liber.

Elley WB (ed) (1994) The IEA study of reading literacy: Achievement and instruction in thirty-two school systems. Oxford: Pergamon.

Emilson-Benoit M, Annell B, Lundberg I (1985) Läs med oss: min egen bok (Read with us: my own book). Stockholm: Natur och Kultur.

Felton RH, Naylor CE, Wood FB (1990) Neuropsychological profile of adult dyslexics. Brain and Language 39: 485–497.

Garlén C (1988) Svenskans fonologi (Swedish phonology). Lund: Studentlitteratur.

Gustafson S (2000) Varieties of reading disability. Phonological and orthographic word decoding deficits and implications for interventions. Doctoral dissertation, Linköpings Universitet, Sweden. Studies from the Swedish Institute for Disability Research, No. 1.

Hoover W, Gough P (1990) The simple view of reading. Reading and Writing: An Interdisciplinary Journal 2: 127–160.

Høien T, Lundberg I (1988) Stages of word recognition in early reading development. Scandinavian Journal of Educational Research 32: 163–182.

Høien T, Lundberg I (2000) Dyslexia: from theory to intervention. Dordrecht: Kluwer.

Johansson E (1987) Literacy campaigns in Sweden. In Arnove RJ, Graff H (eds) National literacy campaigns. Historical and comparative perspectives, pp 65–98. New York: Plenum.

Lundberg I (1985) Longitudinal studies of reading and reading difficulties in Sweden. In MacKinnon GE, Waller TG (eds) Reading research: advances in theory and practice, pp 65–105. New York: Academic Press.

Lundberg I (1991) A decade of reading research in Sweden. Reports from Swedish National Commission for Unesco, No. 1/1991. Stockholm.

Lundberg I (1998) Does language make any difference in reading acquisition? Cross-cultural and crosslinguistic study of reading achievement. In Olofsson Å, Strömquist S (eds) COST A8 – Cross-linguistic studies of dyslexia and early language development, pp 80–92. Luxembourg: Office for Official Publications of the European Communities.

Lundberg I, Linnakylä P (1992) The teaching of reading around the world. The Hague: IEA.

Lundberg I, Frost J, Petersen O-P (1988) Effects of an extensive program for stimulating phonological awareness in preschool children. Reading Research Quarterly 23: 263–284.

Olofsson Å (1998) Ordavkodning: mätning av fonologisk och ortografisk ordavkodningsförmåga (Word decoding: measurement of phonological and orthographic word decoding ability). Östersund, Sweden: Läspedagogiskt Centrum.

Olofsson Å (1999) Early reading problems: a follow up 20 years later. In Lundberg I, Tønnesen FE, Austad (eds), Dyslexia. Advances in theory and practice, pp 197–206. Dordrecht: Kluwer

Olofsson Å, Lundberg I (1985) Evaluation of long term effects of phonemic awareness training in kindergarten: illustrations of some methodological problems in evaluation research. Scandinavian Journal of Psychology 26: 21–34.

Olofsson Å, Niedersøe J (1999) Early language development and kindergarten phonological awareness as predictors of reading problems: from 3 to 11 years of age. Journal of Learning Disabilities 32: 464–472.

Olson RK, Forsberg H, Wise B, Rack J (1994) Measurement of word recognition, ortho-graphic and phonological skills. In Lyon GR (ed) Frames of reference for the assessment of learning disabilities: new views on measurement issues, pp 243–277. Baltimore, MD: Paul H Brookes.

Olsson A (1995) Dyslexi hos barn och ungdomar med beteendeproblem (Dyslexia among children and adolescents with behaviour problems). Unpublished thesis, Umeå University, Sweden.

Plaut DC, McClelland JL, Seidenberg MS, Patterson K (1996) Understanding normal and impaired word reading: computational principles in quasi-regular domains. Psychological Review 103: 56–115.

Raven JC (1960) Guide to the standard progressive matrices. Sets A, B, C, D, and E. London: Lewis.

Samuelsson S, Gustafson S, Rönnberg J (1996) The development of word-decoding skills in young readers. Scandinavian Journal of Educational Research 40: 325–332.

Share D, Stanovich KE (1995) Cognitive processes in early reading development: accommodating individual differences into a model of acquisition. Issues in Education 1: 1–57.

Sigurd B (1970) The status of /ng/ /tje/ and /sje/ in Swedish. In Benediktsson H (ed) The Nordic languages and modern linguistics. Reykjavik: Visindafélag íslendinga.

Stanovich KE, West RF (1989) Exposure to print and orthographic processing. Reading Research Quarterly 24: 402–433.

Strangert E, Hedquist R (1989) Hur svenskar uppfattar och förstår nederländska ord (How Swedes perceive and comprehend Dutch words). Scandinavinan-Dutch language comprehension, Report 4. Department of Linguistics and Nordic Languages, Umeå University.

Tønnessen FE (1997) How can we best define 'dyslexia'? Dyslexia 3: 78–92

Vellutino FR (1979) Dyslexia: theory and research. Cambridge, MA: MIT Press.

Wimmer H (1996) The early manifestation of developmental dyslexia: evidence from German children. Reading and Writing: An Interdisciplinary Journal 8: 171–188.

Wimmer H, Goswami U (1994) The influence of orthographic consistency on reading development: word recognition in English and German children. Cognition 51: 91–103.

CHAPTER 9

Similarities and differences between English- and French-speaking poor spellers

MARKÉTA CARAVOLAS, MAGGIE BRUCK AND FRED GENESEE

Although by definition poor readers and children with developmental dyslexia have extreme difficulties in the acquisition of reading skills, these children are also characterized by their extremely poor spelling skills at all ages. The spelling deficits of dyslexics are well documented in English, where, irrespective of word recognition skills – which may or may not be seriously impaired – spelling problems are inevitable (Frith, 1980; Juel et al., 1986; Bruck and Waters, 1988). Moreover, the spelling deficits observed in dyslexic children tend to persist over time (Bruck, 1990; Snowling et al., 1996). The finding that dyslexics are also poor spellers is not specific to English children; it has also been found for poor readers learning other alphabetic languages. Recent studies by Wimmer and his colleagues have shown that German-speaking dyslexics, who read words quite accurately although very slowly when compared to controls, also fail to acquire spelling skills at the rate of their normally developing peers (Wimmer, 1996; Landerl et al., 1997; Wimmer and Landerl, 1997). Similarly, French-speaking dyslexic children show impaired spelling skills relative to normal peers (Alegria and Mousty, 1994, 1996).

Current explanations concur that difficulties in phonological processing and representation underlie spelling problems as well as the word-recognition difficulties of poor readers and children with developmental dyslexia. Phonological difficulties associated with poor reading skills have been reported for children learning a number of alphabetic writing systems, such as English (Bryant and Bradley, 1985; Hatcher et al., 1994), French (Morais et al., 1984), German (Wimmer, 1993; Landerl et al., 1997), and Italian (Lindgren et al., 1985; Cossu et al., 1988). The general implication of these studies is that, regardless of their spoken language, children who experience difficulty in manipulating and processing phonological units are at risk for alphabetic literacy problems.

The results of a variety of studies across languages and alphabetic writing systems indicate two universal characteristics of dyslexia: a phonological processing deficit and impaired spelling ability. The logical assumption is that these two problems are causally related. There is some evidence from studies of English-speaking children to support this assumption (Rohl and Tunmer, 1988; Bruck and Waters, 1990; Treiman, 1997). However, very few cross-linguistic studies have directly contrasted the spelling skills of dyslexic children from different language backgrounds. Thus, the objective of the present study was to examine whether English- and French-speaking poor spellers showed signs of phonological difficulties in spelling, and whether they manifested these difficulties in the same way. To appreciate how the analysis of dyslexic children's spellings may indicate phonological difficulties, it is necessary to review some of the findings that demonstrate the close connection between alphabetic spelling skills and phonological skills in normally developing children. The description is based primarily on spelling acquisition in English-speaking children, as this language population has been studied most extensively.

Spelling development in English-speaking children

Spelling is a complex skill that requires the integration of a number of component skills (Waters et al., 1988). One such skill is phonological analysis (the ability to 'sound out' all speech sounds in a word) and it is the primary strategy of the beginner speller. In the early stages of alphabetic spelling, children rely on phonological information, attempting to link their knowledge of speech sounds or phonemes to the graphemes of the writing system. This strategy is best exemplified in children's misspellings, which often contain phonologically accurate elements but are orthographically incorrect (Read, 1975; Treiman, 1993). For example, American children often fail to spell the vowel in syllables containing syllabic consonants. Syllabic consonants, such as the /r/ in *girl* and the /l/ in *pencil*, take the role of the vowel as the syllable peak. Accordingly, children often misspell *girl* as grl and *pencil* as pencl. In a study of this phenomenon, Treiman et al. (1993a) found that young spellers omit these vowels because they do not consider syllables with syllabic consonants to contain vowels. Although these spellings are orthographically illegal (because each syllable requires at least one vowel), they nevertheless show children's ability to represent the phonological structure of words with graphemes. If children were relying on a more visual strategy (e.g. memorizing letters or sequences of letters) in the beginning stages of spelling, one would expect these types of phonologically based errors to be less common than they are.

A related example of young English-speaking children's reliance on phonological information for spelling is seen in their greater tendency to omit vowels in unstressed syllables than in stressed syllables. For example, in a word like 'borrow' the second, unstressed, *o* would be omitted more often than the first, stressed, *o*. Moreover, the omissions are even more likely when the unstressed vowel is also reduced to a schwa sound[1] (e.g. the second *o* /ə/ of 'bottom' is more likely to be omitted than the second *o* of 'hollow') because the second *o* in 'bottom' is a reduced vowel (see Treiman et al., 1993b). This pattern of errors reflects the fact that the constituent phonemes of unstressed syllables are perceptually less salient and therefore more difficult to identify than those of stressed syllables. It is hypothesized here that this class of phonological errors may be specific to stress-timed languages such as English, in which lexical stress alternates in a strong-weak pattern (i.e. syllables alternately receive strong and weak emphasis). Vowel omissions may be less frequent in languages that have syllable-timed rather than stress-timed stress patterns. Syllable-timed languages, such as French, do not have an alternating strong-weak stress pattern but rather have fixed stress in one word position; the remaining syllables receive fairly even emphasis. In French, stress typically falls on a word's final syllable, and the differences in emphasis on each syllable (and vowel) constituting a word are much smaller than in English (Delattre, 1981; Halle and Vergnaud, 1987).

The above examples of children's spelling errors, although not exhaustive, demonstrate that many young children are sensitive to the speech sounds that constitute words, and that they use this knowledge as the basis of their developing spelling skill. Their early writing attempts reflect both a limited knowledge of the orthography and a somewhat immature phonological system. As they learn about their writing system, children's spellings become more and more conventional and they reflect the regularities and complexities of the system (Cassar and Treiman, 1997).

Cross-linguistic differences

The above description of children learning to spell in English may not necessarily generalize to learners of other writing systems. This is because the writing systems of languages – even alphabetic ones – can vary considerably in terms of their complexity. A number of terms, such as orthographic depth, transparency, consistency and regularity, have been used to describe and compare alphabetic writing systems. English is considered to be one of the more difficult systems because: (i) the relationship between graphemes and phonemes is often opaque (e.g. the letter '*t*' in 'listen has no corresponding phoneme); (ii) the spelling of phonemes is inconsistent (e.g. although the words 'beef', 'chief' and 'leaf' all contain the same vowel /i/, it is assigned a

---

[1]The schwa is the central vowel sound corresponding to the highlighted vowel letter in words like 'th*e*', 'h*e*llo', 'bott*o*m'.

different spelling in each word); and (iii) many exceptions exist to acceptable orthographic patterns (e.g. the spelling <u>trek</u> violates the rule that word-final /k/ in monosyllabic words with short vowels is spelled with the grapheme *ck*) and in sound-spelling correspondences (e.g. the grapheme *oe* in *does* and the grapheme string *cea* in *ocean* both correspond to exceptional pronunciations). Compared to English, written French is less complex, especially in grapheme-to-phoneme mapping (i.e. reading), although it is still one of the more difficult alphabetic languages, particularly in terms of phoneme-to-grapheme mapping (i.e. spelling) (Ziegler et al., 1996).

Given the differences in complexity among written languages, it is possible not only that some are easier to learn than others, but also that the processes involved in learning to read and spell words may vary as a function of the complexity of the language (Wimmer and Goswami, 1994; Goswami et al., 1998; Sprenger-Charolles et al., 1998). There is some evidence that children acquire general spelling skills more quickly in relatively transparent alphabetic languages. For example, given the same spelling items, first grade Czech children, whose writing system is highly transparent, produced more accurate nonword spellings than same-aged English-speaking children (Caravolas and Bruck, 1993); and German-speaking children in grades 2, 3 and 4 performed better on a word spelling task than same-grade Anglophone peers (Wimmer and Goswami, 1994; Wimmer and Landerl, 1997).

These differences in rates of acquisition have been traced in part to differences in children's ability to spell vowels. For example, Anglophone school beginners find vowel spellings very difficult (Shankweiler and Liberman, 1972; Read, 1975; Stage and Wagner, 1992; Treiman, 1993; Treiman et al., 1993b). Relative to English children, first grade children learning to write in Czech (Caravolas and Bruck, 1993) and French (Alegria and Mousty, 1994; Sprenger-Charolles and Siegel, 1997), as well as German-speaking second graders (Wimmer and Landerl, 1997), do not demonstrate any particular difficulty with this class of phonemes. These between-language differences have been explained in terms of differences in the relative complexity of vowel spellings. As described in the previous section, in English, each vowel can be represented by a number of different graphemes (e.g. *bead*, *seed*, *chief*, *here*), whereas in Czech and German most vowel phonemes are consistently represented by a small range of dedicated graphemes. French vowel spellings are more complex than either Czech or German in that several graphemes may represent a single vowel phoneme (e.g. *o*, *au*, *eau*, *ô* may all represent /o/ as in *rose*, *chaud*, *peau*, *côte*). However, the degree of inconsistency is more restricted in French than in English (Peereman and Content, 1997). Moreover, the grapheme-to-phoneme correspondences of vowels (in reading) are very consistent. Thus one would predict that French-speaking children would acquire spelling skills more quickly than their English-speaking counterparts.

Spelling impairments

In light of the research on normal spelling skill acquisition and on the reading skills of dyslexics, it is reasonable to hypothesize that the phonological processing difficulties of dyslexics prevent them from acquiring the accurate and automatic phoneme-grapheme associations that form the basis of skilled spelling in normally developing children. Research with English-speaking children provides support for this hypothesis. Poor spellers or dyslexic children have more difficulty correctly spelling nonwords than age-matched and spelling-level-matched peers (Bruck, 1988; Rohl and Tunmer, 1988). Nonword spelling is typically used as a measure of knowledge of sound-spelling correspondences, especially when spelling unfamiliar words.

Some researchers have argued that analyses of spelling errors provide evidence that poor spellers do not use phonological information to the same degree as good spellers (e.g. Olson, 1985; Siegel and Ryan, 1988; Lennox and Siegel, 1993). For example, poor spellers may be more likely to misspell 'beef' as bif, whereas good spellers tend to produce errors such as bief or beaf, which are phonologically more accurate. However, these studies considered misspellings that were comparable to normal, younger children's error types (e.g. spelling 'pencil' as pensl, or 'hurt' as hrt) to be nonphonetic. Treiman (1997) has argued that, on balance, the majority of spelling errors even among severely impaired (English) spellers are in fact phonologically motivated and are frequently equivalent to the types of error that are typical of younger, normally developing children whose phonological representations (mental representations of a word's constituent speech sounds) and phonological processing skills are less well-developed.

How the difficulties of English-speaking dyslexics compare with their counterparts learning to spell in other alphabetic languages remains an open question as, to date, very few studies of spelling in dyslexia have been reported in languages other than English. Landerl et al. (1997) carried out a direct cross-linguistic study of dyslexics in which spelling was also examined. In this study, the spelling performance of German-speaking (Austrian) and English-speaking (British) dyslexics aged 11–14 years was compared on a word and a nonword spelling task. (The spelling results are discussed in Lander and Wimmer (2000)). The items were equated across languages for syllable number, and to some extent for phonological content. Although German and English dyslexics made more errors on both word and nonword tasks than the normal spelling control subjects, German-speaking dyslexics spelled both sets of stimuli more accurately than English-speaking dyslexics. The German dyslexics also read words and nonwords more accurately than the English dyslexics.

One hypothesis to account for these differences is that the German dyslexics had less-severe phonological impairments than the English children. However, results from a phonological awareness task cast doubt on this conclusion because both groups performed equally poorly on this task. If both groups of dyslexics showed phonological processing impairments on the oral language task, why did the German-speaking children perform better on nonword spelling? Landerl et al. (1997) suggest that German-speaking dyslexics' better decoding skills in reading (relative to English-speaking dyslexics) enable them to develop better skills in assembling phonological forms in nonword spelling. Although plausible, this hypothesis remains to be tested empirically. An alternative possibility is that some characteristic(s) of the phonological structure of German words enables listeners to analyse the constituent phonemic elements more readily than does the phonological structure of English; in other words, characteristics of the speech input may directly affect nonword spelling ability. This hypothesis will be elaborated below, but first, let us consider what is known about the spelling skills of French-speaking dyslexics.

In two studies of French-speaking dyslexics aged 9 to 14 years, Alegria and Mousty (1994, 1996) found that on words containing highly consistent and context-independent phoneme-grapheme correspondences (e.g. *pour*), dyslexics spelled as accurately as their normally developing, reading-matched peers. Thus, they were able to analyse the phonemic constituents of these words. Their deficits relative to normally developing children were in learning the inconsistencies and irregularities of conventional spelling. That is, whereas normal children demonstrated the ability to learn inconsistent and context-dependent spelling rules as their reading age increased, dyslexic children showed no such developmental pattern. For example, a spelling rule that is readily learned by normally developing children in the early years of schooling is that /g/ is represented by *g* unless followed by *i* and *e*; in order to spell /gi/ and /ge/, *g* must be followed by *u* as in *guitare* and *guêpe*). Dyslexic children in Alegria's studies, however, continued to produce very immature 'one-letter-to-one-sound' types of spellings (e.g. gitare, gepe). The authors (1994) suggested that French dyslexics do not necessarily have impairments in phonological awareness (and analysis) but rather in learning spellings for specific irregular words. They argue that this deficit arises because French dyslexics probably fail to acquire fully specified orthographic representations, as they do not attend to word spellings fully in reading. However, the phonological spelling accuracy of dyslexics and their normally developing peers was not compared in a statistical analysis in either study; rather the units of analysis in these studies were specific graphemes and not whole words. Also, phonological awareness was not assessed. No conclusion can therefore be made about the phonological awareness skills of French dyslexics because, as was shown in the study of Landerl et al. (1997), phonologically accurate spellings do not necessarily rule out phonological awareness or processing difficulties. Nevertheless, the French spelling findings are more in line with those obtained for German-speaking dyslexics than those typically found for Anglophone dyslexics.

In their 1994 study, Alegria and Mousty reported that neither the dyslexic children nor their younger, reading-matched peers had greater difficulty with vowel spellings than with consonant spellings. This finding was replicated by Sprenger-Charolles and Siegel (1997) in a study of normally developing French first grade children. In contrast, English children have particular difficulty in their representation of vowels both in reading and in spelling.

The fact that French- and German-speaking dyslexics appear to have relatively less difficulty in representing the phonological content of words than Anglophone dyslexics, and that they have no particular difficulty with vowel spelling, may reflect differences in orthographic complexity across these languages (Alegria and Mousty, 1994; Wimmer and Landerl, 1997). In their study of first grade French children, Sprenger-Charolles and Siegel (1997) further suggested that phonological factors may underlie these between-language differences. In addition to the effects of a more consistent orthography, they attributed their subjects' relative facility with vowel spellings to the more phonetically/acoustically stable pronunciation of vowels in French (Delattre, 1965; Gottfried, 1984). Sprenger-Charolles and Siegel (1997) argue that the greater stability in speech input (relative to English) makes vowel units more accessible to young spellers, but they did not test this hypothesis directly, either within or across languages. The hypothesis that phonological input has specific effects on children's ability to spell vowels is examined in the present study. However, it is argued that the effect is rooted in supra-phonological characteristics of rhythm and stress assignment in each language, which in turn affects vowel quality (Delattre, 1981). That is, whereas the French syllable-timed stress pattern has a relatively small effect on the quality of spoken vowels, and presumably therefore on children's ability to spell those vowels, the English stress-timed stress pattern has a strong effect on spoken vowel quality, and presumably children's ability to spell vowels varies as a function of the type of stress associated with them.

The present study

A cross-linguistic study of English- and French-speaking third grade poor spellers was carried out. Children's spellings of words and nonwords were compared to those of age-matched and language-matched good spellers.

The present analyses were motivated by a body of research which suggests that, for English-speaking children, spelling is a phonological task involving the ability to accurately segment the target word into its component phonemes and then to accurately assign graphemes (letters or groups of letters) to these phonological units (e.g. Read, 1975; Treiman, 1993). Thus, in addition to assessing whether the children could spell words correctly, their misspellings were further evaluated to assess the extent to which poor spellers of English and French represent phonological information. First, the children's spelling errors were examined for their phonological accuracy. For example, the misspelling beaf for 'beef' would be considered phonologically accurate, whereas the misspelling bafe would be categorized as phonologically inaccurate. Such analyses reflect the degree to which children use phoneme-grapheme information to spell words that are in their lexicon.

A 'phonological skeleton' measure was devised to assess the more fundamental skill of phonemic segmentation of words. On this measure, if children's misspellings contained the same sequence of consonant and vowel graphemes (i.e. the same consonant-vowel structure) as the phonological (oral) structure of an item, then it was considered to have preserved the phonological skeleton. For example, the misspelling machac for the word 'magic' accurately reflects the consonant-vowel structure of the word, whereas the misspelling magisk does not.

Children's spellings of nonwords were also examined. They were included here because nonword spelling provides a measure of children's knowledge of sound-spelling correspondences, especially when spelling unfamiliar words. Moreover, in the present study, they provided a validation measure for the word test. That is, if French and English children performed differently from each other on the word test, this might reflect true between-language differences in poor spellers' abilities and/or strategies in spelling. On the other hand, it may simply be an artefact of differences between the difficulty of the French versus the English words. If, however, both language groups demonstrate similar patterns of performance on both the word and nonword tests, this would support the generalizability of the findings beyond the specific set of words used in each language.

The analyses were designed to address several hypotheses. First, in line with previous findings that the complexity of an alphabetic writing system differentially affects spelling development (Lindgren et al., 1985; Caravolas and Bruck, 1993; Wimmer and Landerl, 1997), French-speaking poor spellers, whose orthography is more consistent, were expected to spell more words correctly than English poor-spellers. Both poor-speller groups were nevertheless expected to make more errors than good spellers.

Second, on the assumption that dyslexics suffer from a universal core deficit in phonological processing, both groups of poor spellers were expected to show poorer ability to accurately represent phonological content in their spellings as compared to their normal peers. Specifically, they were expected to produce more phonologically inaccurate misspellings on nonwords and to have fewer phonologically acceptable misspellings of words.

Third, in line with the phonological input hypothesis, language-specific differences in phonology were expected to differentially affect French and English children's ability to represent the phonological structure of words, with English children making more omissions of segments than French children.

Fourth, the cross-linguistic differences in lexical stress were expected to affect French and English children's relative ability to represent vowels. Briefly, as discussed above, English is a stress-timed language in which syllables alternately receive strong and weak emphasis. This prosodic pattern has a direct effect on the quality of all segments, but particularly on vowels, such that vowels in unstressed syllables are perceptually less salient than those in stressed syllables. Also, English has a high proportion of syllables with closed structure, which in turn means that frequently, vowels are coarticulated with the ensuing consonant. Associated with this stress pattern and with the tendency to closed syllables is the tendency, in English, to reduce vowels in unstressed syllables.[2] In contrast, French has a 'syllable-timed' stress pattern, with primary stress on the final syllable. This means that each syllable preceding the last syllable in a spoken word is assigned approximately equal emphasis, but the main emphasis always falls on the last syllable. Also, the predominant syllable structure of French is open, hence without a final consonant. The combined effects of prosodic and structural (and articulatory) characteristics of French result in a lesser degree of vowel reduction (Delattre, 1981). On the basis of these considerations, it was predicted that English poor spellers would omit vowels in unstressed, reduced syllables (and hence misrepresent the phonological structure of words) more frequently than their Francophone peers, whose language contains fewer and less-reduced vowels.

Method

Participants

English- and French-speaking groups of good and poor spellers were selected from a cohort of 73 monolingual Anglophone grade 3 children, and from a

---

[2]Vowel reduction is in fact influenced by several additional factors. However, an in-depth discussion of this topic is beyond the scope of this chapter. Interested readers are referred to Delattre (1981).

cohort of 66 monolingual Francophone children respectively. All children were participants in a larger longitudinal study (described in Bruck et al., 1997) which tracked their progress in the acquisition of literacy skills from kindergarten to grade 3. The English children were sampled from six public schools and the French children from two public schools. The schools were in middle-class suburban neighbourhoods of Montreal. Each group was instructed in their native language. The mean age of each cohort at testing in grade 3 was 8.9 years (range 8.3 to 9.8 years) in the English group, and 9.0 years (range 8.4 to 9.6 years) in the French group.

The subgroups examined in the present study were selected on the basis of their spelling scores on a word-spelling test (described below) administered at the end of grade 3. In both language groups, any child who scored less than one standard deviation below the group mean on two- and three-syllable items of the word-spelling test was designated a poor speller.[3] Similarly, a child who scored one standard deviation above the mean on word spelling was designated a good speller. This procedure yielded the following results. In English, nine children were classified as poor spellers and 12 children were classified as good spellers. In French, there were nine poor spellers and ten good spellers.

Additional confirmation that the poor spellers had experienced pervasive difficulties with the acquisition of literacy skills was provided by analyses of variance of the children's reading skills in first, second and third grade. These analyses showed that already, in first grade, both groups of French and English poor spellers read words and nonwords significantly less well than their good speller peers, and this discrepancy held through to the third grade.

Tasks

At each grade level, all participants were administered a battery of cognitive, phonological and literacy tests. Only the tests relevant to the present paper are described here.

Nonverbal IQ
In order to ascertain that any ensuing between-language differences on the spelling measures were not due to significant IQ differences between French and English children, all participants were given the Raven's Coloured Progressive Matrices, a culture-fair test of analogical reasoning and visuospatial organization (Raven and Summers, 1986), in kindergarten and again in grade 3. The results of an analysis of variance showed that in kindergarten, the children did not differ in terms of non-verbal IQ either by language group

---

[3]Children's performance on one-syllable words was not considered in this selection because a ceiling effect was obtained for these items in the French word test.

or by spelling ability. In third grade, both French and English poor spellers obtained slightly, but significantly, lower non-verbal IQ scores than good spellers. Importantly, however, no differences emerged between language groups.

Word spelling test

A word spelling test, containing one-, two- and three-syllable items was administered in grade 3. Parallel English and French versions of each test were created. Despite attempts at equating all test forms, minor differences existed. The English word test contained 25 words, of which 13 were monosyllables, six were bisyllables and six were trisyllables. The French word-spelling test contained 26 items, of which 13 were monosyllables, seven were bisyllables and six were trisyllables. The stimuli were selected in each language such that: (i) they represented the spelling patterns typically taught in first to third grades in each language; (ii) all items contained regular spelling patterns; (iii) all items were equated in French and English for the number of letters and number of syllables; and (iv) the items in each language were as similar as possible in terms of syllable structure (e.g. CVC: 'big' and 'lac'; CVCC: 'hard' and 'verte'; CVCVC: 'magic' and 'musique') and number of graphemes (e.g. *dramatic* and *bricolage* both have eight graphemes).

Attempts were made to equate the French and English word stimuli as closely as possible. However, this was not always possible due to inherent differences in English and French orthography. Specifically, 16 words in the French and English lists had the same syllable structure, and 24 words in the French and English lists had the same number of graphemes. However, because many words in French contain silent letters (e.g. *vert, tard, pont*), only 19 of the words on both lists had the same number of phonemes. Generally, when items were not fully equated, the French stimuli contained more letters, whereas the English stimuli contained more phonemes (See Table 9.1).

Nonword spelling test

A nonword spelling test analogous to the word-spelling test was also administered. The nonword stimuli were derived from the word items by substituting one to three consonants. As a result, the distribution of one-, two- and three-syllable items was identical to the word test in each language, as was the number of English and French items having the same syllable structure (i.e. 16 of 25 and 26 items respectively). The number of English and French items having the same number of phonemes was also virtually identical to the word-spelling test (i.e. 20 items). Equating French and English stimuli for the number of letters was not relevant on this test because unlike real words, nonwords have no conventional spellings. That is, in both languages, many phonemes may be represented by a variety of graphemes. Moreover, the silent letters that are present in many French words need not be represented in nonwords. Thus, on the assumption that both English and French writing systems represent each phoneme by (at least) one grapheme, French and English stimuli were matched in terms of the essential number of graphemes on 20 items.

Procedures

Both tests (word and nonword) were administered as dictations to groups of three or four children. In each language, the items of the word-spelling test were presented first in isolation, then in a carrier sentence, then in isolation once more. Children were instructed to wait until they heard the full sentence before attempting to write the target word. For the nonword stimuli, the experimenter repeated each item three times. Word and nonword tests were administered in counterbalanced order on separate days.

Results

The following analyses examine not only accuracy of spellings of words and nonwords, but also the degree to which phonological information was used in spelling. Unless specified otherwise, the data were analysed by analyses of variance in which the independent variables were language group (English versus French) and spelling ability (good versus poor). Significant interactions were followed up by Spjøtvoll-Stoline HSD tests for unequal sample sizes. Separate analyses were conducted on the word and nonword data. In this chapter, we do not report the details of the statistical tests; however, graphs with errors bars are included. Only statistically significant results are reported.

Spelling accuracy

Correct spelling of two- and three-syllable words
Scoring: the first analysis examined spelling accuracy on the two- and three-syllable items of the word test. The scoring of the word data was straightforward. One point was awarded for each correct spelling of the two- and

Table 9.1 Examples of English and French word and nonword items

French word	English word	French nonword	English nonword
lac	big	dac	hig
verte	hard	lerte	bard
musique	magic	tusique	fagic
journal	pencil	sourmal	hencil
bricolage	dramatic	tricomage	bracatic
transplanter	transparent	planscranter	planscarent

three-syllable items. Recall that one-syllable items were not considered in the word accuracy analysis, although the whole-word set was analysed in subsequent analyses. (A number of the one-syllable words were too easy, especially in French, and this obscured poor spellers' difficulties on polysyllabic words. So, for purposes of group selection we looked only at the more difficult items, i.e. two- and three-syllable words.) The total score was expressed as a percentage of the total number of items. Because this measure was used for selection of good and poor spellers, differences were expected between ability groups. However, it was not known whether differences would occur between English and French groups.

Results: this analysis showed, as expected, that good spellers were significantly better at spelling words than poor spellers. In addition, however, both good and poor French spellers produced more correct spellings than their English counterparts. Moreover, the discrepancy between good (M = 80%) and poor (M = 6%) English spellers was much greater than that between good (M = 97%) and poor (M = 50%) French spellers. Thus, relative to their age-matched controls, the English poor spellers were more impaired than their French counterparts. The analysis also indicated that the French poor spellers were at ceiling on the word test.

Spelling accuracy on all words and nonwords

The percentages of correct word spellings for the full set of word items (including one-syllable words) were analysed next, as were the percentages of correctly spelled nonwords according to the constrained system. The scoring system for words is as described above. For nonwords, it was carried out as follows. One point was awarded to each item that was phonologically and orthographically acceptable. In previous work, this scoring system has been termed 'phonologically accurate according to a constrained system' (Bruck and Waters, 1988; Bruck et al., 1998). This system has been found to best reflect spelling ability.

Specifically, one point was given if a nonword spelling was phonologically acceptable and respected the positional and sequencing constraints of the orthography in each language. For example, the spelling <u>trive</u> for the nonword /traiv/ (derived from the word 'drive') was considered correct because: (i) it could be pronounced like the target nonword by application of grapheme-phoneme correspondences; and (ii) it respected positional constraints (i.e. the constraint that a certain grapheme is related to a specific pronunciation by virtue of its physical position in the word and by the surrounding graphemes). However the spelling <u>triv</u> was not correct because in English orthography the grapheme v is not permissible in the word-final position (it must be followed by e) and because the grapheme i in this context corresponds to the phoneme /ɪ/ and not to /ai/. Also, the nonword

/meɪpɹ/ (derived from 'paper') spelled as <u>maypr</u> was not scored as a correct nonword, because although phonologically plausible, the lack of a vowel in the second syllable is illegal in the English orthography. Similarly the French spelling <u>lerte</u> for the nonword */lɛʁt/* (derived from the word 'verte') was acceptable, whereas the spelling <u>lertte</u> was not because in French orthography consonant letters do not double within syllables when following another consonant.

Results: the analyses of correct word and of nonword spellings showed the same pattern of results (see Figure 9.1). First, as expected, good spellers were more accurate than poor spellers on word and nonword measures. Second, French children were more accurate on words and nonwords than their English counterparts. Third, the discrepancy between good and poor English spellers was greater than that between good and poor French spellers. Thus, again English poor spellers showed a greater degree of impairment than French poor spellers.

This pattern of results is consistent with the hypothesis that orthographic transparency affects the rate at which children learn about the conventions of their orthographic system. Importantly, it also appears that poor spellers learning an inconsistent and complex orthography (i.e. English) are significantly more handicapped by the writing system than their counterparts learning a more consistent orthography (i.e. French).

Phonological accuracy of misspellings

The following analyses allowed an examination of the degree to which children used phonological information (phoneme-grapheme correspondences) despite the fact that their spellings of words or nonwords did not

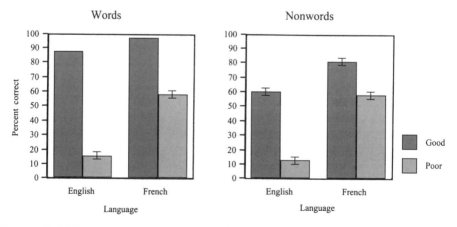

Figure 9.1 Mean percent correct on word and nonword spelling of two- and three-syllable items as a function of language and spelling level.

include conventional (or word-specific) orthographic patterns. This system of scoring errors has been referred to as 'phonologically unconstrained' (see Bruck et al., 1998 for full details).

Scoring of words: according to this system, a misspelling of a word was considered phonologically plausible if all phonemes were represented by corresponding plausible graphemes; and a phonologically accurate misspelling did not have to respect the positional and sequencing rules of the orthography. For example the spelling of 'drive' as <u>driv</u> was awarded one point because each grapheme could conceivably represent the constituent phonemes /d/-/r/-/ai/-/v/ when positional and sequencing rules regarding graphemes were ignored. Similarly, 'paper' spelled as <u>papper</u> was considered phonologically acceptable because when considered on a grapheme-by-grapheme basis, and independently of spelling rules, each grapheme could represent a phoneme of the target word. In contrast, the spelling <u>hrde</u> for the word 'hard' was not considered as phonologically acceptable because the vowel /ɑ/ was not represented at all. Although this type of error may be phonologically motivated, reflecting a child's use of a letter-name spelling strategy (i.e. /aːr/ can be represented by the letter name of R) (see Treiman, 1994), the attempt nevertheless fails to represent the full segmental CVCC structure of the word 'hard'. A more flexible approach was taken with the subset of English words (and nonwords) containing the syllabic consonants /r/ and /l/ in unstressed syllables because the phonological status of vowels in such syllables is questionable (Kenyon, 1950; Treiman et al., 1993a). Four words ('paper', 'pencil', 'cleverness' and 'surprising') fell into this category. Spellings that reflected the phonological content of these words but lacked a vowel grapheme corresponding to the schwa /ə/ preceding the syllabic consonant were considered phonologically acceptable (for example spellings such as <u>papr</u>, <u>pencl</u>, <u>clevrness</u> and <u>srprising</u> were accepted). In French, the misspelling <u>vert</u> for 'verte' (/vɛʀt/) was acceptable by the unconstrained system because the graphemes v, e, r, t corresponded to the phonemes /v/, /ɛ/, /r/, /t/. Similarly, the misspelling <u>trout</u> for 'trou' (/tru:/) was accepted because the final grapheme t may appear as a word-final silent grapheme in words such as 'tout' (/tu/) and 'goût' (/gu/), for example.

Scoring of nonwords: this evaluation was similar to the second unconstrained evaluation of the word items. The spellings did not need to respect the legal constraints of English or French orthography. For example, the spellings <u>triv</u> and <u>maypr</u> were now each awarded a point because the phonological forms /traiv/ and /meɪpr̩/ could be derived from these spellings if each grapheme was considered independently of the orthographic rules of English. In this evaluation, the omission of vowels preceding syllabic consonants was permissible if the spelling was otherwise phonologically plausible. In French, the misspelling <u>lertte</u> was now awarded one point. Also a spelling like <u>mesu</u> for the nonword /mǝsy/ (derived from 'reçu') was phonologically acceptable even though according to contextual rules, an intervocalic *s* is pronounced as /z/.

Results: the proportions of children's phonologically acceptable misspellings of words and of nonwords were examined. Because six children in the French good-speller group made no errors on the word-spelling task, their data were eliminated from the word analysis, leaving only four children in the group. However, the performance of the four remaining children was highly variable. Moreover, their results on this measure were not very informative because they produced very few errors (on average, one). Thus, if a child misspelled only one word and this misspelling was not phonologically plausible, he or she obtained 0% on the phonologically acceptable misspelling measure. This proportion is much less telling, of course, than that of a child who made 12 errors of which 0% were phonologically acceptable. Consequently, the results of the French good spellers were not considered in the word test error analyses. Because all children made at least one error on the nonwords spelling task, no subjects were excluded from the nonword analyses.

The results of the word analysis (see Figure 9.2) showed that English poor spellers produced significantly fewer phonologically plausible spellings than English good spellers and French poor spellers. The nonword results (which are based on the results of all children) showed that both groups of poor spellers produced significantly fewer phonologically acceptable misspellings than good spellers. The difference between the English and French poor spellers' rates of phonologically acceptable spellings was not statistically significant.

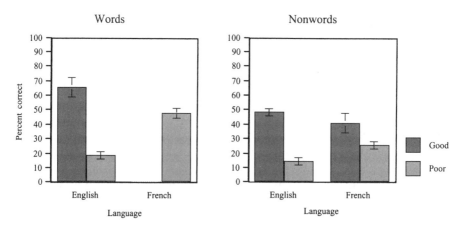

Figure 9.2 Mean percent correct on word and nonword phonologically acceptable misspelling as a function of language and spelling level.

The results of the nonword spelling task suggest that when they misspell words, French children are not more likely to produce a phonologically acceptable spelling than English children; this is despite the fact that French children demonstrated generally better knowledge of conventional spelling than English children. The more important finding is that poor spellers of both English and French produce fewer phonologically acceptable spelling attempts than their skilled peers. This result supports the hypothesis that regardless of the language they speak, poor spellers have more difficulty than skilled peers in representing the phonological content of words in alphabetic scripts.

Analyses of phonological structure of misspelled items

In this set of analyses, we examined whether language-specific and ability-specific differences existed in children's ability to represent words at the more basic segmental (skeleton) level.

Scoring of words and nonwords: the phonological acceptability of spellings was not relevant in this evaluation. Rather, each misspelling was examined to determine if the basic segmental structure of consonant(s) and vowel(s) – referred to here as the phonological skeleton – was preserved. To illustrate, the skeleton of the word 'hard' is CVCC (in Canadian English). Any spelling containing the CVCC structure for the target word 'hard' was awarded one point, even if the phonemes did not correspond to /h/, /ɑ/, /r/, /d/ (e.g. hord and harb were misspellings that preserved that phonological skeleton of *hard*). A spelling like had was not acceptable because it corresponded to a CVC structure. For the four English words containing syllabic consonants in unstressed syllables, the phonological skeleton was acceptable if it reflected the full CV structure or if it reflected all but the vowel preceding the syllabic consonant. For example, both the spelling papper (i.e. CVCVC) and papr (CVCC) were considered to reflect the phonological skeleton of 'paper'. According to the same criteria, the spelling bricoulag for the French word 'bricolage' was awarded one point for preserving the skeleton, whereas the spelling bicolage did not. The same procedure was carried out for misspellings of nonwords.

Results: as in the previous analysis, the results of the French good spellers were not considered in the word test analysis. As shown in Figure 9.3, the English poor spellers were significantly worse at preserving the phonological structure of words than English good spellers and French poor spellers. The French poor spellers were as accurate on this measure as English good spellers. In the nonword analysis, English poor spellers showed the same pattern of performance as on the word test. In contrast, although the French poor spellers produced slightly fewer acceptable skeleton spellings than French and English good spellers, these three groups were not statistically different from each other.

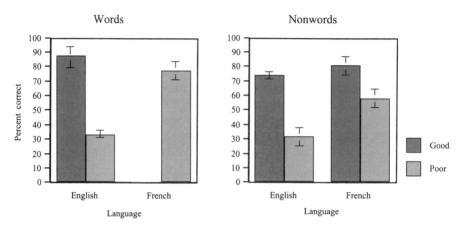

Figure 9.3 Mean percent of misspellings with preserved phonological skeleton on word and nonword spelling as a function of language and spelling level.

Thus a somewhat different pattern emerged for this analysis. When French poor spellers misspelled words and nonwords, their spellings were more accurate at the segmental level than those of their English counterparts. Moreover, French poor spellers did not perform significantly worse than English good spellers or French good spellers on the nonword task. English poor spellers, on the other hand, showed considerable impairments relative to all other groups.

Consonant and vowel omissions

In order to explore the basis of English children's poorer ability to represent the phonological structure of words and nonwords, the ensuing analyses focused on vowel versus consonant omissions in their misspellings. Omissions of vowels and consonants would result in inaccurate representations of the phonological skeleton. On the basis of previous work showing that English-speaking children make most errors on the spelling of vowels (Read, 1975; Stage and Wagner, 1992; Treiman, 1993), it was expected that English children would omit vowels at a higher rate than they omitted consonants. In contrast, one study with French-speaking children showed that consonants are more often misspelled than vowels (Sprenger-Charolles and Siegel, 1997). We examined whether the same (misspelling) patterns extended to consonant and vowel omissions.

Scoring: the number of word and nonword spellings in which a child omitted the consonant was counted (e.g. <u>dive</u> for 'drive' and <u>potehtef</u> for 'protective'), as was the number of vowel omissions (e.g. the spelling of <u>dremdik</u> for 'dramatic' contained one vowel omission, the medial *a*). Because omission errors were evaluated relative to conventional spellings, the omission of vowels preceding syllabic consonants (in four English words and nonwords) were counted as errors. The percentage of omitted consonants was calculated for words and nonwords respectively. Similar scores were calculated for vowel omissions.

Results: because both English and French good spellers made virtually no errors of omission (up to a maximum of 1%) on words and nonwords, their data were dropped from the analyses. Thus in the following analyses, English poor spellers are directly compared to French poor spellers.

As shown in Figure 9.4, English poor spellers made relatively more errors of omission on both vowels and consonants than the French poor spellers on both word and nonword analyses. In fact, the French poor spellers made very few errors with slightly (but not significantly) more omissions of consonants than of vowels. In addition, on both words and nonwords, English poor spellers omitted vowels approximately twice as often as they omitted consonants.

Omission of stressed versus unstressed vowels
The final analyses further examined the source of English children's difficulties with vowel spelling. It was hypothesized that lexical stress, and particularly stress-related vowel reduction in English, might specifically affect children's vowel spellings. That is, vowels in unstressed syllables may be more prone to omission than vowels in stressed syllables because the former are less salient than the latter. The hypothesis that French children do not experience difficulties with vowel spelling as a result of lexical stress is confirmed by the above finding that even French poor spellers rarely omit vowels. Consequently, the stress hypothesis was only tested on the data of English poor spellers. The vowel omission rates were compared in stressed

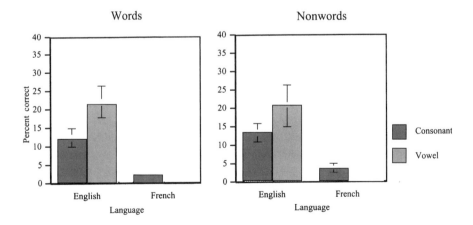

Figure 9.4 Mean percent of consonant versus vowel omissions on word and nonword spelling as a function of language.

versus unstressed syllables of the 12 polysyllabic words and nonwords respectively. To illustrate, the word 'magic' has a stressed vowel /æ/ in the first syllable and an unstressed vowel /ɪ/ in the second.

If vowel reduction in unstressed syllables affects children's ability to spell vowels, then English poor spellers (whose language is stress timed) should have greater difficulty in spelling unstressed than stressed vowels. Consistent with this hypothesis we found that English poor spellers omitted stressed vowels of words and nonwords 22% and 23% of the time respectively. In unstressed vowels, their omission rates were almost twice as frequent, with omissions of 40% in words and 36% in nonwords.

Discussion

In this study, the spelling skills of English and French poor spellers were compared relative to each other and to age-matched and language-matched skilled spellers. Both language groups were given a word test as well as a nonword test. The latter task was included to provide a more stringent measure of children's phoneme-grapheme knowledge, and as a validation measure of the word task. In addition to comparing spelling accuracy, children's ability to represent the phonological content and the phonological structure of words was examined. Finally, the source of language-specific differences in poor spellers' ability to represent phonological structure was examined on consonant and vowel omissions.

The comparison of nonword spellings that were phonologically accurate and respected the spelling conventions (i.e. the constrained spellings) revealed that relative to good spellers, both French and English poor spellers had greater difficulty learning the conventions of their orthography. This result replicates the findings for French (Alegria and Mousty, 1994, 1996), German (Landerl et al., 1997) and English (Bruck and Waters, 1988; Rohl and Tunmer, 1988) dyslexics.

There was also support for the hypothesis that orthographic complexity specifically affects the rates at which children acquire spelling skill. That is, both good and poor French groups spelled words and nonwords more accurately than their respective Anglophone peers. Moreover, on both tests, French poor spellers showed less impairment than English poor spellers. This is in line with the findings of Landerl et al. (1997) for German-speaking dyslexics relative to same-age English dyslexics.

In addition to the differences in spelling ability that may be attributed to the writing system itself, analyses of phonological accuracy in misspelled words and nonwords suggested that poor spellers have particular difficulty in representing the phonological content of words regardless of their language. That is, both groups of poor spellers produced fewer phonologically plausible errors than their skilled peers. Thus, the present results support the hypothesis that difficulties with phonological processing are associated with children's spelling difficulties across alphabetic languages. They do not support the suggestion of Alegria and Mousty (1994) that French dyslexics may not have difficulties in representing phonology in spelling.

Language-specific patterns of performance were obtained on analyses of poor spellers' rudimentary ability to represent the phonological skeleton of words. Specifically, English poor spellers showed significantly greater problems with this level of representation than French poor spellers, who, in turn, showed little sign of impairment on this aspect of spelling.

When these phonological skeleton errors were examined in terms of omissions of consonant and vowel graphemes, language-specific differences emerged that replicated earlier findings for French (Alegria and Mousty, 1994, 1996) and English (Read, 1975; Stage and Wagner, 1992; Treiman, 1993) children. First, it was found that good spellers in both languages omitted segments extremely rarely (up to 1%). This was also true of the French poor spellers whose omission rates for vowels were less than 1%, and slightly (but not significantly) higher for consonants. In contrast, English poor spellers produced omission rates of approximately 13% for consonants and 22% for vowels. Thus, whereas both French and English poor spellers experience difficulties in representing the phonological content of words, English spellers demonstrate an additional deficit in representing the phonological structure of words, particularly with vowels.

It is important to note that omission errors cannot simply be explained in terms of a more complex orthography, as there is no logical reason why phonemes with more complex grapheme mappings should lead to higher omission rates. The hypothesis put forward at the beginning of the chapter was that the ability to represent the speech segments in words may be specifically related to patterns of lexical stress. This hypothesis was supported by the finding that English poor spellers were significantly more likely to omit vowels in unstressed syllables that contained reduced vowels than those in stressed syllables.

The present study had several limitations. First, the number of poor spellers in each group was small, thus possibly reducing the reliability of the finding. Second, the French good-speller group performed at ceiling on the word test, which precluded meaningful comparisons with that group on that task. Third, the spelling tests administered were not standardized and thus the possibility exists that despite all attempts at equating the French and English test forms, the tests were not of equal difficulty. Despite these limitations, which need to be redressed in future work, a number of findings in this study are compelling. First, the general patterns of results were replicated in all but one analysis on both word and nonword tests. This suggests that between-language differences, especially between poor spellers, reflected language-specific difficulties and not inequalities between French and English test versions. Second, although both groups of poor spellers demonstrated difficulties at the level of phonology, English poor spellers were clearly more impaired in their ability to represent the phonological structure of words, which in turn requires good phonemic segmentation skills. Finally, the differences in omission rates between the two poor speller groups, as well as the finding that vowel omission rates varied as a function of stress type in English poor spellers, indicate that the relative differences between English and French poor spellers cannot be attributed solely to factors of orthographic complexity. Phonological characteristics of languages also affect the types of difficulty that children experience in their literacy skills.

References

Alegria J, Mousty P (1994) On the development of lexical and non-lexical spelling procedures of French-speaking normal and disabled children. In G Brown, N Ellis (eds), Handbook of spelling: theory, process and intervention, pp 211–226. Chichester: John Wiley & Sons.

Alegria J, Mousty P (1996) The development of spelling procedures in French-speaking, normal and reading-disabled children: effects of frequency and lexicality. Journal of Experimental Child Psychology 63: 312–338.

Bruck M (1988) The word recognition and spelling of dyslexic children. Reading Research Quarterly 23: 51–69.

Bruck M (1990) Word recognition skills of adults with childhood diagnosis of dyslexia. Developmental Psychology 26: 439–454.

Bruck M, Waters G (1988) An analysis of the spelling errors of children who differ in their reading and spelling skills. Applied Psycholinguistics 9: 77–92.

Bruck M, Waters G (1990) Effects of reading skills on component spelling skills. Applied Psycholinguistics 11: 425–437.

Bruck M, Genesee F, Caravolas M (1997) A cross-linguistic study of early literacy acquisition. In B Blachman (ed), Foundations of reading acquisition and dyslexia: Implications for early intervention, pp 145–162. Mahwah, NJ: Lawrence Erlbaum Associates.

Bruck M, Treiman R, Caravolas M, Genesee F, Cassar M (1998) Spelling skills of children in whole language and phonics classrooms. Applied Psycholinguistics 19: 669–684.

Bryant PE, Bradley L (1985) Children's reading problems. Oxford: Blackwell.

Caravolas M, Bruck M (1993) The effect of oral and written language input on children's phonological awareness: a cross-linguistic study. Journal of Experimental Child Psychology 55: 1–30.

Cassar M, Treiman R (1997) The beginnings of orthographic knowledge: children's knowledge of double letters in words. Journal of Educational Psychology 89: 631–644.

Cossu G, Shankweiler D, Liberman IY, Katz L, Tola G (1988) Awareness of phonological segments and reading ability in Italian children. Applied Psycholinguistics 9: 1–16.

Delattre P (1965) Comparing the phonetic features of English, French, German and Spanish. Heidelberg: Julius Groos Verlag.

Delattre P (1981) Studies in comparative phonetics: English, German, Spanish, and French. Heidelberg: Julius Groos Verlag.

Frith U (1980) Unexpected spelling problems. In U Frith (ed) Cognitive processes in spelling, pp 495-515. Toronto: Academic Press.

Goswami U, Gombert J-E, de Berrera LF (1998) Children's orthographic representations and linguistic transparency: nonsense word reading in English, French and Spanish. Applied Psycholinguistics 19: 19-52.

Gottfried T (1984) Effects of consonant context on the perception of French vowels. Journal of Phonetics 12: 91-114.

Halle M, Vergnaud J (1987) An essay on stress. Cambridge, MA: MIT Press.

Hatcher P, Hulme C, Ellis AW (1994) Ameliorating early reading failure by integrating the teaching of reading and phonological skills: the phonological linkage hypothesis. Child Development 65: 41-57.

Juel C, Griffith P, Gough P (1986) Acquisition of literacy: a longitudinal study of children in first and second grade. Journal of Educational Psychology 78: 243-255.

Kenyon JS (1950) American pronunciation, 10th edn. Ann Arbor: George Wahr.

Landerl K, Wimmer H (2000) Deficits in phoneme segmentation are not the core problem of dyslexia: Evidence from German and English children. Applied Psycholinguistics 21: 243-262.

Landerl K, Wimmer H, Frith U (1997) The impact of orthographic consistency on dyslexia: a German-English comparison. Cognition 63: 315-334.

Lennox D, Siegel L (1993) Visual and phonological spelling errors in subtypes of children with learning disabilities. Applied Psycholinguistics 14: 473-488.

Lindgren S, De Renzi E, Richman L (1985) Cross-national comparisons of developmental dyslexia in Italy and the United States. Child Development 56: 1404-1417.

Morais J, Cluytens M, Alegria J (1984) Segmentation abilities of dyslexics and normal readers. Perceptual and Motor Skills 58: 221-222.

Olson R (1985) Disabled reading processes and cognitive profiles. In D Gray, J Kavanagh (eds) Biobehavioral measures of dyslexia, pp 215-243. Parkton: York Press.

Peereman R, Content A (1997) Orthographic and phonological neighborhoods in naming: not all neighbors are equally influential in orthographic space. Journal of Memory and Language 37: 382-410.

Raven JC, Summers B (1986) Manual for Raven's Progressive Matrices and Vocabulary Scales (Research supplement no. 3). London: Lewis.

Read C (1975) Children's categorizations of speech sounds in English (NCTE Research Report Number 17). Urbana, IL: National Council of Teachers of English.

Rohl M, Tunmer W (1988) Phonemic segmentation skill and spelling acquisition. Applied Psycholinguistics 9: 335-349.

Shankweiler D, Liberman IY (1972) Misreading: a search for causes. In JF Kavanagh, IG Mattingley (eds), Language by ear and by eye: the relationships between speech and reading, pp 293-317. Cambridge, MA: MIT Press.

Siegel L, Ryan E (1988) Development of grammatical sensitivity, phonological, and short-term memory skills in normally achieving and learning disabled children. Developmental Psychology 24: 28-37.

Snowling M, Goulandris N, Defty N (1996) A longitudinal study of reading development in dyslexic children. Journal of Educational Psychology 88: 653-669.

Sprenger-Charolles L, Siegel L (1997) A longitudinal study of the effects of syllabic structure on the development of reading and spelling skills in French. Applied Psycholinguistics 18: 485-505.

Sprenger-Charolles L, Siegel L, Bonnet P (1998) Reading and spelling acquisition in French: the role of phonological mediation and orthographic factors. Journal of Experimental Child Psychology 68: 134-165.

Stage S, Wagner R (1992) Development of young children's phonological and orthographic knowledge as revealed by their spellings. Developmental Psychology 28: 287-296.

Treiman R (1993) Beginning to spell: a study of first grade children. New York: Oxford University Press.

Treiman R (1994) Use of consonant letter names in beginning spelling. Developmental Psychology 30: 567-580.

Treiman R (1997) Spelling in normal children and dyslexics. In B Blachman (ed) Foundations of reading acquisition and dyslexia: implications for early intervention, pp 191-218. Mahwah, NJ: Lawrence Erlbaum Associates.

Treiman R, Berch D, Tincoff R, Weatherston S (1993a) Phonology and spelling: the case of syllabic consonants. Journal of Experimental Child Psychology 56: 267-290.

Treiman R, Berch D, Weatherston S (1993b) Children's use of phoneme-grapheme correspondences in spelling: Roles of position and stress. Journal of Educational Psychology 85: 466-477.

Waters G, Bruck M, Malus-Abramowitz M (1988) The role of linguistic and visual information in spelling: a developmental study. Journal of Experimental Child Psychology 45: 400-421.

Wimmer H (1993) Characteristics of developmental dyslexia in a regular writing system. Applied Psycholinguistics 14: 1-33.

Wimmer H (1996) The early manifestation of developmental dyslexia: evidence from German children. Reading and Writing 8: 171-188.

Wimmer H, Goswami U (1994) The influence of orthographic consistency on reading development: word recognition in English and German children. Cognition 51: 91-103.

Wimmer H, Landerl K (1997) How learning to spell German differs from learning to spell English. In C Perfetti, L Rieben, M Fayol (eds) Learning to spell: research, theory, and practice, pp 81-96. Mahwah, NJ: Lawrence Erlbaum Associates.

Ziegler JC, Jacobs AM, Stone GO (1996) Statistical analysis of the bidirectional inconsistency of spelling and sound in French. Behavior Research Methods Instruments and Computers 28: 504-515.

Chapter 10
The spelling errors of Norwegian good and poor decoders: a developmental cross-linguistic perspective

BENTE E HAGTVET AND SOLVEIG-ALMA H LYSTER

Knowledge of normal reading and spelling development is, to a large extent, based on English-speaking individuals. English orthography differs from many other alphabetic orthographies in terms of its low phoneme–grapheme consistency (e.g. Venezky, 1970). In a series of recent studies, variations in spelling and reading development across orthographic systems have been investigated extensively (Wimmer and Hummer 1990; Wimmer and Goswami, 1994; Cossu et al., 1995; Treiman and Cassar, 1997; Valtin, 1997). A number of these studies have compared the reading abilities of English-speaking children acquiring English orthography with children acquiring other orthographies, especially German (Wimmer and Goswami, 1994; Goswami et al., 1995; Landerl, 1997; Landerl et al., 1997). These studies suggest that the degree of regularity and complexity of the different orthographies influence both the manner and the speed with which children learn to read and spell. German-speaking poor readers, for example, have been documented to read even nonwords accurately, although slowly, in contrast to English-speaking poor readers who typically show severe problems in reading nonwords (Wimmer and Frith, 1994).

Most of the studies comparing the development of literacy in different orthographies have been concerned with reading development. There are, however, important exceptions to this. Valtin (1997) and Wimmer and Landerl (1997) evaluated German-speaking children's spelling development. They found that German-speaking children at the end of first grade generally produced phonemically acceptable word spellings and showed few signs of phonologically based spelling errors. In other words, German-speaking children appear to break the alphabetic code relatively easily and depend less on an inadequate logographic strategy than English-speaking children in the early grades. The authors explain these differences with reference to the transparency and complexity of the two orthographies, and differences in reading instruction in British and Austrian schools. The German orthography is more transparent than English, and beginning reading instruction in both Austria and Germany places heavy emphasis on phonics as well as focusing on regular words with one-to-one grapheme–phoneme correspondences. On these grounds, greater knowledge of how literacy development takes place in orthographies other than English appears important to our understanding of how children come to terms with the alphabetic code and how we understand reading problems, which in turn has implications for effective teaching strategies.

The present study focuses on spelling development in Norwegian. We compare spelling errors made by a group of good readers with those made by a group of poor readers to establish whether the spelling development of these two groups differs in degree or kind. The results will be related to similar studies in other orthographic and school contexts. Spelling development in Norwegian has rarely been studied and, is, for this reason alone worth increased attention (but see Gjessing, 1986; Wiggen, 1990; Elsness, 1991; Thygesen, 1993; Bråten, 1994). In a comparative perspective, it is interesting for a number of reasons. First, on a continuum of transparency where Portuguese and Finish would be considered highly regular (one-to-one relation between phonemes and graphemes) and English would be considered extremely irregular (one-to-many relations between phonemes and graphemes), Norwegian lies in an intermediate position, but with a substantially more transparent orthography than English (Elley, 1992). Second, instruction in Norwegian schools is generally more phonically oriented than is the case in British schools, but generally not so consistently phonically oriented as Austrian and German instruction (see also Hagtvet and Lyster, 1998). Knowledge of Norwegian children's spelling development should therefore shed light on the importance of orthography and instruction for literacy development.

The Norwegian orthography

Norwegian, like English and German, is an alphabetic script. The Norwegian phonological system comprises approximately 40 phonemes, and the Norwegian alphabet has 29 letters. Children in the present study came from the Oslo area. The sound structure and the orthography are more transparent in the Oslo dialect than in some other Norwegian dialects (Thygesen, 1993) (see note 1). Most phonemes are represented by graphemes consisting of one letter. Only one Norwegian grapheme has three letters, *skj* for /ʃ/. The phoneme /ʃ/ is represented by *skj* in most words, but can also be represented by *s*, *sk*, *sj* and *rs*, and in loan words by *sch* (*schæfer*), *ch* (*charm*), *g* (*geni*), j (*journalist*) and *sh* (*shorts*). Relatively few phonemes are represented by two letters, for example /ʈ/ is written *rt*, /ŋ/ is written *ng*, /ɳ/ is written *rn*, /ɖ/ is written *rd* and /ç/ is written *kj*, or *k* when preceding the sounds /iː/, /i/, /yː/ and /y/, or in a small number of words *tj*.

While the main principle that governs Norwegian orthography is phonemic, there are exceptions related to morphology. Morphemes are spelled the same even if pronounced differently in different but related words. The word *trygt* /trykt/ (neutral for 'safe') is, for example, spelled with a *g* even though the /g/ sounds like a *k* because the root is spelled *trygg* /tryg/. Norwegian also has many long compound words that are hard to read unless one identifies the morphemes instead of using sequential decoding of single graphemes.

Spelling strategies

Learning to spell is a complex task and involves the integration of a number of skills: phonological, syntactic and semantic knowledge; analogical reasoning on the basis of orthographic patterns in visual memory; and knowledge of orthographic rules and conventions (e.g. Bradley and Bryant, 1981; Henderson and Templeton, 1986; Bruck and Treiman, 1990; Gough et al., 1992). Given that a script represents an approximation of the sound structure of a language, the characteristics of children's phonological systems and metalinguistic knowledge would be expected to be reflected in their spellings. Studies by Read (1971) and Treiman (1993), among others, have shown that a child learning to read and spell in an alphabetic script constructs a theory of how speech sounds relate to graphemes. This constructive process involves forming, testing and modifying hypotheses about sound–letter relationships and the orthographic system. This process and the strategies the child adopts are, however, often hidden. The most revealing window on this process is provided by the child's spelling errors and how they change with development.

The driving force behind this development is presumably an interaction between the child's underlying skills, the structure of the orthography and the environmental input. The more a child reads and writes, the faster and more automated will be the transition from sounds to graphemes in spelling and from graphemes to sounds in reading (Stanovich and West, 1989). However, we know that individual differences in developing reading and writing skills are considerable. While some children appear to develop from a pre-alphabetic competence to fluent spelling rapidly, other children struggle to master basic skills.

Much of what is known about early spelling development derives from children with precocious spelling skills while less is known about the various roads to conventional spelling taken by average to poor spellers (but see Lennox and Siegel, 1994; Frost, 1998). A core problem in poor readers appears to be a reduced sensitivity to the phonological structure of language (e.g. Perfetti, 1985; Snowling, 1987; Wagner and Torgesen, 1987; Stanovich, 1988; Lundberg and Høien, 1989; Olson et al., 1990). Lennox and Siegel (1994) studied poor and good English spellers in grade 2 and found that the two groups made more or less equal proportions of 'visual errors'. However, in grade 3, the good spellers made use of phonological strategies, while the poor spellers continued to rely on visual memory skills when spelling difficult words (see note 2). These differences persisted until the children reached a spelling level of grade 6. Such findings corroborate other results from English-speaking communities, where poor spellers appear to rely more on visual memory skills when spelling (e.g. regular and long words) than do good spellers, who typically make use of phonemic strategies (Frith, 1985; Henderson and Templeton, 1986).

German-speaking children, on the other hand, seem to rely heavily on phonological coding and grapheme–phoneme correspondences with the support of articulation right from the beginning (Valtin, 1997, p 190): 'The long logographic phase that has been proclaimed by Frith for English-speaking children seems not to be typical for German children. Only poor readers and spellers who have not yet grasped the alphabetic principle have been observed to use this strategy', and in most cases it disappears during grade 1. In a longitudinal study of German-speaking first graders, Klicpera and Gasteiger-Klicpera (1993) focused on this developmental difference between good and poor readers. Good readers showed little evidence of logographic reading during their first months in school, while the persistently poor readers started with logographic strategies and showed no evidence of phonological recoding before the middle of the school year.

Thus, the picture emerging is that English-speaking children start as mainly logographic readers and spellers, and while most of them develop into phonological readers and spellers as time goes by, poor readers continue to rely heavily on visual memory skills. German-speaking children on the other hand, generally depend on phonological coding right from the beginning in both reading and spelling. The exceptions are persistently poor readers who read logographically until the middle of the first year when they get a better hold of phonologically-based strategies. However, this picture is not universally accepted. Research on English-speaking beginning spellers is inconsistent with respect to the dominance of logographic reading in the early years of schooling. Some have suggested that beginning spellers primarily use phonological cues and as they become more experienced, memory for visual chunks and analogies are more frequently used (e.g. Barron, 1980; Bryant and Bradley, 1980; Ehri and Robbins, 1992; Treiman,

1994). One possible explanation of this apparent inconsistency presumably reflects the fact that the 'beginning spellers' may vary in chronological age and print experience in different studies.

While a fair amount of attention has been paid to the potential role that the orthographic system pays to individual differences in spelling development, less systematic research interest has addressed the possible contribution made by reading and spelling methods (but see Landerl, 2000, Chapters 2, 4, and 5 in this volume). Teaching practices may play a role in determining patterns of normal development and the patterns of difficulties displayed in learning to read and spell. In Austrian and German schools – as is typically also the case in other countries where reading and spelling is taught via fairly consistent orthographic systems, such as Finnish, Italian, Dutch and Portuguese – reading and spelling is typically taught via straightforward phonic teaching methods. Perhaps this is because accumulated experience has guided teachers in their preference for these methods. On the other hand, English-speaking children are, as a rule, exposed to a combination of whole-word and phonic methods – often with a priority given to whole words. The complexity of the English orthographic system might well be responsible for the extensive use of whole-word teaching approaches in English-speaking countries, where children are also often encouraged to read books from the very beginning of reading instruction (Goodman, 1967; Smith, 1978). This 'look-and-say' method in English and American schools may in turn foster logographic strategies on the part of their children (Valtin, 1997).

We have limited knowledge of the dual effects that orthography and teaching methods have on literacy development. Recent research, however, indicates that it may be larger than previously assumed (see for example Landerl, 1997). A study by Wimmer and Goswami (1994) found that children aged 7, 8 and 9 years learning to read in English and German had similar reading speed and error rates on a word-reading task, but the German- speaking Austrian children showed a big advantage in reading nonwords compared to the English children. This suggests that young German-speaking children made use of a phonologically-based reading strategy, while the English-speaking children to a larger extent used a logographic (partial visual recognition) approach. The different approaches adopted by the Austrian and English children were interpreted by Wimmer and Goswami as a combined effect of the different orthographies and teaching methods in the two countries.

Norwegian reading instruction has traditionally been dominated by phonic teaching methods. In the 1970s, Ulrika Leimar introduced the language experience approach to the Scandivavian scene (Leimar, 1974). She emphasized the importance of language experience and the use of texts composed by children and dictated to the teacher as the material for reading. This focus on the child's own experience and interest has had a considerable impact on Norwegian teaching practices in the past two decades. However, while the language experience approach has been widely accepted in many classrooms, much attention continues to be paid to phonics. Therefore, if the combined effect of orthography and teaching method is as influential as suggested by the studies on German-speaking children, Norwegian children would be expected to develop their reading and spelling more in line with German- than English-speaking children.

Spelling development

On the assumption that children's non-standard spellings reflect their developing sense of the linguistic properties of words, developmental descriptions of misspellings of young children have been prolific (Read, 1971, 1975, 1986; Gentry, 1978; Henderson and Beers, 1980; Ehri, 1985). A common basis for these descriptions is the idea that spelling errors provide an index of children's metalinguistic understanding and that children move through distinct stages of spelling (Ellis, 1994). This does not mean that a child makes use of only one strategy at a time. Rather, one and the same child typically operates with mixed strategies cutting across a number of the stages mentioned below. However, at each point in time a child's spelling appears to be dominated by one strategy more than by others, and the developmental sequence observed appears to be fairly similar across different ages of formal introduction to the alphabetic script and across different orthographies, including English (Henderson and Beers, 1980; Bear and Templeton, 1998), Spanish (Ferreiro and Teberosky, 1983); Norwegian (Hagtvet, 1989), Danish (Frost, 1998) and German (Scheerer-Neumann, 1993; Spitta, 1993; Valtin, 1997). The general developmental pattern is typically characterized as a process of continuous changes from prephonetic via semiphonetic and phonemic spellings to phonemic spelling with integration of orthographic regularities and finally conventional spellings (see for example Ellis, 1994).

Previous Norwegian studies replicate the general descriptions of developmental stages of English-speaking children (Hagtvet, 1989; Elsness, 1991), but they do not in any systematic fashion study the non-standard spellings of children moving from semiphonetic to conventional spellings. Lyster (1995), however, found that Norwegian children after eight to nine months in grade 1 made very few errors when spelling complex regular words such as *elektrisk* (electric), *struts* (ostrich) and *nifst* (scary) and nonwords such as *prakto*, *fakati* and *burt*. This is in line with knowledge about phoneme–grapheme correspondences found in German-speaking children early on in grade 1.

In the present study, we examine the possible differences in strategies adopted by poor and good readers in grade 1 when moving from semiphonetic to conventional spelling, with an explicit focus on similarities and differences between Norwegian-, English- and German-speaking children.

Method

Participants

Sampling

The sample consisted of 60 children from families where at least one of the parents had current or previous reading problems. (This sample is a subsample of a larger sample of children from dyslexic families and their controls; Hagtvet et al., 1998.) Subjects were recruited via the media, the Norwegian Dyslexia Association, local newspapers and community health clinics in the Oslo and Akershus county.

Age of assessment

The children in the present study were on average 8-years-old at the time of assessment at the end of grade 1. They had by then had nine months of formal instruction in reading and writing.

Intelligence

Intelligence was assessed at age 5 using the Wechsler Pre-school and Primary Scale of Intelligence (WPPSI). Only children with a non-verbal score of 85 and above (52 out of 60 children) were included in this study (average IQ at age 5 on WPPSI was 105 with a range of 85–133).

Schooling

All children attended different schools and were taught reading by different combinations of phonic and whole-language instruction, but with a strong emphasis on phonics. The educational system in Norway, from an international perspective, would be described as of good quality and teaching the children to read and write is given top priority in the first grades in all schools (see note 3). The participants had been assessed annually for our research project since they were 5 years old. In addition to general language, problem-solving and motor abilities, the assessments focused on different aspects of linguistic awareness, in particular phonological awareness. Since these assessments were usually observed by one of the parents, they presumably learnt about the strengths and weaknesses of their child, and also about the importance we saw in the mastery of different aspects of oral language. We shall not neglect the possible impact this awareness may have had on the activities taking place in the children's homes.

Parental reading disorders and socioeconomic background

Preliminary analyses indicated that the affected parents fell within the category of 'dyslexic', but that their current difficulties varied depending on the degree of the original problem and quality of the education they had received. Socioeconomically the families cut across the whole span of educational levels and occupations. Most – including the dyslexic parents – had finished nine years of compulsory education and also had some occupational training. However, only a few of the affected parents had a college degree at the Bachelor level, while a greater number of the non-affected parents had. Generally, the parents showed a high degree of knowledge, awareness and concern about their children, which is typically associated with middle-class and upper-middle-class values. It is likely that this is partly a consequence of the way the families were recruited to the project.

Procedures

Subgrouping

The children were given a range of reading and spelling tasks nine months after starting school, i.e. between the ages of 7:5 and 8:4. The basis for subgrouping the children was a standardized word-reading task, consisting of 20 words (Nasjonalt læremiddelsenter (The National Centre for Teaching Aids), 1995). The children were asked to match a written word to a picture (out of a selection of four). The testing was timed, and 23 children, i.e. 44% of the sample, answered all the items correctly. These children were grouped as 'good readers'. In a national standardization, 69% of the 1300 children (the same age range as for our group) tested at the age of 8 years got all items correct. At the lower end, 21 children, i.e. 41% of the children included in the analyses, fell under the critical score of 17, which in the Norwegian standardization was the cut-off score at the 22nd percentile below which children were considered 'at risk'. These 21 children were classified as poor readers. These children of dyslexic parents thus have approximately twice as many poor readers among them as would be expected in a representative sample. They also have a smaller number of good readers.

Materials

Word and nonword spelling were assessed. Word spelling was tested using a short form of the Norwegian version of the Aston index (Sivertsen, 1986); it consists of 30 familiar words varying in length, regularity and graphemic complexity (see Appendix A). Nonword spelling was assessed by a short form of a Norwegian reading test designed by Klinkenberg and Skar (1994). It consists of 16 nonwords varying in length, regularity and graphemic complexity (See Appendix A). The children were told to write each word and nonword according to the experimenter's dictation. Each item was presented twice, and a context was given for the words to ensure that the child understood the word's meaning.

Results and discussion

Reading and spelling in good and poor readers

According to their word-reading performance, the good and poor readers had reached very different levels of automatization of reading ability. We therefore concluded that a comparison of the non-standard spellings made by these two groups would shed light on the challenges facing reading-disabled children learning to read and spell, and also on the stages involved in developing a mastery of Norwegian orthography.

The correlation between word reading and spelling was found to be 0.77, suggesting that most poor readers were also poor spellers. This corroborates other findings underscoring a strong relationship between spelling and reading in the early stages of learning (Juel et al., 1986; Cataldo and Ellis, 1988). It also legitimizes our methodological approach of studying how children come to terms with the alphabetic system by studying the non-standard spellings made by poor and good readers. Yet we should also note that with a correlation of 0.77, there may still be children who are good readers but poor spellers and vice versa.

A series of analyses of variance were run to assess the differences between poor readers and good readers on word reading, spelling and intelligence. The results are presented in Table 10.1.

As may be seen in Table 10.1, no differences were found between the poor and good readers for verbal and performance IQ. This confirms our

Table 10.1 Word reading, word spelling, nonword spelling and intelligence for good and poor readers

Measure	Good readers (n = 23)		Poor readers (n = 21)		F	p
	Mean	s.d.	Mean	s.d.		
Word reading (max = 20)	20	–	12.67	3.61	95.12	< 0.000
Word spelling (max = 30)	26.32	3.85	20.52	6.54	12.68	< 0.001
Nonword spelling (max = 16)	12.64	3.06	10.52	4.80	2.99	n.s.
WPPSI, performance IQ	111.17	13.56	105.10	11.32	2.58	n.s.
WPPSI, verbal IQ	103.00	10.57	97.76	10.40	2.74	n.s.

s.d., standard deviation; n.s., not significant.

expectation based on the criteria for subgrouping the children, that the low scores of the poor readers and spellers cannot be explained by low intellectual ability. The problems of these poor readers therefore are likely to be the ones commonly associated with specific reading problems (dyslexia).

Since reaching ceiling was a criterion for being classified as a good reader, the mean score for word reading in the group of good readers equalled the maximum score of 20. The poor readers on the other hand read an average of only 12 of the words correctly. As most of these words are short and highly frequent, this result reflects a fairly low reading level. For word spelling, the difference between the groups is also highly significant, while no statistically significant difference was observed for nonword spelling. The difference in results between word spelling and nonword spelling may partly be explained by differences in orthographic complexity and irregularity. Some of the words in the word spelling test are irregular and some words have multiple-letter graphemes, while the nonwords are generally regular and somewhat less phonologically and orthographically complex.

It is notable that even the poor readers had broken the alphabetic code as demonstrated by their spelling of words and nonwords. After only nine months of formal education even poor readers were able to segment the phonemes correctly when the phonemic structure was regular. They could also connect the phonemes to the relevant graphemes. Only two poor readers had problems at this most elementary level, and even they were capable of partial segmentation by spelling the first and last phonemes correctly. However, as will become evident in the next section, the poor readers had great problems in spelling irregular words and words containing complex letter–sound relationships.

Qualitative analyses of spelling errors

Table 10.2 shows the degree to which the good and poor readers mastered a selection of 15 words and five nonwords. These words and nonwords were selected because they illustrate well the kinds of words that were easy or difficult for the two groups.

The first 11 words in Table 10.2 are spelled regularly, while the following four are irregular (in the dialect spoken by our children). The regularly spelled words are semantically familiar yet not so frequent that there is a high probability that they may be spelled logographically. (The one possible exception to this is the first word, *sol*, which is used in all textbooks for beginning readers.) The regular words vary in degree of phonological and orthographic complexity. (Words with consonant clusters (*seks*, *bamse*) are phonologically complex, while words that contain phonemes represented by two-letter graphemes (digraphs) are orthographically complex.) The irregularly spelled words vary in degree of irregularity and frequency/

Table 10.2 Percent correct spellings of words and nonwords in poor and good readers

Words/ Nonwords		Poor readers (n = 21) %	Good readers (n = 23) %
Words			
1	sol /su:l)/ (sun)	100	100
2	fem /fem/ (five)	86	100
3	rose /ru:sə/ (rose)	86	100
4	sile /si:lə/ (filter)	86	100
5	lese /le:sə/ (read)	86	96
6	seks /seks/ (six)	81	91
7	bamse /bamsə/ (teddybear)	81	96
8	damer /da:mər/ (ladies)	67	96
9	gøy /gœy/ (fun)	48	83
10	bort /buʈ/ (away)	52	96
11	lenger /leŋər/ (longer/any more)	10	74
12	med /me:/ (with)	29	87
13	det /de:/ (it/that)	33	70
14	jeg /jæi/ (I)	70	96
15	seg /sæi/ (himself, herself) themselves)	24	70
Nonwords			
16	båf /bɔ:f/	67	70
17	gål /gɔ:l/	76	78
18	pøvy /pœ:vy/	57	52
19	bnof /bnu:f/	67	82
20	skjang /ʃaŋ/	0	18

familiarity. The words *jeg* and *seg* are the most irregular ones in this sample of words. However, they are also among the most frequently used, but *jeg* more so than *seg*. Therefore, the extent to which these two words are conventionally spelled is presumably suggestive of the influence of 'sight reading', and also of the ease with which a possible orthographic spelling of *jeg* is generalized to the less frequent word, *seg*. The nonwords are regularly spelled, but vary in degree of phoneme–grapheme complexity. The word *sjang* is the most complex since both /ʃ/ and /ŋ/ are represented by multiple letters.

As can be seen in Table 10.2, both the poor and the good readers made very few mistakes on the first seven words, which are all spelled regularly (good readers > 90% correct, poor readers > 80% correct). These included two phonologically complex words containing a consonant cluster (*seks* (6), *bamse* (7)). When the distinctiveness of phonemes is less clear, as in *damer* (8) and *gøy* (9), the poor readers made more mistakes than did good readers (*damer* (8) was mastered by 67% of the poor readers, and *gøy* (9) by 48%). The good readers in general (> 80%) continued to produce standard spellings. (The plural *-er* in 'damer' contains an unstressed vowel /ə/, and this was omitted by many poor readers, as in <u>damr</u>, presumably because it is represented by the letter name for /r/. The diphthong, *øy* in *gøy* representing /œy/ 'sounds like' /œi/ or /œj/, and many poor and good readers spelled this diphthong in a phonetically correct manner.

When the words contained phonemes represented by multiple-letter graphemes (*bort* (10) and *lenger* (11)), the good readers still spelled more than 70% of the words correctly, while poor readers made more mistakes. The *-rt* in *bort* represents a retroflex sound in the Oslo area and was spelled conventionally by 52% of poor and 96% of good readers respectively. The *-ng-* in *lenger* represents the nasal /ŋ/, and was spelled conventionally by 10% and 74% of poor and good readers respectively.

Frequent irregular words (e.g. *jeg* /jæɪ/ (14)) were on the whole mastered better than less frequent words (e.g. *seg* /sæi/ (15)) by poor as well as by good readers. As many as 70% of poor and 96% of good readers spelled *jeg* conventionally, while only 24% of poor and 70% of good readers spelled *seg* conventionally. This difference is important because *jeg* and *seg* are similar in all respects other than familiarity – in pronunciation (/jæi/ /sæi/), in grammatical category (both are pronouns) and in spelling pattern. Still they apparently pose very different demands on the children at this age.

The number of times a word has been seen appears to be an extremely influential variable in learning irregular spelling patterns. It is noteworthy that this is the case even in a fairly regular orthography like Norwegian – and is apparently more important than learning to spell by analogy on the basis of similarity of grammatical category and pronunciation, at least at this age. Familiarity, in fact, appears to be more important than degree of regularity, as words with only minor irregularities, e.g. *med* (12) and *det* (13) were mastered less well than the highly familiar, but also highly irregular *jeg* (14). (The only irregularity of *med* and *det* is that the pronunciation leaves the final phonemes silent /me:/ and /de:/.)

The nonwords in Table 10.2 also confirm the pattern of difficulty that we have seen for the words. The short and regular nonwords (*båf* (16) and *gål* (17)) were mastered equally well by poor and good readers. This underscores the ease with which Norwegian children in general break the alphabetic code. When a consonant cluster is involved, as in *bnof* (19), the poor readers made more mistakes than the good readers, and this tendency was even more obvious for the word *sjang* (20), where none of the poor readers and only 18% of the good readers mastered the task. (The nonword *sjang* has the most complex orthographic pattern of the nonwords, since both /ʃ/ and /ŋ/ are represented by multiple letters *skj/sj* and *ng*.)

To sum up, the relative difficulty in spelling different words and nonwords was surprisingly similar in poor and good readers, even though the overall level of performance was better in the good readers. Both groups mastered short and regular words and nonwords, indicating that almost all children mastered the alphabetic code and were able to apply it correctly in spelling even for phonologically complex words. When a word had a more complex orthographic pattern (e.g. a digraph) or was spelled irregularly, it became more challenging for both good and poor readers, but more so for the poor readers. Thus, on the basis of these findings, three variables stand out as potential explanations of the observed differences in spelling performance: the regularity of the script; the complexity of the orthographic system; and the degree of familiarity of the individual word. Familiarity was particularly crucial for irregularly spelled words (*jeg* versus *seg*). This observation, in addition to the observation that overall performance was so much higher for the good readers (who had presumably had more exposure to written words) for words that were only slightly irregular (*med*) or words which contained digraphs (*bort, lenger*), speaks for the importance of familiarity. These observations contribute to the explanation of the finding in Table 10.1 that there were statistically significant differences between poor and good readers for words, but not for nonwords. Children who were good readers had seen these more challenging words more often, and therefore presumably had a better grasp of their spelling. On the other hand, nonwords, which may be spelled phonologically, did not cause a great problem for either the good or the poor readers.

These Norwegian data therefore suggest that the spelling performance of poor readers (who are genetically at risk for dyslexia) are not qualitatively different from those of good readers. Furthermore, both groups appear to master the alphabetic system at an elementary level, even when dealing with phonologically rather complex words. The performance of both good and poor readers is, however, strongly influenced by characteristics of the orthographic system (regularity and complexity), but this effect is more pronounced for the poor readers.

These findings invite us to explore further the hypothesis that the differences between good and poor readers were of degree rather than of kind. The non-standard spellings were therefore classified according to the degree to which the phonological structure of the words was preserved. The ability to transform the sound pattern of a word into a graphemic pattern involves manipulating the phonological structure of a word, and this, according to much recent research, is a primary problem for many children with reading problems (e.g. Snowling, 1987; Lundberg and Høien, 1989). The non-standard spellings produced by our 52 children were therefore classified into 12 categories, and these were summarized in the four following types (the 12 subcategories with examples are presented in parentheses and Appendix B):

A Correct phonemic spelling, including phonemic spellings in combination
   with letter names.
B Phonemic spelling with a reduced, but correct phonemic representation
   involving omissions.
C Phonemically inaccurate spellings involving substitution, reversal or
   addition of phonemes.
D Unclassifiable spellings (see note 4).

The distribution of error types across reading groups is presented in Table
10.3.

The majority of the "errors" for words made by the good readers reflect a
'correct phonemic structure' (category A). As many as 78% of their non-
standard spellings of words were of this kind, while the other "errors" were
more or less evenly distributed in the other categories. For nonwords, 48% of
their "errors" reflected a correct phonemic structure (category A), 23%
reflected a 'partial phonemic structure' (category B), another 20% reflected
an 'inaccurate phonemic structure' (category C) and only 10% were

Table 10.3 Non-standard spellings for words and nonwords in good and poor readers

		Good readers		Poor readers	
Category		No of "errors"[a]	%	No of "errors"[b]	%
A Correct phonemic structure					
	words	64	78	106	56.1
	nonwords	40	47.6	27	23.9
B Partial phonemic structure					
	words	6	7.3	36	17
	nonwords	19	22.6	28	24.8
C Inaccurate phonemic structure					
	words	9	11	14	7.4
	nonwords	17	20.2	11	9.7
D Unclassifiable					
	words	3	3.7	33	17.5
	nonwords	8	9.5	47	41.6

[a]Total number of "errors" in good readers = 82 for words and 84 for nonwords.
[b]Total number of "errors" in poor readers = 189 for words and 113 for nonwords.

'multiple/unclassifiable', i.e. responses that indicate a serious breakdown of the phonological structure.

The non-standard spellings made by the poor readers showed a slightly different pattern. For words, most "errors" (56%) reflected a 'correct phonemic structure' (category A), 17% reflected a 'partial phonemic structure' (category B), 18% were 'multiple/unclassifiable' (category D) and only 7% were classified as 'inaccurate' (category C). For nonwords as many as 42% of the "errors" were 'multiple/unclassifiable' (category D), while 25% reflected a 'partial phonemic structure' (category B) and 24% a 'correct phonemic structure' (category A). Fewer of the "errors" of the poor readers, therefore, reflected a correct phonemic structure. However, this does not mean that the poor readers were 'spelling by sight'. Rather, they appeared to apply a phonological strategy, but in an imprecise or flawed manner. This may be deduced from the observation that the poor readers only produced three cases of spellings that contained elements that were clearly influenced by print, e.g. jge for jeg (/jei/). Also, as many as 49% of the "errors" made when spelling nonwords and 73% of the "errors" for real words may be explained phonologically with no trace of using visual strategies (categories A and B). (Comparable figures for the good readers were 70 and 85%.) Most of the regular words and nonwords were conventionally spelled (see Table 10.2), but in the face of irregular words and digraphs, the poor readers lost track of the phonological structure of the words (42% of the "errors" for nonwords in poor readers reflect a breakdown of the phonological structure (category D)). When unable to go by the rule, 'write as you speak', children with little reading experience and therefore presumably with reduced ability to recognize orthographic patterns visually, appear to be at a loss, and the phonological structure of spelling breaks down. This is in contrast to the good readers whose "errors" in similar cases appeared to be 'inaccurate' rather than 'multiple', i.e. less severely disrupted. It is also in contrast to the spelling of words in which the orthographic structure is more visually familiar. In this case only 18% of the poor readers' "errors" involved multiple or unclassifiable errors.

It should be emphasized that 10% of the good readers' "errors" for nonwords were also of this kind. And along the same lines of argument, 20% of the good readers' "errors" represented an inaccurate or disrupted phonemic structure. This suggests that even with good readers, attempts to represent the phonemic structure of challenging words occasionally failed, but this occurred less often and was less severe than was the case for poor readers. The good readers more typically substituted, added or reversed the position of phonemes, while the poor readers tended to make many mistakes in the same word, or they gave up completely. Again we observe degrees of difference rather than differences in kind, since all types of "errors", with one exception, were observed in both groups. The one exception is the category 'inability to spell' (which is categorized as unclassifiable). The good readers never completely failed to attempt a spelling.

Discussion and conclusions

We have analysed the spellings of beginning readers on the assumption that their spellings – and in particular their non-standard spellings – reveal their notions of speech sounds and how they relate to the orthographic system. By comparing the spellings of poor and good readers we gained insight into individual differences in both reading and spelling.

We found that, with two exceptions, all children independent of reading ability had broken the alphabetic code. Furthermore, poor readers spelled nonwords and regularly spelled words almost as well as did good readers. This is a surprising finding given that, in general, poor readers in English-speaking samples have problems when expected to manipulate the phonological structure of language. We should also remember that the children in this study constituted the poorest readers in a sample that was genetically at risk for developing difficulties with the written language. They were average to above-average in intelligence, and they scored below the 22nd percentile compared to a normal group of Norwegian children unselected for IQ. The only words that caused problems for the Norwegian poor readers were the low-frequency, irregularly spelled words and words with complex orthography, i.e. words with multiple-letter graphemes representing one phoneme. These were the very same words that in rare cases also caused problems for the good readers, as well as the same words that may typically cause problems for older reading-disabled children. This suggests that differences between normal and poor literacy development are a matter of degree rather than kind, or a reflection of a developmental lag rather than deviancy.

The qualitative analysis of non-standard spellings substantiated these findings. Most of the non-standard spellings by poor as well as good readers could be explained phonologically, and contained few signs of influence from orthographic patterns. (Both groups in fact produced only three cases of non-standard spellings that were influenced by orthography.) Rather, when making mistakes, both groups tended to be over-reliant on the use of a phonological strategy, even when tackling nonwords and irregular words, where orthographically based strategies would be the more appropriate alternative. However, poor readers tended to adhere more rigidly to a phonological strategy than did the good readers. These findings contrast with studies of English-speaking children's difficulties with the written language. Lennox and Siegel (1994) found that '...poor spellers, because of poor phonological skills, are more likely to successfully use their visual memory skills for the form of the words in their spelling. ...Our research suggests that good and poor spellers use different strategies to spell . . . . . . poor spellers display a deviant developmental pattern in learning to spell, rather than a developmental lag or immaturity' (Lennox and Siegel, 1994) (cf. also Juel et al., 1986). In contrast, our Norwegian results corroborate reports describing the spelling strategies of German-speaking children, e.g. those of Valtin (1997) and Landerl et al. (1997). These studies suggest – as did our study – that poor readers have relatively few difficulties applying the phonological principle. Both good and poor readers appear to make use of phonological strategies when spelling, but the good readers are better at it. Even though the phonological system of poor readers appeared intact at one level, they had problems in applying the system in linguistically demanding contexts.

In a cross-linguistic perspective, these findings indicate that variables like 'regularity' and 'complexity of the orthographic system' represent challenges that invite flexibility and variability in the use of spelling strategies. When mastery of a strategy is limited or shallow, it is a commonly observed phenomenon in cognitive psychology that behaviour regresses to a less advanced level of performance (e.g. Karmiloff-Smith, 1979, 1986). This is exactly what happened to the performance of the poor readers in our study when faced with irregular or complex spelling patterns. Their spellings did not reveal the phonemic structure of the spoken word as they did with the regular words and nonwords, but contained severe spelling errors. This indicates that the child either failed to represent the phonological structure of the word or was unable to perform a correct analysis of the phonemic structure when the structure became complex. In contrast, the good readers did not experience a breakdown of the phonemic structure to the same extent, but showed milder forms of disruption to the phonemic structure of the word. On this basis we would assume that a writing system with few or no digraphs or multi-letter graphemes is easier to learn than a writing system with many digraphs (cf. also Treiman, 1993). There thus appears to be an interaction between individually based phonological weaknesses and degree of linguistic challenge, which underscores the importance of context and environment for the development of reading problems, including the importance of teaching methods. In our study, the influence of teaching method could not be separated from the influence of orthography when comparisons were made cross-linguistically. What we can conclude is that the orthographic system, as well as teaching method, may increase or reduce the cognitive–linguistic challenges that reading and spelling impose on the child, and that the phonological weakness of a child will therefore manifest itself differently in different linguistic and educational contexts. Presumably, the more irregular or complex the orthographic system is, the more the teaching method used with beginning readers must shed light on the phonemic structure of words for the child to discover it. Landerl's (2000) comparative study of German- and English-speaking children suggests that both groups take advantage of a teaching method that emphasizes the phonemic structure of words by focusing on regular words, i.e. words with a transparent orthography. This is not to say that German-speaking children do not face problems with written language. They appear, however, to have less-marked problems than are reported for English-speaking children, and their problems are primarily with reading speed rather than reading accuracy. Cross-linguistic, longitudinal investigations of the interaction between an individual's mastery of the phoneme structure of words and teaching method in use should be a priority for future research.

Even though correlation is not evidence for causation, the high correlation between reading and spelling (r = 0.77) suggests that experience with reading is an important contributor to good spelling performance: good readers were able to spell words with a complex orthographic structure. As pointed out by Treiman (1993), behind children's capabilities in both early reading and spelling, there is a growing awareness of 'print as a means of representing all the words in their language'. When reading, the child experiences that some phonemes are represented by multiple letters. To be able to spell digraphs correctly, the child has to use his or her stored knowledge of correspondences between sounds and spellings. Treiman argues that for this aspect of spelling, reading influences spelling and not vice versa. Our data support Treiman's argument on this point, since there were no differences between good and poor readers' spelling of regular words and nonwords, but there were differences in the spelling of digraphs. The educational implications of this accord with the idea presented by Frith (1985) that reading and writing influence the development of literacy differently at different stages in development. When breaking the alphabetic code, spelling appears to be important for the child to discover the phonemic structure in language. When coming to terms with irregularities and digraphs, the child has to be familiar with the written form of words, which comes from reading. On this point Treiman (1993, p 289) is crystal clear: 'My results suggest that, although writing is important, the "write first, read later" view should not be pushed to extremes. Much of the raw material children use to form and test hypotheses about the links between sounds and spellings and about the properties of printed words comes from experience with reading. ...Children benefit from their reading experience to learn things they have not been explicitly taught.' Our data support this view.

The fact that most good readers were also good spellers came as no surprise, as spelling–sound rules are used in both reading and spelling (cf. also Nelson and Warrington, 1974; Joshi and Aaron, 1991), although there were exceptions to this tendency. However, only one child classified as a good reader could be considered a poor speller – a phenomenon which in the literature has been labelled developmental spelling retardation (Nelson and Warrington, 1976), unexpected spelling problems (Frith, 1980) or spelling only retardation (Jorm, 1983). This good reader was among the 8% poorest word spellers in the total sample and is a clear exception. Two poor readers were among the 16% best spellers in the total sample. A wide range of individual differences may cause these exceptions. Studies focusing on such exceptional cases should shed light on individual differences in spelling and reading development. However, the general developmental pattern is not invalidated by these few exceptions, and only two of the poor readers had more severe spelling problems with only five and six of the 30 words spelled correctly.

We have argued that the difference between good and poor readers is of degree rather than kind, and the developmental path we hypothesize develops from phonologically driven spelling to gradually more orthographically driven spelling for both good and poor readers. We have speculated that the driving force behind this strategic shift is the activity of reading, as indicated by the good readers' advanced ability to handle irregular words and digraphs. Along this developmental path from prephonetic to conventional spellings we observed some characteristic spelling "errors", presumably reflecting different depths of insight into the phonological structure. We should underscore, however, that all the observed "errors", except for 'giving up', were found in both poor and good readers. On these grounds the developmental sequence we observed in the Norwegian 8-year-olds may be described as follows:

1 Prephonetic spellings, manifested in tendency to 'give up' or to attempt aspects which could be recognized logographically (observed in only two poor readers)
2 Semiphonemic spellings, characterized by three depths of insight into the phonemic structure:
   (a) shallow insight, as indicated by many errors in the same word (multiple errors), in particular errors that disrupt the phonemic structure of the word to the point that the phonemic structure is hardly recognizable (most typically among poor readers)
   (b) 'disrupted' or 'inaccurate' insight, as indicated when one phoneme is substituted, added or reversed, while the rest of the word is spelled correctly (most typically among good readers)
   (c) partial insight, as indicated when part(s) of the phonemic structure is deleted, but the rest of the structure is phonemically correct (more typically among poor readers, but also observed in good readers, in particular with nonwords).

3 Phonemic spellings, characterized by errors with a complete phonemic structure (more typical in good than poor readers, but also observed in poor readers, particularly for common words).
4 Conventional spellings.

There is one clear difference in this pattern from that observed in English-speaking communities, namely the lack of orthographically based spelling errors. This may be explained by the words used in our study, which may have been too short, too simple or too regular for the orthographic spelling patterns to show up. The difference may also be explained by the children's age. The children were, on average, 8 years old, and this may be too late for logographic spelling and too early for orthographically based spellings in a Norwegian educational setting. We would, however, also like to underscore that we have based our developmental description on non-standard spellings, and that this does not take into consideration the strategies used by the children when spelling conventionally. Presumably spelling digraphs and irregular words conventionally make demands on orthographic knowledge, and the good readers were the ones who mastered these aspects correctly.

Acknowledgement

This work was financed by a grant 132365/520 from The Norwegian Research Council.

References

Barron RW (1980) Visual and phonological strategies in reading and spelling. In U Frith (ed) Cognitive processing in spelling, pp 195–213. Toronto: Academic Press.

Bear DR, Templeton S (1998) Explorations in developmental spelling: Foundations for learning and teaching phonics, spelling, and vocabulary. The Reading Teacher 52: 222–242.

Bradley L, Bryant P (1981) Visual memory and phonological skills in reading and spelling backwardness. Psychological Research 43: 193–199.

Bråten I (1994) Learning to spell. Training orthographic problem-solving with poor spellers: a strategy instructional approach. Oslo: Scandinavian University Press.

Bruck M, Treiman R (1990) Phonological awareness and spelling in normal children and dyslexics: the case of initial consonant clusters. Journal of Experimental Child Psychology 50: 156–178.

Bryant P, Bradley L (1980) Why children sometimes write words which they do not read. In U Frith (ed) Cognitive Processes in Spelling, pp 355–370. Toronto: Academic Press.

Cataldo S, Ellis N (1988) Interactions in the development of spelling, reading and phonological skills. Journal of Research in Reading 11: 86–109.

Cossu G, Gugliotta M, Marshall JC (1995) Acquisition of reading and written spelling in a transparent orthography: two non-parallel processes? Reading and Writing 7: 9–22.

Ehri LC (1985) Sources of difficulty in learning to spell and read. Advances in Developmental and Behavioural Paediatrics 7: 121–195.

Elley WB (1992) How in the world do students read? Hamburg: The International Association for the Evaluation of Educational Achievement.

Ellis NC (1994) Longitudinal studies of spelling development. In GDA Brown, NC Ellis (eds) Handbook of spelling. Theory, processes and intervention, pp 155-177. New York: Wiley.

Elsness TF (1991) 'Meningsfylte tekster' og den grunnleggende lese-og skriveopplæringen. In I Austad (ed) Mening i tekst (Meaning in text). Oslo: Cappelen. 15-51.

Ferreiro E, Teberosky A (1983) Literacy before schooling. London: Heinemann

Frith U (1980) Unexpected spelling problems. In U Frith (ed) Cognitive processes in spelling, pp 495-515. Toronto: Academic Press.

Frith U (1985) Beneath the surface of developmental dyslexia. In KE Patterson, JC Marshall, M Coltheart (eds) Surface dyslexia. London: Lawrence Erlbaum Associates. pp 301-330.

Frost J (1998) Phonemic awareness, spontaneous writing, and reading and spelling. Difficulties from a preventive perspective. Reading and Writing 14: 487-513.

Gentry JR (1978) Early spelling strategies. The Elementary School Journal 79: 88-92.

Gjessing HJ (1986) Function analysis as a way of subgrouping the reading disabled: clinical and statistical analyses. Scandinavnian Journal of Educational Research 30: 95-106.

Goodman K (1967) Reading: a psycholinguistic guessing game. Journal of the Reading Specialist 6: 126-135.

Goswami UC, Gombert JE, Fraca de Barrera L (1998) Children's orthographic representations and linguistic transparency: nonsense word reading in English, French and Spanish. Applied Psycholinguistics 19: 19-52.

Gough PB, Juel C, Griffith P (1992) Reading, spelling and the orthographic cipher. In P Gough, L Ehri, R Treiman (eds) Reading acquisition, pp 35-48. Hillsdale, NJ: Lawrence Erlbaum Associates.

Hagtvet BE (1989) Emergent literacy in Norwegian six-year-olds. From pretend writing to phonemic awareness and invented writing. In F Biglmaier (ed) Reading at the crossroads, pp 164-179. Conference proceedings, the 6th European Conference on Reading, Berlin.

Hagtvet BE, Lyster SAH (1998) Literacy teaching in Norway. In V Edwards, D Corson (eds) Encyclopedia of Language and Education, vol 2. Literacy, pp 225-233. The Netherlands: Kluwen Academic Press.

Hagtvet BE, Horn E, Lassen L, Lauvås K, Lyster S, Misund S (1998) Developing literacy in families with histories of reading problems. Preliminary results from a longitudinal study of young children of dyslexic parents. Journal of Special Needs Education 2: 29-39.

Henderson EH, Beers JW (eds) (1980) Developmental and cognitive aspects of learning to spell: a reflection of word knowledge. Newark, DE: International Reading Association.

Henderson EH, Templeton S (1986) A developmental perspective of formal spelling instruction through alphabet, pattern and meaning. The Elementary School Journal 186: 305-316.

Jorm AF (1983) The psychology of reading and spelling disabilities. London: Routledge & Kegan Paul.

Joshi RM, Aaron PG (1991) Developmental reading and spelling disabilities: are these dissociable? In RM Joshi (ed) Written language disorders. Neuropsychology and cognition, vol 2, pp 1-24.The Netherlands: Kluwer.

Juel C, Griffith PL, Gough PB (1986) Acquisition of literacy: a longitudinal study of children in first and second grade. Journal of Educational Psychology 78: 243-255.

Karmiloff-Smith A (1979) Language development after five. In R Fletcher, M Garman (eds) Language acquisition. Studies in first grade development. Cambridge, MA: Cambridge University Press.

Karmiloff-Smith A (1986) From meta-processes to conscious access. Evidence from children's metalinguistic and repair data. Cognition 23: 94–147.

Klicpera C, Gasteiger-Klicpera B (1993) Lesen und Schreiben. Entwicklung und Schwierigkeiten (Reading and writing; development and difficulties). Bern: Hans Huber.

Klinkenberg JE, Skar E (1994) Non-ord diktat i kartlegging av teknisk leseferdighet (Reading test). Hole kommune.

Landerl K (1997) Word recognition in English and German dyslexics. In CK Leong, RM Joshi (eds) Cross-language studies of learning to read and spell, pp 121-137. The Netherlands: Kluwer Academic Publishers.

Landerl K (2000) Influences of orthographic consistency and reading instruction on the development of nonword reading skills. European Journal of Psychology of Education 15: 239-257.

Landerl K, Wimmer H, Frith U (1997) The impact of orthographic consistency on dyslexia: a German-English comparison. Cognition 63: 315-334.

Leimar U (1974-76) Leseinnlæring bygd på barnas eget språk (Reading based on children's dictations). Oslo: Tanum.

Lennox C, Siegel LS (1994) The role of phonological and orthographic processes in learning to spell. In GDA Brown, NC Ellis (eds) Handbook of spelling. Theory, processes and intervention, pp 93-109. New York: Wiley.

Lundberg I, Høien T (1989) Phonemic deficits: a core symptom of developmental dyslexia? The Irish Journal of Psychology 10: 579-592.

Lyster SAH (1995) Preventing reading and spelling failure. Doctoral dissertation, University of Oslo, Institute for Special Needs Education.

Nasjonalt læremiddelsenter (1995) The National Centre for Teaching Aids. Leseprove for 2 klasse (Reading Test grade 2) Oslo.

Nelson HD, Warrington EK (1974) Developmental spelling retardation and its relation to other cognitive abilities. British Journal of Psychology 65: 265-274.

Nurss J (1988a) Development of written communication in Norwegian kindergarten children. Scandinavian Journal of Educational Research 32: 33-48.

Nurss J (1988b) Written language environments for young children: comparison of Scandinavian, British, and American kindergartens. International Journal of Early Childhood 20: 45-53.

Olson RK, Wise B, Conners F, Rack J (1990) Organization, heritability, and remediation of component word recognition and language skills in disabled readers. In TH Carr, BA Levy (eds) Reading and its development: component skills approaches, pp 261-322. New York: Academic Press.

Perfetti CA (1985) Reading ability. New York: Oxford University Press.

Read C (1971) Preschool children's knowledge of English phonology. Harvard Educational Review 41: 1-34.

Read C (1975) Children's categorization of speech sounds in English. Urbana, IL: National Council of Teachers of English.

Read C (1986) Children's creative spelling. London: Routledge & Kegan Paul.

Scheerer-Neumann G (1989/1993) Rechtschreibschwäche im Kontext der Entwicklung (Difficulties of spelling seen in the context of development). In I Naegele, R Valtin (eds) LRS in den Klassen 1-10. Handbuch der Lese-Rechtscreibschwierigkeiten (Dyslexia in grades 1 to 10. Handbook of reading and spelling difficulties), pp 25-35. Weinheim: Beltz.

Sivertsen R (1986) Norsk standardisering av Aston Index (Norwegian stanardization of Aston Index). Oslo: Vigga Forlag.

Smith F (1978) Reading. Cambridge: Cambridge University Press.

Snowling MJ (1987) Dyslexia: a cognitive developmental perspective. Oxford: Basil Blackwell.

Spitta G (1993) Kinder entdecken die Schriftsprache (Children detect written language). In R Valtin and I Naegele (eds) Schreiben ist wichtig! Grundlagen und Beispeiele für kommunikatives Schreiben (lernen) (Writing is important: foundations and examples for (learning) communicative writing), pp 67-83. Frankfurt: Arbeitskreis Grundschule.

Stanovich KE (1988) Explaining the differences between the dyslexic and the garden-variety poor reader: the phonological-core variable-difference model. Journal of Learning Disabilities 21: 590-604.

Stanovich KE, West RF (1989) Exposure to print and orthographic processing. Reading Research Quarterly 24: 402-433.

Thygesen R (1993) Språknormkonflikt og skrivevansker. Dissertation. Trondheim: Institute of Education, University of Trondheim. Mimeo.

Treiman R (1993) Beginning to spell: a study of first-grade children. New York: Oxford University Press.

Treiman R (1994) Sources of information used by beginning spellers. In GDA Brown, NC Ellis (eds) Handbook of spelling. Theory, processes and intervention, pp 75-91. New York: Wiley.

Treiman R, Cassar M (1997) Spelling acquisition in English. In CA Perfetti, L Rieben, M Fayol (eds) Learning to spell, pp 61-80. Mahwah, NJ.: Lawrence Erlbaum.

Valtin R (1997) Strategies of spelling and reading of young children learning German orthography. In CK Leong, RM Joshi (eds) Cross-language studies of learning to read and spell. Phonological and orthographic processing, pp 175-193. Dordrecht: Kluwer.

Venezky RL (1970) The sound structure of English orthography. The Hague: Mouton.

Wagner RK, Torgesen JK (1987) The nature of phonological processing and its causal role in the acquisition of reading skills. Psychological Bulletin 101: 192-212.

Wiggen G (1990). Språksosiologogiske aspekt ved rettskrivingsavvik hos norske barneskoleelever. Frederikshaun, Denmark. Dafolo Forlag.

Wimmer H, Frith U (1994) Reading difficulties among English and German children: same cause - different manifestation. Paper presented at the European Science Foundation Workshop, Written Language and Literacy, Nice, September.

Wimmer H, Goswami U (1994) The influence of orthographic consistency on reading development: word recognition in English and German children. Cognition 51: 91-103.

Wimmer H, Hummer (1990) How German-speaking first graders read and spell: doubts on the importance of the logographic stage. Applied Psycholinguistics 11: 249-368.

Wimmer H, Landerl K (1997) How learning to spell German differs from learning to spell English. In CA Perfetti, L Rieben, M Fayol (eds) Learning to spell. Mahwah, NJ: Lawrence Erlbaum.

Notes

1   The Norwegian orthographic system:
    • graphic markers for vowels: short vowel sounds may be represented by
      the doubling of the following consonants: *b, d, f, g, k, l, m, n, p, r, s, t*
    • the phoneme /ʃ/may be represented by *skj, sj, sk, rs*, as well by *sch, sh,
      ch, g, j* in different words adopted from other orthographies
    • the phoneme /ç/ may be represented by *k, kj* and *tj*
    • the phoneme /j/ may be represented by *j, g, gj, hj* and *lj*
    • following a short vowel /l/ may be written *ll, ld, lv* or *lg* and /n/ as *nn*
      or *nd*
    • the phonemes /ŋ/,/ʈ/, /ɳ/ and /ɖ/ are written *ng, rt, rn* and *rd* respec-
      tively
    • the phonemes /b/, /d/, /g/ are represented by *p, t* and *k*, respectively,
      following /s/ in the beginning of words
    • the phonemes /i/, /i/, /y/, /y:/, /œ/, /œ:/, /ʉ/, /ʉ:/, /a/ and /a:/ are
      always written *i, y, ø, u* and *a* respectively
    • the phoneme /e/ is always written *e* while /e:/ corresponds to both *e*
      and *æ*.
    • the phoneme /æ/ is always written *e* while /æ:/ corresponds to both *æ*
      and *e*
    • the phoneme /ʉ:/ is always written *o* while /ʉ/ corresponds to both *o*
      and *u*
    • the phonemes /ɔ:/ and /ɔ/ both correspond to either *å* and *o*. Vowel
      length, specific orthographic rules, e.g. that /ɔ:/ is often written *o*
      when preceding /v/ and /g/ and the morphemic system will help the
      writer to decide which letter to choose
    • the diphthongs /æi/, /œy/ and /æʉ/ are mostly written *ei, øy* and *au*
      respectively, but /ei/ is written *eg* in a few high frequency words such
      as *jeg* (I), *deg* (you) and in a few low frequency words. The diphthongs
      /ai/ and /ɔy/ are always written *ai* and *oi* respectively and are only
      found in foreign words and loanwords such as in *haike* (hitch hike)
      and *konvoi* (convoy)
    • a small group of consonants are 'silent' in special positions in some
      orthographic structures. No vowels are silent, but /ə/ which is always
      part of a syllable without stress is difficult to analyse in the dialect
      focused in this study.
2   The visual memory skills (logographic skills) drawn on by poor readers
    should not be confused with the skills used by advanced spellers who use
    orthographic cues by drawing lexical analogies on the basis of well-
    known orthographic patterns (orthographic reading).
3   Norwegian children have by tradition started school at age 7. In 1997,

school entrance age was reduced to 6, but with the understanding that grade 1 should be play-oriented, inviting the child to explore and discover the written language in literacy-stimulating environments and informal activities, while more formal introductions to reading and writing should not take place until grade 2. By tradition there is furthermore a strong tendency among Norwegian kindergarten teachers as well as parents not to stimulate written language either formally or informally before children start school. While this tendency has changed considerably over the past five years, the tendency is still to give priority to social, motor, oral language and creative abilities in nursery schools (e.g. Nurss, 1988a,b). The children in this study entered school before the 1997 reform.

4 Category D is 'mixed', and contains errors which share few similarities beyond being unclassifiable in categories, A, B and C. Some of the errors in category D in fact reflect a phono/orthographic representation which may be described as 'advanced' mistakes, implying that the child is approaching a more orthographically driven spelling stage (see for example Frith, 1985; Treiman and Cassar, 1997). However, such phono/orthographic errors were few (we observed only four and three errors of this kind in good and poor readers respectively). Also it is hard to interpret the representational basis for such errors without developmental data. What unifies category C is that all the errors reflect a serious breakdown of the phonological structure.

Appendix A: Words and nonwords

Words (Sivertsen, 1986)

is
sol
ola
fem
mor
lim
lese
mil
rose
sile
mus
låven
jeg
tre
noen

damer
her
seks
bamse
gøy
mat
det
bade
dem
med
natt
seg
bort
de
lenger

Nonwords (Klinkenberg, 1995)

dæ
ma
vy
lø
båf
gål
pyn
år
pøvy
bine
bnofr
krøt
vryg
flin
skjang
glypte

Appendix B: Types of errors

We do not include the nonwords in this overview as they do not add to the information given by the examples presented. The spellings of the children are written in capital letters.

A Correct phonemic spellings

- Correct phonemic spelling e.g. gøi or gøj for 'gøy', iæi or jæj for 'jeg' and me for 'med'.
- Correct phonemic spellings with imprecise phonemic representation e.g. lesse for 'lese' and gøjj for 'gøy'.
- Phonemic spelling in combination with letter names, e.g. fm for 'fem', lsc for 'lese', damr for 'damer', sx for 'sex' and lengr for 'lenger'.

B Phonemic spelling with a reduced, but correct phonemic representation involving omissions

- Omission of one phoneme, e.g. rce for 'rose', em for 'fem', sil for 'sile', ses for 'seks', base for 'bamse', leer for 'lenger', jæ, iæ for 'jeg' and sæ for 'seg'.
- More than 50% of phonemic structure correctly represented, e.g. dmr for 'damer' and ler for 'lenger'.
- 50% or less of phonemic structure correctly represented, e.g. ro for 'rose', ls for 'lese', bs for 'bamse' and g for 'gøy'.

C Phonemically inaccurate spellings involving substitution, reversal or addition of phonemes

- Substitutions, e.g. fen for 'fem', banse, danse for 'bamse', bot for 'bort', leger, lener, lemer for 'lenger.
- Reversal of phonemic sequence, e.g. RSO for 'rose' and ILSE for 'sile'. Additions, e.g. deit for 'de'.

D Unclassifiable spellings

- Phonemic spelling in combination with orthographic pattern, e.g. ded for 'det', gej, jg, geg, edg for 'jeg', and sejg for 'seg'.
- Multiple mistakes e.g. lenir, leem for 'lenger'.
- Other.
- Missing data caused by inability to spell.

CHAPTER 11

Dyslexia in Hebrew

DAVID L SHARE

This chapter reviews the available evidence on developmental dyslexia in the Hebrew language. The first of four sections provides an overview of the unique features of the Hebrew language and orthography, with special emphasis on Semitic morphology (the 'root-plus-pattern' system) and the consonantal alphabet in both its 'pointed' (fully vowelled) and 'unpointed' (partly vowelled) forms. The next section reviews several cross-sectional and longitudinal studies investigating sources of individual differences in reading ability. The third section looks at studies examining the characteristics of diagnosed dyslexics. The chapter concludes with a consideration of the continuities and discontinuities between dyslexia in Hebrew and contemporary English language research on dyslexia.

Aspects of Hebrew morphology and orthography

Morphology

The most characteristically Semitic feature of Hebrew is its derivational morphology (Berman, 1985). Almost all content words consist of a primarily consonantal 'root' and vocalic 'pattern'. The root is the semantic core of a word and usually consists of three (but occasionally four) consonants. Indeed, the entire Hebrew vocabulary (some 50,000 to 100,000 words) is based on only some 2000 roots. Specific words are produced only when a root is embedded into a pattern consisting of vocalic infixes, and mostly syllabic prefixes and/or suffixes. For example, verb forms derived from the triconsonantal root קלט = **KLT** include: קָלַט = **KaLaT** (he grasped) נִקְלַט = ni**KLaT** (was grasped/absorbed), הִקְלִיט = hi**KLiT** (he recorded) הוּקְלַט = hu**KLaT** (was recorded). (All root letters appear in boldface type in this and the following example.) Noun forms operate on the same root-plus-pattern principle. Nouns derived from the KLT root include: קְלִיטָה = **KLiT**a (absorption) מִקְלָט = miKLaT (shelter) הָקְלַטָה = haKLaTa (recording), מַקְלֵט = maKLeT (receiver), תַקְלִיט = taKLiT (record). While some noun patterns represent semantic categories (for example, the form CaCaC[1] is characteristic of professions: KaTaV – journalist, NaGaR – carpenter, SaPaR – barber), others are highly unpredictable. The contribution of morphological knowledge to Hebrew reading acquisition is apparent in findings showing that: (i) children are more accurate reading aloud pseudowords that conform to regular noun patterns (Birnboim, 1995); (ii) unpointed pseudowords are assigned pronunciations that conform to regular noun vowelling patterns (Rothschild-Yakar, 1989); and (iii) incorrectly vowelled items tend to be read in accordance with regular vowelling patterns (Rothschild-Yakar, 1989).

Morphological knowledge is likely to be a source of individual differences in reading ability because roots are phonologically highly opaque, manifest at the surface level in a variety of syllable forms with many combinations of vowels (e.g. KaLaT (he grasped), yiKLoT (he will grasp), KaLTu (they grasped), etc.). Although English is not always morphophonologically transparent (e.g. *electric/electricity/electrician*), the root morpheme (because it comprises both consonants and stem-internal vowels) is often preserved at the surface level as an integral unit. Indeed, most root morphemes in English can actually be 'heard', whereas Hebrew roots (e.g. KLT) are uniformly unpronounceable. This problem is further compounded in the orthography by extensive usage of prefixes and suffixes. Not only are tense, person, number, etc., usually indicated by inflecting roots, but many prefixed prepositions, conjunctions and articles (so called 'clitics' such as *to, from, in, and, the*, etc.), as well as suffixed pronouns, possessives and even direct objects (*my, them, your, him*, etc.) are frequently affixed to nouns and pronouns. For example, the two-word sentence נאכל בבוקר (NOKHAL BABOKER) translates into six English words 'We will eat in the morning'. This morphological density demands considerable 'unpacking' on the part of the reader and creates an additional source of homography.

As already noted, the semantic core of a word (the root) is usually consonantal, with vowels (and certain additional consonants) indicating grammatical inflections such as person, number and gender. Possibly for this reason, Hebrew orthographies from the earliest times until the present day have been predominantly consonantal systems with either no vowels or vowels represented in a subsidiary manner. The major drawback of such a system, however, is the abundance of homographic words, words that have the same spellings. Homographic words can be either homophonic (the words sound similar) or heterophonic (the words sound different), all deriving from the

---

[1]Here and elsewhere, the upper case letter 'C' refers to a root consonant; the lower case letter 'a' refers to the vowel /a/ as in 'bun'.

same consonantal root (Bentin et al., 1984; Navon and Shimron, 1984). For example, כתב (KTV) could represent 'journalist', 'orthography', 'he wrote', and more. In fact, a single unpointed consonantal string can represent up to a dozen different words. Shimron and Sivan (1994) estimate that almost one quarter of the words appearing in regular unpointed text are homographic when presented out of context.

Two separate systems of vowelling exist today. The first, and oldest, system of vowelling – called 'mothers of reading' – employs four of the consonantal letters (אהוי) to serve the dual function of signifying vowels as well as consonants. Apart from the ambiguity caused by using the same letter to represent both a vowel and a consonant (e.g.עוֹל(AVEL) 'injustice',עוֹל(OL) 'burden'), this system is both inconsistent and incomplete (Yanay and Porat, 1987; Shimron, 1993). Standard printed Hebrew appearing in today's books, newspapers and magazines is partly and inconsistently vowelled by means of the mothers of reading.

A second system of vowelization employs diacritical marks or points (*nekudot*). So-called pointed Hebrew is largely restricted to poetry, sacred texts and children's books.[2] In contrast to the mothers of reading, this diacritical system provides a complete and virtually unambiguous representation of the vowels by means of tiny dots and dashes appearing mostly under, but sometimes also above and between the letters. For example: דִ = /di/, דוֹ = /do/, דֻ = /du/, דַ = /da/, דֶ = /de/. There is, however, considerable duplication in this system in that each sound has between one and four representations marking phonetic distinctions that no longer exist. Indeed, most proposals for orthographic reform centre on simplifying this diacritical system whose visuospatial complexity is often claimed to be a source of reading difficulties for beginners (Feitelson, 1988; Lamm, 1989). Although the evidence is clear that adding vowel diacritics helps young readers resolve the ambiguity of unpointed text when reading aloud[3] (Shimron and Navon, 1981–82; Eshel, 1985; Ravid, 1996), diacritics remain a source of difficulty as witnessed by the fact that most reading errors even in pointed text are vowel errors (Rothschild-Yakar, 1989; Birnboim, 1995).

Children learn to read in pointed Hebrew, which has almost perfect grapheme-to-phoneme correspondence; both consonants and vowel diacritics have a single unambiguous pronunciation (Navon and Shimron,

---

[2]It is generally accepted that skilled readers do not require pointed texts for fluent reading. Poetry and sacred texts are the exceptions to this rule, probably because the identification of exact phonological form is considered essential in these genres.

[3]The developmental data on the role of pointing when reading words silently in meaningful context suggests a diminished, or even negligible role for vowel diacritics (Kahn-Horowitz, 1994; Even, 1995).

1984). From the point of view of grapheme-to-phoneme translation, there are no phonologically irregular words in pointed Hebrew. Probably owing to the shallow orthography, decoding is mastered very rapidly (Geva and Siegel, 1991; Geva et al., 1993; Birnboim, 1995; Shatil, 1997). Indeed, the accuracy of decoding pointed Hebrew in grade 1 matches the level achieved in English only in grade 5 (Geva et al., 1993). Unlike grapheme-to-phoneme correspondences, phoneme-to-grapheme relationships are frequently variable, with a number of pairs of (once phonemically distinct) graphemes now representing the same phoneme. As a result, the vast majority of Hebrew words contain consonants and vowels that could be spelled by alternate letters. Not surprisingly, attaining spelling proficiency is a much greater challenge than learning to decode and consistently lags behind that of English (Geva et al., 1993).

As the name 'square alphabet' suggests, letter architecture, relative to the Latin alphabet, is more uniformly block-like, with more horizontal and vertical strokes and fewer curves and diagonals than English. Slower letter recognition times relative to English may be attributable to this uniformity (Shimron and Navon, 1981). Not only are letters less distinctive, but word length and word shape are also quite uniform; the former attributable to the ubiquitous three-letter root and the latter to the paucity of ascenders and descenders.

Although some influential scholars (e.g. Gelb, 1963) have claimed that early (unpointed) Semitic scripts were not true alphabets but syllabaries, contemporary Israeli scholars are agreed that regular, unpointed Hebrew is a consonantal alphabet (Navon and Shimron, 1984; Frost and Bentin, 1992; Share and Levin, 1999), with graphemes representing individual consonant phonemes. Owing to its distinctive morphology, full representation of vowels in Hebrew, at least for the skilled reader, may well be unnecessary in contrast to Indo-European languages such as English, which use vowel distinctions to mark basic morphemic contrasts and for which the graphemic representation of vowels may be more critical (consider BUT, BET, BAT, BIT, BOAT, BEAT, etc.). Not only is vowel information less critical for the Hebrew speaker, who often exchanges vowels when pronouncing words (Ravid, 1996), but this information is far more easily inferred in printed Hebrew owing to simple and predictable syllable structures which consist almost exclusively of CV and CVC structures (Berman, 1969)

The psycholinguistic precedence of consonants over vowels is also apparent in the fact that kindergarten children more easily identify and isolate (spoken) consonant phonemes than vowel phonemes (Lapidot et al., 1995–96; Tolchinsky and Teberosky, 1998). They also tend to produce consonant letters earlier than vowel letters in their early writing (Levin and Korat, 1993; Levin et al., 1998), and most reading errors among beginning readers are vowel errors not consonant errors (Rothschild-Yakar, 1989; Birnboim, 1995).

Sources of individual differences in Hebrew reading ability

A modest number of Hebrew language studies have examined factors associated with individual differences in reading skill across a range of ability. Although these studies have not directly examined the characteristics of Hebrew-speaking dyslexics, they are, nonetheless, an invaluable source of data regarding reading difficulties for at least two reasons. First, it is becoming increasingly clear that dyslexia does not represent a unique, qualitatively distinct syndrome, but rather lies on the normal continuum of reading ability (Stanovich, 1991; Shaywitz et al., 1992; Fletcher et al., 1994; Aaron, 1997). Moreover, the available evidence suggests that this is also true in Hebrew (see for example Lamm, 1990). Thus studies that compare preselected groups at designated ability levels (disabled/non-disabled, good/ poor readers, etc.), and correlational studies encompassing a range of ability are addressing one and the same issue. Second, and consistent with the previous proposition, the Hebrew language studies reviewed in this section on factors associated with individual differences in reading ability essentially converge with the findings emerging from studies of selected groups of diagnosed dyslexics.

Predictive/longitudinal studies of reading development

A small number of studies have investigated preschool cognitive and psycholinguistic factors accounting for early individual differences in the ability to read pointed (fully vowelled) script.

A longitudinal study by Meyler and Breznitz (1998) examined the role of visual and verbal short-term memory (STM) in early reading. Sixty-three kindergarten children were administered tests of verbal memory (digit span, letter span and nonsense-syllable span) and visuospatial memory (Stanford-Binet Object and Bead Memory). Factor analysis of these six tests in kindergarten produced two clear-cut visual and verbal factors. Both visual and verbal STM in kindergarten predicted significant variance in grade 2 decoding skills even after controlling for IQ, although visual STM was more consistent. In addition, WISC-R block design in kindergarten also correlated significantly with later decoding ($r = 0.47$).

The most comprehensive study to date of the cognitive and psycholinguistic predictors of early reading achievement is Shatil's (1997) longitudinal study of a representative sample of over 300 children. In the final months of kindergarten, a battery of 30 measures was administered covering four domain-specific sets of variables (visuospatial processing, phonological awareness, phonological memory and early literacy,[4] and three domain-general sets (general intelligence, metacognitive functioning and oral language). Word recognition (speed and accuracy of oral word reading) and reading comprehension were assessed at the end of grade 1. Collectively, the domain-general block explained a borderline 5% of the variance in word-recognition skill attesting to what Shatil termed the 'cognitive modularity' of decoding. In contrast, the same domain-specific factors collectively explained a significant 33% of the variance in word recognition. Both domain-specific and domain-general blocks contributed significant and substantial portions of variance to the prediction of grade 1 reading comprehension (51% and 44% respectively).

Individual domain-specific sets of variables each accounted for significant amounts of decoding variance (visuospatial processing – 11%, phonological awareness – 11%, phonological memory – 16%, and early literacy – 19%). With the exception of phonological awareness, all these sets made a significant and unique individual contribution to the prediction of grade 1 decoding after the variance from the other sets was partialled out.

Of particular interest in the present context is the confirmation of Meyler and Breznitz's finding that visuospatial factors significantly predicted early reading in Hebrew. Included in this set were the Stanford–Binet Bead Memory test, the Witkin Embedded Figures test, and a 'memory-for-symbol-strings' task. Although no research to date has empirically addressed the question of why visuospatial factors predict early reading, a number of possibilities have been raised (see Shatil, 1997; Meyler and Breznitz, 1998), including the visuospatial complexity of the diacritical system, the relative lack of orthographic redundancy, the potential difficulties parsing multimorphemic strings into constituent morphemes, and the highly confusable letter shapes and word forms.

Phonological awareness

Several predictive/longitudinal and training studies have demonstrated that phonological awareness is an important determinant of individual differences in Hebrew reading acquisition, and furthermore, that the connection is causal.

The first study of phonological awareness to appear in Hebrew (Bentin and Leshem, 1993) assessed the phonemic segmentation abilities of over 500 kindergarten children. The lowest-scoring 100 children were then randomly assigned to one of four training groups (n = 25) matched for age, phonemic

---

[4]The early literacy measures included letter and word naming, Clay's test of print concepts, parental print exposure and invented spelling.

awareness and general intelligence. Interventions consisted of phoneme segmentation alone (recognizing and segmenting phonemes), phoneme segmentation plus letter identity, general language skills and non-specific training (additional regular kindergarten activities). A fifth no-treatment control group included 17 children scoring at the top end of the phoneme segmentation distribution. Training spanned a period of 10 weeks and consisted of two half-hour sessions per week with groups of up to four children. At the conclusion of training, both groups trained in recognizing and segmenting phonemes, but not the other groups, had improved significantly in phonemic segmentation and, by post-test, matched the initially high-scoring segmenters on phonemic segmentation ability. Word and pseudoword reading were tested in the middle and end of grade 1. At both follow-ups, the two groups trained in phonemic awareness were well ahead of the other groups in reading. In fact, these two groups read almost twice as many words correctly (65% and 61%) as the control groups (34% and 38%) and, moreover, were not significantly different from the initially high-scoring group (73%). Correlations between kindergarten phoneme segmentation and grade 1 reading for a group of 60 children who did not undergo intervention of any kind indicated a strong positive association in the middle of the year ($r = 0.55$), but a weaker association ($r = 0.35$) at the end of the year.

Kozminsky and Kozminsky (1993–94) randomly assigned two entire kindergarten classes (n = 35) in a lower middle-class area to experimental and control groups. Pre-intervention evaluation of phonemic awareness at the beginning of kindergarten established that these two groups were similar in age and phonemic awareness. Over the next eight months, both groups received two weekly (whole-class) training sessions each lasting 20 minutes, plus two daily five-minute booster (revision) sessions. Training in the experimental group focused on syllabic, subsyllabic and phonemic awareness, while the control class received a programme of visuomotor integration. A series of post-training phonological awareness tests showed a clear advantage for the experimental group following intervention. Furthermore, these gains were maintained through to the end of grade 1. Most importantly, the group trained in phonological awareness demonstrated significantly superior reading comprehension not only at the end of grade 1 but also when assessed again three years later at the end of grade 3.

Lapidot et al. (1995–96) examined the ability of kindergarten phonological awareness to predict grade 1 reading difficulties in an upper-middle class group of 100 children. The kindergarten measures included a variety of phoneme-level tasks – identification, matching, isolation and elision, as well as rhyme recognition and production. Grade 1 reading difficulty was defined as a score of 55% or below on oral word-reading accuracy; the criterion for poor phonological awareness was set at 40% or less on total kindergarten phonological (phoneme and rhyme) awareness. Of the 18 children with poor kindergarten phonological awareness, nine were correctly classified as having reading difficulties in grade 1. All 79 children who scored above the kindergarten cut-off were correctly classified as having no reading problem in grade 1.

These few longitudinal investigations of phonological awareness in Hebrew concur with the English language findings: difficulty in accessing phonemes was a significant predictor of later reading difficulties and, when trained, has a significant and durable impact on later reading ability. But is the relationship as powerful at that observed in English?

In her longitudinal study, Shatil (1997) included a number of tests of phonological awareness in her kindergarten battery: rhyme identification, rhyme production, word production on the basis of initial consonant-plus-vowel (CV), initial consonant matching, initial consonant isolation and phoneme blending. Correlations with decoding and comprehension at the end of grade 1 were consistently significant but substantially smaller (ranging from 0.31 to 0.42, with a median of 0.36) than those reported in the English literature (cf. Stanovich et al., 1984; Yopp, 1988). Indeed, Shatil's correlations were very similar to those reported both by Bentin and Leshem (1993) at the end of grade 1 (0.35). In a sample of Hebrew–English bilinguals, Geva et al. (1993) found the correlation between grade 1 syllable and phoneme deletion (the Rosner test) and grade 1 Hebrew word recognition to be significantly weaker (0.32) than between the Rosner and English word recognition (0.62).

If, indeed, phonemic awareness is a weaker predictor of early reading in Hebrew compared to English, several factors may be responsible. The first simply suggests that most children have attained mastery in decoding by the end of grade 1, hence the correlation is attenuated by the greater range restriction in reading scores. This account is consistent with the strong correlation (0.55) reported by Bentin and Leshem (1993) in the middle of grade 1, at which point, it seems reasonable to assume that the variance in decoding is considerably greater, as most children are still learning basic letter–sound correspondences. As noted in the introduction, the developmental trajectory of Hebrew decoding far outstrips that of English. It might be speculated that Hebrew decoding skills in the middle of grade 1 may be more comparable to those of English speakers later in the year. This implies that the contribution of phonological awareness to individual differences in reading may be equally strong in both languages, the only difference being one of timing.

Alternatively, language- and orthography-specific features may be responsible for an intrinsically attenuated relationship. Candidates include the highly consistent orthography and the language's relatively simple syllable structure discussed above. Either or both of these factors may reduce the cognitive complexity involved in learning to decode pointed Hebrew script.

Morphology

Levin et al. (1998) examined the longitudinal relationships between early writing and knowledge of morphological structures that are characteristic of high-register written language in a sample of 40 preschoolers followed from kindergarten to the end of grade 1. Children were asked to write dictated words that were then scored according to four levels: random letter strings, basic phonetic spelling (some consonantal phonemes correctly transcribed), advanced phonetic spelling (most consonantal phonemes correctly transcribed) and conventional spelling. Morphology and writing were correlated both in kindergarten and at grade 1 around the 0.50 mark. Moreover, kindergarten morphology predicted grade 1 writing (median r = 0.45) and remained a significant predictor even after controlling for kindergarten writing. These data suggest that morphology may be an important source of individual differences in early spelling. Other data reviewed in the next section confirm that morphological knowledge is a particularly important factor in explaining both reading and writing difficulties in the Hebrew language (Ben-Dror et al., 1995; Cohen et al., 1996).

Characteristics of diagnosed dyslexics

Morphological awareness among dyslexics

Ben-Dror et al. (1995) compared the semantic, phonological and morphological skills of fifth grade disabled readers to both chronological age-matched normal readers and a younger vocabulary-matched group of normal readers. (In this study, the reading-disabled group scored well below both control groups on the reading measure – pseudoword naming.) Children were asked to judge phonemic identity, semantic relatedness and morphological relatedness. The strongest differences between the groups were obtained on the morphological task in which children decided whether two words shared a common root. Reading-disabled children were significantly poorer than the vocabulary-matched group, who in turn were poorer than the age-matched group. In other words, the differences in morphological knowledge faithfully reflected the relative reading ability of all three groups. On the phonological and semantic tests, however, the reading-disabled group was consistently inferior only to the age-matched group.

A study by Cohen et al. (1996) further confirms that morphological deficits are endemic to Hebrew dyslexics. Cohen et al. examined the spoken and written storytelling of 45 reading-disabled children in grades 3 to 6 and 41 matched non-disabled readers. Children were shown a series of pictures depicting a story and asked to tell the story orally and in writing. Oral and written narratives were coded for morphological, syntactic and narrative richness,[5] false starts (oral story only) and text length. There were significant differences between disabled and normal readers on all measures in both oral and written productions, with the greatest differences observed in the written mode.

The findings from both the Cohen et al. and Ben-Dror et al. studies, as well as the Levin et al. longitudinal investigation, all converge on the conclusion that morphological deficiencies appear to play a causal role in reading and writing difficulties in Hebrew. To date, however, no experimental training study in morphology has yet been conducted.

Phonological skills among Hebrew dyslexics

The few studies that have examined the pseudoword reading skills of disabled readers clearly show that, as a group, dyslexics show severe deficits as in the English language research literature.

Breznitz (1997a) compared pseudoword reading and phonological awareness performance of 52 grade 3 dyslexic and 52 normal grade 1 readers individually matched for gender, IQ, handedness, word recognition accuracy and reading comprehension. Dyslexics were far inferior on pseudoword reading accuracy and speed (despite being matched solely on the basis of word recognition accuracy[6] and reading comprehension) as well as on several measures of phonological awareness. The pseudoword reading and phonological awareness deficits in these groups are consistent with the view that Israeli dyslexics as a group are, like English language dyslexics, characterized by severe phonological deficits.

The Ben-Dror et al. (1995) study, referred to earlier, selected 20 grade 5 children from a population of diagnosed reading-disabled children. The children included in this study were selected on the basis of at least 50% errors reading a list of pseudowords. (A majority of the population sampled fell below this cutoff (Ben-Dror, personal communication, 1999).) Control groups consisted of 20 grade 5 normal readers and a second vocabulary-matched group consisting of grade 3 normal readers. The authors reported that although they attempted to include a younger reading-age matched

---

[5]The assessment of: (a) morphological, (b) syntactic and (c) narrative richness was based on the use of: (a) construct forms, bound possessives and subject–verb agreement, (b) subordinate clauses and (c) number of story elements.

[6]Because dyslexics were considerably slower than the grade 1 readers (Z Breznitz, personal communication, 1999) it was not possible to match these two groups on word-recognition speed as well as accuracy.

control group '...our attempts failed because we were unable to find children with such low [pseudoword] reading scores after first grade, whereas children in first grade could not take the morphologic tests' (p 881). The grade 3 vocabulary-matched normal readers committed less than half as many pseudoword reading errors as the grade 5 disabled readers, a finding very similar to that reported by Breznitz (1997a). Disabled readers were also significantly slower and less accurate than both control groups on a phoneme identification test. On a phonological production task (supplying as many words as possible in 30 seconds beginning with a given phoneme), reading-disabled children again performed more poorly than both control groups.

Brande (1997) administered a host of reading and cognitive tasks to two groups of adolescent (age 15) and pre-adolescent (age 11) dyslexics and their chronological-age (CA) matched normal readers. Overall, the differences between controls and dyslexics on phonological abilities (e.g. pseudoword reading, phonological awareness and rapid serial naming) tended to be stronger and more consistently significant statistically than other variables such as orthographic processing (e.g. identifying words embedded in longer letter strings, lexical decision). Brande also examined developmental differences in the cognitive profiles of the dyslexics at the different ages by comparing relative effect sizes for dyslexics and controls. Smaller differences were obtained at the older age level on several measures related to meaning, comprehension and orthographic processing. The gap between disabled and non-disabled readers did not narrow, and in certain cases actually widened in the case of oral reading time, pseudoword reading, phoneme segmentation and serial naming. These data accord with the English language findings demonstrating weakness in phonological processing co-existing with relative strengths in orthography and meaning (Stanovich and Siegel, 1994; Share 1995; Siegel et al., 1995). This pattern of phonological weakness and relative orthographic strengths has also been confirmed both behaviourally and electrophysiologically in a small number of neuropsychological studies of Hebrew-speaking dyslexics.

Speed of processing (SOP)

Breznitz (2001a) undertook a series of studies investigating the sources of reading-rate differences between dyslexic and normal readers. She hypothesized that speed of processing within and/or between the information-processing subsystems involved in word recognition may be a key factor in reading rate and create the differences observed in word recognition between dyslexic and normal readers. This first study examined both the behavioural and electrophysiological (ERP[7]) correlates of phonological and orthographic processing. Participants were 20 dyslexic and 20 normal college students. While the adult dyslexics achieved almost perfect decoding accuracy, reading speed, both silent and oral, was slow and comprehension poor. In a series of experiments, subjects were required to make both orthographic decisions (judging whether two heterophonic homographs, words with identical spellings but different pronunciations, shared the same consonantal string) and phonological decisions (judging homophony and rhyme).

Behaviourally, dyslexics displayed slower reaction times on the phonological but not on the orthographic tasks. Dyslexics also committed significantly more errors on rhyme judgements. Dyslexics showed significantly slower ERP latencies on phonological decisions but not orthographic decisions.

Employing these same subjects, Breznitz and Meyler (2001) went on to examine speed of processing for low-level linguistic and non-linguistic stimuli presented in each modality separately and also cross-modally. Auditory and visual choice reaction time tasks required subjects to detect target tones (non-linguistic) and consonant sounds (linguistic), visual symbols (non-linguistic) and printed letters (linguistic). In a second task, tones and light flashes were presented simultaneously or with small interstimulus intervals in a cross-modal (non-linguistic) task in which subjects were required to determine whether the two stimuli were presented simultaneously or not. Behaviourally, the dyslexics were less accurate on both auditory tasks (tones and phonemes) but not the visual tasks. There were no differences on any of the four measures of behavioural reaction times. On the cross-modal task, while response accuracy was almost perfect for both groups, dyslexics were slower when auditory stimuli (tones) preceded the visual stimuli (flashes) and also when the two stimuli occurred together (but not when visual stimuli preceded auditory tones). Electrophysiologically, many ERP latencies were delayed for all stimulus types, although delays on

---

[7]ERP (event-related potential) recording is a technique for mapping cognitive activity based on brain electrical activity (electroencephalogram) data recorded on-line in response to a given event, such as the presentation of a printed word. ERPs consist of discrete components, or brain waves, that are related to different stages of information processing in terms of amplitude or latency. These components are usually designated by their polarity (P – positive, N – negative) and by the latency of their maximum amplitudes, or peaks, in milliseconds. For example, the P300 wave refers to a positive component peaking around 300 milliseconds after an event. Areas of brain specialization can be identified by observing variations of amplitude and latency in ERP components at different scalp locations. For example, the left side of the brain (hemisphere) is normally more prominent in the processing of linguistic information, whereas the right hemisphere is more active in the processing of visuospatial information.

the auditory tasks tended to occur earlier (at N100). On the cross-modal integration task, when the two stimuli occurred together, latencies among dyslexics were later for each of the four ERP components.

Breznitz suggested that dyslexics suffer from a general speed-of-processing deficit that is most pronounced in the auditory/phonological domain.[8] She also speculated that integration of phonological and visual/orthographic information may fail among poor readers owing to excessive separation ('asynchrony') of faster visual processing and slower auditory processing.

In a third study, Breznitz (2001b) went on to investigate whether the gap between the rates of processing for auditory–phonological and visual–orthographic stimuli among dyslexics accounts for their poorer word recognition. The sample, in this case, were uncompensated dyslexic children compared to chronological age-matched controls. These young dyslexics were significantly slower and less accurate on a host of reading achievement and reading-related variables, such as naming speed, phonological processing, orthographic processing, WISC Symbol Search and same/different judgements for consonant–vowel–consonant (CVC) pairs separated by 80 ms inter-stimulus intervals, but not simple motoric reaction time (pressing a button in response to a light flash). On the experimental task, dyslexics were slower on all low-level auditory and visual tasks as well as the higher-level phonological and orthographic decisions. Response accuracy was also lower on all measures except low-level non-linguistic visual stimuli (visual symbols).

Electrophysiological analyses focused on P200 and P300 components. For both the lower-level and higher-level auditory and visual tasks,[9] both these latencies were significantly later among dyslexics compared to controls, with significantly greater differences on the auditory task. For both phonological and orthographic decisions, dyslexics' ERP latencies were delayed, but again with greater differences on the phonological tasks. Dyslexics also had significantly greater latency 'gaps' between auditory and visual tasks for each of the linguistic, non-linguistic and homophone–homograph tasks. Stepwise

---

[8]While these data show a reliable low-level deficit in auditory processing (tone detections), the evidence for a low-level visual deficit is questionable, since both the 'visual' tasks were based on either letters or letter-like symbols. In the latter case, the symbols were the English letters 'L' and 'T' in unconventional rotations and likely to be familiar to college dyslexics literate in English. More recently, however, Breznitz (unpublished data) has replicated these findings using non-verbal visual symbols suggesting that the lower-level visual deficit is a genuine non-verbal deficit.

[9]Although children at this age (dyslexics included) are learning to read and write English in school, these data strengthen the case for a low-level speed-of-visual-processing deficit, since 10-year old children are less likely than adults to perceive these letter-like symbols as verbal stimuli.

multiple regression was then used to determine which independent variables best accounted for decoding ability in the two groups. Results indicated that the best predictors of decoding ability were the gaps in phoneme detection-minus-grapheme detection tasks for both ERP latencies (P200 and P300) and simple P300 latencies for homophone judgements. Discriminant analyses revealed that subjects could be classified with 100% accuracy as dyslexics or normal readers on the basis of the P300 phoneme-minus-grapheme latency gap and also P300 latencies for the rhyming task.

In her discussion, Breznitz argued for the predominance of a domain-specific phonological SOP deficit within the context of a general SOP deficit. She also proposed that a fundamental SOP asynchrony between visual and auditory modalities may constitute the underlying cause of dyslexia.

Verbal weaknesses and non-verbal strengths

Two other neuropsychological studies of Hebrew dyslexics also emphasized the primacy of left-hemisphere, verbal/linguistic deficits together with relative strengths in right-hemisphere, visuospatial functioning.

Barnea et al. (1994) examined event-related potentials for 14 dyslexics (aged 9 to 13) and 16 chronological-age (CA) controls. Subjects performed a Sternberg memory-scanning task in which they were required to memorize several items and were then presented with a test item and required to decide whether the test item was a member of the memorized set. Stimuli were either familiar verbal symbols (digits 1 to 9) or unfamiliar non-verbal symbols (mostly Greek letters). Response accuracy was consistently lower among dyslexics for both types of items. However, response latencies yielded a true crossover interaction: normals were faster on digits and slower on non-verbal items, whereas dyslexics were faster on non-verbal symbols and slower on digits. Among dyslexics, ERP amplitudes (P300) were larger for the digits than for the non-verbal stimuli, with the opposite pattern observed for normals. Brain activity was more prominent over the left hemisphere for normals, but over the right hemisphere for dyslexics.

Harness et al. (1984) assessed 108 dyslexics (ages 8 to 15) referred to a reading disability clinic on a battery of visuospatial ('right hemisphere') tasks and verbal/sequential ('left hemisphere') tasks. All but three of the 108 children performed better on the right hemisphere tasks averaging half a standard deviation above age norms. Left hemisphere performance was depressed to the same extent with average right-plus-left performance close to the overall population average.

It should be remarked that both these neuropsychological studies of predominantly older dyslexics would appear to contradict the two longitudinal studies cited earlier pointing to the role of visuospatial factors in early decoding (Shatil, 1997; Meyler and Breznitz, 1998). It may be possible to resolve this apparent contradiction by postulating that while most dyslexics, young and old alike, have verbal/phonological deficits, a significant minority of younger but not older dyslexics have selective deficits in the visual domain.[10] Unfortunately, all studies reviewed thus far have emphasized the commonalities of dyslexics as a group, without addressing the possibility of subtypes. However, there is at least one Hebrew language study (Lamm and Epstein, 1994) that has expressly searched for subtypes of dyslexia. The results provide some support for the notion that substantial numbers of Hebrew dyslexics may indeed fit a non-verbal subtype.[11]

Subtypes of dyslexia

In a large-scale study of diagnosed dyslexics, Lamm and Epstein (1994) investigated the dichotic listening[12] performance of 320 children from grades 3 to 10 referred to a private clinic. Of particular interest in this study was a subtype analysis statistically derived from the cluster analysis of reading and cognitive performance of these children.

A battery of reading (accuracy and speed), spelling and cognitive (verbal/serial and visuo-spatial) measures was administered.[13] Four groups emerged from the cluster analysis. In contrast to English language subtyping work (Castles and Coltheart, 1993; Manis et al., 1996; Stanovich et al., 1997; Castles et al., 1999), the largest group – almost half the sample (43%) – were classified not as phonological dyslexics but as 'surface/lexical' dyslexics. In this subgroup, at least 75% of the oral reading errors consisted of incorrect pronunciations of vowel diacritics. The proportion of these errors was reduced by at least 50% when reading fully vowelled (pointed) versions of the same text. The latter designation was based on the assumption that 'the

---

[10]The Shatil (1997) and Meyler and Breznitz (1998) data all related to grade 1 children reading pointed Hebrew with its complex diacritics, whereas the Harness et al. (1984) and Barnea et al. (1994) samples consisted of substantially older groups (grades 3 to 12) reading unpointed script. Lamm (1990) has suggested that a visuomotor subtype of dyslexia is quite common among young dyslexics who are learning to read pointed script, but less common after grade 3, when diacritics are dropped. It is hoped that future subtyping work with representative unselected (i.e. non-clinic) samples may help to clear up this issue.

[11]Unfortunately, ages were not reported separately for the different subtypes emerging in this study.

[12]Dichotic listening is a technique for evaluating hemispheric specialization based on the presentation of auditory events to a single ear only and thereby to only one side of the brain. For example, superior performance in 'right ear' processing of speech information is assumed to indicate greater specialization of the left (contralateral) hemisphere for language.

[13]Pseudoword reading and phonemic awareness were not examined in this study.

significant decrease of pure vowel errors in reading vowellized as compared with unvowellized text originated in the greater ability of such subjects in utilizing phonological cues compared with their ability of direct orthographic decoding' (p 763). Spelling errors were solely homophone confusions. This group also demonstrated inferior performance on verbal/serial cognitive measures relative to visuospatial measures – the latter being in the normal range. Lamm and Epstein observed that these reading/spelling profiles suggest developmental delay rather than deficit (cf. Manis et al., 1996; Stanovich et al., 1997), as such profiles are typical of younger normal beginning readers tested with texts at higher levels.

The next largest group (25%) were labelled 'visuomotor' dyslexics. In this group, at least 45% of the oral reading errors were classified as 'visual' (confusion of visually similar letters and words), and 35% of writing difficulties as 'visuospatial' (poor letter spacing, line alignment, letter repetitions and omissions). Cognitive performance on the visuospatial tests was also poor in this group.

Perhaps the most surprising outcome of the Lamm and Epstein subtype analysis was the very small proportion (4.4%) classified as 'phonological' dyslexics. This group displayed severe difficulties in grapheme–phoneme translation; 30% of oral reading errors and 35% of spelling errors were consonant errors. Lamm and Epstein described this group as having 'an extraordinarily severe reading deficit … resembling illiterates with only a vague conception of the relations between phonology and orthography … almost total inability to read and write' (p 763). (The remaining 28% of the sample could not be classified into any of the preceding groups and were labelled 'non-specific'.)

External validity for these subgroups was provided by the results of the dichotic listening tests. Dichotic performance of dyslexics was compared to a control group of normal readers (mostly from the same classes) who were matched for age, gender and IQ. Total performance (percentage of items correctly reported from both ears) was lowest in the phonological group and next lowest in surface/lexical dyslexics and non-specifics, with the best performance observed among visuomotor dyslexics. Phonological dyslexics were the most discrepant vis-à-vis controls, followed by the surface group, while visuomotor dyslexics were on a par with controls. The dichotic data, therefore, essentially validate the results of the cluster analysis with regard to verbal/non-verbal profiles.

Lamm and Epstein's findings present several intriguing results. Fully one quarter of the dyslexic sample were classified as visuomotor dyslexics. This group did not differ from matched controls on any dichotic measure, nor were they better readers than either 'surface' or 'non-specific' dyslexics, hence reading level cannot explain these differences. Lamm and Epstein concluded that the reading difficulties in this group cannot be traced to any basic deficit in auditory–verbal processing. Although these data diverge from the current picture emerging from English language research regarding the paucity of a visual or visuospatial subtype of dyslexia (see for example Rayner et al., 1995), they converge with the Hebrew language findings regarding the importance of visuospatial factors in early reading (Shatil, 1997; Meyler and Breznitz, 1998).

The most surprising outcome of this subtyping study was the rarity of phonological dyslexics. Elsewhere, Lamm (1989) has claimed that Hebrew has few phonological dyslexics because systematic phonics instruction is virtually universal in grade 1, and because of the fact that pointed script is so highly regular. However, studies directly investigating phonological factors in reading ability (Bentin and Leshem, 1993; Kozminsky and Kozminsky, 1993–94; Ben-Dror et al., 1995; Lapidot et al. 1995–96; Brande, 1997; Breznitz, 1997a; Shatil, 1997; Meyler and Breznitz, 1998) have, in each and every case, converged on the conclusion that substantial portions of early reading variance are attributable to phonological factors.

It is possible to reconcile Lamm and Epstein's seemingly conflicting data within the recent reconceptualization of surface dyslexia as a mild phonological deficit (Manis et al., 1996; Stanovich et al., 1997; Castles et al., 1999). Although Lamm and Epstein did not directly test either pseudoword reading or phonemic awareness, several features of their group data are consistent with such a view. First the verbal/serial deficits evident in tasks such as Digit-Span are likely to depend on phonological codes in STM. Second, the pattern of developmental delay as opposed to developmental deviance/deficit is characteristic of English language surface dyslexics. In addition, Lamm and Epstein noted several parallels between their surface dyslexics' neuropsychological profiles and a subgroup of dysphonetic dyslexics with poor phonetic attack skills reported by Cohen et al. (1992), who also showed poorer verbal performance relative to spatial performance as well as poor Digit-Span. Thus, the 'surface' dyslexics may represent the expression of mild or moderate phonological deficits in a regular orthography. The presence of subtle phonological deficits when learning to read a highly regular orthography taught via systematic phonics methods may permit a child to attain a relatively high level of decoding accuracy (relative to English) if not speed, yet with difficulties in developing the orthographic representations typical of surface dyslexia. These surface or lexical deficits appear to be attributable not to visual deficits (Lamm and Epstein's data did not indicate any visual/spatial processing deficits in this group), but to higher-order aspects of decoding that require the string of decoded elements to be efficiently synthesized and integrated with lexical and morphological knowledge. Elsewhere, Lamm (1989) observes that most 'surface/lexical' dyslexics seem unable to make the transition from bottom-up, letter-by-letter phonological recoding (*kriya metzarefet*) to direct automatic visual/orthographic recognition. He speculates that problems of lexical retrieval prevent this transition with the result that children fail to progress beyond the level of effortful, bottom-up phonological decoding.

The subtle phonological deficit hypothesis regarding these Hebrew surface/lexical dyslexics gleans some support from several case studies of acquired surface dyslexia that directly examined phonological processing (Birnboim, 1995; Birnboim and Share, 1995). In many, but not all respects, these acquired surface dyslexics resembled Lamm's surface/lexical dyslexics in their profiles of bottom-up, non-lexical (phonological) reading and relative insensitivity to surface orthography (e.g. homophone confusions). As a group, they were able to read most pseudowords presented and, in most cases, successfully identified matching initial and final phonemes. However, in all but one case, performance on both pseudowords and phonemic analysis fell at least a full standard deviation below the level achieved by normal controls, pointing to phonological weaknesses.

An alternative account of Lamm and Epstein's surface/lexical dyslexics (but one that fails to resolve the inconsistency with other Hebrew language studies of phonological processing) relates to morphology. A morphological deficit account would cohere with both the Ben-Dror et al. (1995) and Cohen et al. (1996) data. Indeed, it is widely agreed that skilled Hebrew word recognition of unpointed script requires direct access to tri-consonantal roots, which are the semantic core of words. Lamm (1990) notes that surface/lexical dyslexics often show up clinically only around grades 3–4, at the time of transition from pointed to unpointed text.

Recently, Lamm (in preparation) found evidence that Hebrew surface dyslexics may have both subtle phonological deficits and lexical/morphological deficits. This study examined the naming of unpointed tri-consonantal words and pseudowords in a group of 24 adult surface dyslexics, all of whom had attained normal-for-age text reading levels. Such consonant strings, when presented in isolation, can be assigned any one of a variety of different sound (vowelling) patterns, although the most common by far (50% of all Hebrew words) is the CaCaC pattern. These adult surface dyslexics were more likely than controls to pronounce the strings in accordance with the common 'default' CaCaC pattern even when lexical factors such as frequency in the case of real words, or bigram probabilities in the case of pseudowords, favoured a non-default vowelling pattern. These data support the view that Hebrew surface dyslexics suffer a reduced sensitivity to both lexical and morphophonological constraints in word decoding.

Before leaving Lamm and Epstein's subtyping work, it should be added that the subtyping data obtained from a clinic-referred sample may not necessarily reflect the true prevalence of these subtypes in the general population owing to the problem of referral biases. A large-scale survey of an unselected sample would go a long way towards validating the findings from Lamm and Epstein's clinical sample.

Remediation of diagnosed dyslexics

Only a single researcher appears to have undertaken controlled empirical research with direct implications for the remediation of diagnosed dyslexics. The work of Breznitz on reading rate acceleration also reaffirms the existence of a basic phonological dysfunction among dyslexics.

In a series of studies (Breznitz, 1987, 1990, 1993, 1997a,b; Breznitz and Share, 1992), Breznitz examined the effects of accelerating the reading rates of normal and disabled readers. Rate of acceleration was individually adapted for each child by first assessing their natural reading rates in each of six short passages read at the child's spontaneous (self-paced) reading rate. From the separate per-letter reading rates, the highest per-letter rate was designated as the presentation rate for the accelerated reading rate condition. In accelerated rate presentation, text is erased letter by letter at this designated 'fast-paced' rate that typically averages around 20% above a child's self-paced mean. Across several hundred novice grade 1 readers in both Hebrew and English, rate acceleration was found to result in reliable gains in both decoding accuracy and reading comprehension. Gains appear to be attributable to several factors including reduced distractibility (Breznitz, 1988), greater convergence between the vocal output of oral reading and stored pronunciations (Breznitz, 1990), and enhanced STM functioning (Breznitz and Share, 1992). Poor readers, in particular, benefited from this fast-paced manipulation (Breznitz, 1987).

Breznitz (1997b) also examined the effects of accelerated reading in a group of 23 diagnosed dyslexics (average age 9). Reading rate acceleration resulted in significant and substantially increased reading accuracy and comprehension. A series of experimental manipulations examined item order recall, primacy versus recency effects and memory for exact wording as opposed to meaning. Findings suggested that STM functioning among disabled readers was facilitated only when reliance on context was feasible, in contrast to an earlier study with normal novice readers that showed STM gains to be independent of context (Breznitz and Share, 1992). Normal second graders improved detection of wording changes under fast-paced conditions more so than semantic changes, while the opposite occurred for dyslexics. Recall of primacy items but not recency items improved among dyslexics, whereas normal readers improved more on recency items. Breznitz concluded that accelerated reading improves the efficiency of STM-related processes involved in the utilization of contextual information consistent with Stanovich's (1980) interactive compensatory model. These data are also consistent with the view that for normal readers, the fast-paced manipulation works partly by enhancing phonological processes in STM, whereas for dyslexics, the benefits were derived more through the enhanced utilization of contextual information and less by way of phonological processes.

Breznitz (1997a) investigated the effects of acceleration and auditory interference among 52 grade 3 dyslexic and 52 grade 1 control readers. The effects of fast-paced reading relative to self-paced reading were compared with and without accompanying auditory interference (a familiar melody). Breznitz predicted that auditory interference would impair reading performance for normals but benefit dyslexics by suppressing reliance on inefficient phonological processes and increasing reliance on alternative non-phonological (visual–orthographic and contextual) sources of information. Under conditions of auditory interference, fast-paced reading was found to improve the reading comprehension of both groups, but the effects were significantly greater among dyslexics. Dyslexics, but not controls, decreased reading errors in this manipulation. In self-paced conditions, auditory interference led to faster reading times for dyslexics but not control readers. Among dyslexics, the strongest performance gains were recorded when both rate acceleration and interference were combined. For normal readers, the larger gains were apparent during fast-paced reading in the absence of auditory masking. Like the 1997b study, these data suggest that rate acceleration is beneficial for dyslexics not because of enhanced phonological processing as in the case of normal readers (Breznitz and Share, 1992), but by promoting greater reliance on non-phonological processing strengths such as top-down contextual and visual–orthographic information (cf. Brande, 1997).

Difficulties negotiating the transition from pointed to unpointed orthography

As stated earlier, children begin learning to read with pointed text, but are gradually exposed to unpointed text in a systematic manner around grade 3. By grade 4, a child is expected to be competent in both scripts. Only two studies appear to have addressed the unique difficulties associated with the transition from pointed to unpointed script.

Bentin et al. (1990) hypothesized that some poor readers may have difficulties making this transition owing not to inadequate knowledge of grapheme–phoneme correspondences (sufficient for reading pointed text) but because of weaknesses in exploiting contextual information hypothesized to be critical for reading the phonologically ambiguous unpointed text. Bentin et al. selected a subgroup of 19 disabled readers (aged 11 years) based on poor decoding ability of both pointed pseudowords and the ability to use sentence context to identify ambiguous (unpointed) homographs. These disabled readers were compared to a younger control group consisting of 15 good readers (aged 9). A third group, labelled 'poor context' readers (also aged 9), matched the good readers on accuracy of decoding pointed pseudo-words and IQ, but were poorer at using sentence context to identify ambiguous homographs.

Sensitivity to syntactic context was examined by presenting subjects with short, spoken sentences containing a noise-masked target word that was either syntactically congruent or syntactically incongruent with the sentence. The authors hypothesized that if either the disabled or 'poor context' readers have impoverished syntactic knowledge or are less able to use this knowledge efficiently, then the effect of syntactic congruity should be attenuated relative to good readers. Bentin et al. also examined the extent to which syntactically incongruent targets were 'corrected' to conform to the context. Several months later, subjects heard the same spoken sentences and were asked to correct the violation (syntactic correction task).

Both older disabled and younger normal readers correctly identified more targets in congruent as opposed to incongruent contexts, but the difference was significantly smaller among disabled readers. When identifying target words, good readers also committed significantly more syntactic 'corrections' than disabled readers. Finally, the explicit syntactic correction task also revealed significant differences between the two groups both in judging syntactic integrity and in correcting violations. The authors attributed these results to inferior sensitivity among disabled readers to basic syntactic structures.

In contrast, the 'poor context' group showed the same syntactic congruity effect as the good readers. However, the percentage of syntactic 'corrections' was higher among controls. Although these two groups did not differ when explicitly identifying syntactic violations (syntactic judgment), the good readers were better at repairing the violations. Thus, both groups were equally sensitive to deviant syntactic structures but differed in their ability to correct these violations. Since all sentences were very short (three to four words) and all children were able to repeat all test sentences verbatim, Bentin et al. ascribed the performance deficits among disabled readers to a genuine linguistic deficit. With regard to the 'poor context' group, the deficits in syntactic correction were attributed to impairments not in sensitivity or knowledge of basic syntactic structures, but to an inability to use syntactic knowledge in a productive way.

In a follow-up study using the same auditory presentation of noise-masked targets in congruent and incongruent contexts, Deutsch and Bentin (1996) replicated the earlier finding of a reduced context effect among disabled readers with a view to teasing out the relative contribution of inhibitory and facilitatory processes. Differences between the groups were found to be attributable primarily to performance differences in syntactic incongruity: the differences between the groups were significant only in the congruent and neutral conditions, but not in the incongruent condition. A second experiment examined the locus of this effect, focusing on how the inhibition of syntactically incongruent targets interacts with reading ability. The use of context-based expectations was discouraged by blocked presentation of ungrammatical sentences. The authors found decreased inhibition for good readers, while disabled readers were significantly less affected by this manipulation owing, according to the authors, to the reduced efficiency of an attention-based inhibitory component of contextual processing.

Both these studies of syntactic processing, together with Cohen et al.'s (1996) findings, are important in suggesting that some children experience difficulties bridging the gap between pointed and unpointed text because of inadequate syntactic knowledge and/or inefficient use of this knowledge.

It seems likely, however, that problems in exploiting syntactic context are critical only for decoding unpointed text. Shatil's longitudinal study found a negligible relationship between two measures of syntax in kindergarten (syntactic correction, $r = 0.21$ and oral cloze, $r = 0.16$) and first graders' decoding of pointed script. It appears that unpointed, but not pointed, script imposes considerable demands on contextual processing (see also Frost and Bentin, 1992).

As discussed above, another source of difficulty in negotiating the transition to the deeper unpointed orthography may be a failure to acquire the root-based orthographic representations necessary for efficient reading in unpointed script owing possibly to deficient lexico-morphological knowledge. A reader who has difficulties establishing orthographic representations in memory may still cope satisfactorily with pointed print, albeit in a strictly bottom-up (surface) manner, but would be at a relative loss in unpointed script. The transition from pointed to unpointed orthography would appear to be an important topic for future research.

Summary and conclusions

This chapter has highlighted both universal and language-specific aspects of developmental reading difficulties in the Hebrew language. Essential continuities between the data emerging from correlational (predictive and cross-sectional) studies of individual differences and investigations into the characteristics of diagnosed dyslexics provide cross-linguistic support for the view that dyslexia does not represent a qualitatively distinct syndrome but, like other reading problems, lies on the normal continuum of reading ability. The Hebrew data also converge with the findings from other languages, indicating that phonological skills are a universal source of individual differences in learning to read. The phonological deficiencies that characterize Hebrew poor/disabled readers' and the data emerging from experimental training studies showing that deficits in early phonological awareness lead to later reading failure, collectively affirm that phonology is central to becoming literate. In Hebrew, as in English, deficiencies in phonology are counterbalanced by relative strengths in non-phonological aspects of reading such as contextual and orthographic processing that have important implications for remediation. Alongside these continuities, however, there exists a certain discontinuity with regard to the magnitude and/or timing of the relationship between phonemic awareness (and phonological factors generally) and early reading owing perhaps to the highly regular orthography (taught via systematic phonics instruction) that may diminish the cognitive complexity of early decoding.

Several studies converge on the conclusion that morphological deficiencies have a special significance in understanding reading problems in Hebrew. Awareness of structural regularities across lexical items would seem to be especially important in view of both the high degree of morphemic density of written Hebrew and a writing system uniquely designed to convey the abstract consonantal roots that constitute the semantic core of Hebrew words. The diacritical system, therefore, seems well adapted to the task of marking vowels while preserving the orthographic integrity of consonantal roots.

Unfortunately, the diacritical system seems to be relatively inefficient in that the incidence of diacritical errors exceeds consonantal errors even in pointed script. One possible source of these inefficiencies may be the considerable demands imposed by Hebrew diacritics on the processing of spatial location. Evidence consistent with this speculation can be found in the predictive value of preschool visuospatial abilities, as well as the large number of subjects defined in Lamm and Epstein's subtyping study as visuomotor dyslexics.

The potentially problematic transition from the shallow, pointed script to the deeper, unpointed script represents another issue requiring further attention. Data on homograph confusions and the difficulties certain readers seem to experience in utilizing context to resolve lexical ambiguity suggest that the transition from the shallower, pointed script to the deeper, unpointed script represents another potential pitfall, particularly for children with weak syntactic abilities.

References

Aaron PG (1997) The impending demise of the discrepancy formula. Review of Educational Research 67: 461–502.

Barnea A, Lamm O, Epstein R, Pratt H (1994) Brain potentials from dyslexic children recorded during short-term memory tasks. International Journal of Neuroscience 74: 227-237.

Ben-Dror I, Bentin S, Frost R (1995) Semantic, phonologic, and morphologic skills in reading disabled and normal children: evidence from perception and production of spoken Hebrew. Reading Research Quarterly 30: 876-893.

Bentin S, Leshem H (1993) On the interaction of phonologic awareness and reading acquisition: it's a two-way street. Psychological Science 2: 271-274.

Bentin S, Bargai N, Katz L (1984) Orthographic and phonemic coding for lexical access: Evidence from Hebrew. Journal of Experimental Psychology: Learning, Memory and Cognition 10: 353-368.

Bentin S, Deutsch A, Liberman IY.(1990) Syntactic competence and reading ability in children. Journal of Experimental Child Psychology 48: 147-172.

Berman RA (1969) The predictability of vowel patterns in Hebrew. Glossa 3: 127-145.

Berman R (1985) Hebrew. In DI Slobin (ed) The crosslinguistic study of language acquisition. Hillsdale, NJ: Erlbaum.

Birnboim S (1995) Acquired surface dyslexia: the evidence from Hebrew. Applied Psycholinguistics 16: 83-102.

Birnboim S, Share DL (1995) Surface dyslexia in Hebrew: a case study. Cognitive Neuropsychology 12: 825-846.

Brande S (1997) Ifyunei meyumanuyot hakriya bekerev dislectim bogrim behashva'a ledislectim tze'irim (Characteristics of reading skills among adult dyslexics in comparison to dyslexic children). Unpublished master's thesis, University of Haifa.

Breznitz Z (1987) Increasing first graders' reading accuracy and comprehension by accelerating their reading rates. Journal of Educational Psychology 79: 236-242.

Breznitz Z (1988) Reading performance of first graders: the effects of pictorial discractors. Journal of Educational Research 82: 47-52.

Breznitz Z (1990) Vocalization and pauses in fast-paced reading. Journal of General Psychology 117: 153-159.

Breznitz Z (1993) Short-circuiting phonological limitations in dyslexia: the beneficial effect of accelerated reading pace. In P Tallal, AM Galaburda, RR Llinas, C von Euler (eds) Temporal information processing in the nervous system: special reference to dyslexia and dysphasia. Annals of the New York Academy of Sciences 682: 321-322.

Breznitz Z (1997a) Enhancing the reading of dyslexic children by reading acceleration and auditory masking. Journal of Educational Psychology 89: 103-113.

Breznitz Z (1997b) Effects of accelerated reading rate on memory for text among dyslexic readers. Journal of Educational Psychology 89: 289-308.

Breznitz Z (2001a) Speed of phonological and orthographic processing as a factor in dyslexia: electrophysiological evidence. Brain and Language (submitted).

Breznitz Z (2001b) Asynchrony of visual-orthographic and auditory-phonological word recognition processes: an underlying factor in dyslexia. Reading and Writing (in press).

Breznitz Z, Meyler A (2001) Speed of lower-level auditory and visual processing as a basic factor in dyslexia: electrophysiological evidence. Brain and Language (submitted).

Breznitz Z, Share DL (1992) The effect of accelerated reading rate on memory for text. Journal of Educational Psychology 84: 193-199.

Castles A, Coltheart M (1993) Varieties of developmental dyslexia. Cognition 47: 149-180.

Castles A, Datta H, Gayan J, Olson RK (1999) Varieties of developmental reading disorder: genetic and environmental influences. Journal of Experimental Child Psychology 72: 73-94.

Cohen A, Schiff R, Gillis-Carlebach M (1996) Hashva'at ha'osher hamorfologi, hatachbiri vehanarativi bein yeladim hamitkashim bekriya levein yeladim yod'ei kro (Complexity of morphological, syntactic and narrative characteristics: a comparison of children with reading difficulties and children who can read). Megamot 37: 273-291.

Cohen M, Hynd G, Hugdahl K (1992) Dichotic listening performance in subtypes of developmental dyslexia and a left lobe brain tumor contrast group. Brain and Language 42: 187-202.

Deutsch A, Bentin S (1996) Attention factors mediating syntactic deficiency in reading-disabled children. Journal of Experimental Child Psychology 63: 386-415.

Eshel R (1985) Effects of contextual richness on word recognition in pointed and unpointed Hebrew. Reading Psychology 6: 127-143.

Even D (1995) Trumat hanikud lehavanat hanikra velemehirut hakri'a etsel talmidim mekitot bet vedalet halomdim beshitot hora'a shonot. (The contribution of diacritical marks in Hebrew script to reading comprehension and reading speed among Grade 2 and Grade 4 pupils taught by two different instructional methods). Unpublished master's thesis, University of Haifa.

Feitelson D (1988). Facts and fads in beginning reading. New York: Ablex.

Fletcher JM, Shaywitz SE, Shankweiler DP, Katz L, Liberman IY, Stuebing KK, Francis DJ, Fowler AE, Shaywitz BA (1994) Cognitive profiles of reading disability: comparisons of discrepancy and low achievement definitions. Journal of Educational Psychology 86: 6-23.

Frost R, Bentin S (1992) Reading consonants and guessing vowels: visual word recognition in Hebrew orthography. In R Frost, L Katz (eds) Orthography, phonology, morphology, and meaning. Amsterdam: North Holland.

Gelb IJ (1963) A study of writing, 2nd edn. Chicago: University of Chicago Press.

Geva E, Siegel L (1991) The role of orthography and cognitive factors in the concurrent development of basic reading skills in bilingual children. Paper presented at the meeting of the International Society for the Study of Behavioral Development, Minneapolis, MN.

Geva E, Wade-Woolley L, Shany M (1993) The concurrent development of spelling and decoding in two different orthographies. Journal of Reading Behavior 25: 383-406.

Harness BZ, Epstein R, Gordon HW (1984) Cognitive profile of children referred to a clinic for reading disabilities. Journal of Learning Disabilities 17: 346-352.

Kahn-Horowitz J (1994) Megamot hitputchutiot shel hama'avar lekri'at tekstim lo minukadim. (Developmental trends in the transition to reading unpointed texts). Unpublished master's thesis. University of Haifa.

Kozminsky L, Kozminsky E (1993-94) Hahashpa'a shel ha'imun bemudaut fonologit begil hagan al hahatslacha berechishat hakri'a bevet hasefer (The effects of phonological awareness training in kindergarten on reading acquisition in school). Chelkat Lashon 15-16: 7-28.

Lamm O (1989) Dislexia hitpatxutit vehora'at kri'a - ha'omnam hapitaron hu bektse haxotem?] Developmental dyslexia and the teaching of reading. Issues in Special Education and Rehabilitation 6: 13-26. (In Hebrew)

Lamm O (1990) Developmental dyslexia and the dynamics of psychomotor skills acquisition. In G Hales (ed) Meeting points in dyslexia, pp 108-113. London: British Dyslexia Association.

Lamm O (in press) Surface dyslexia: Is it a lexical–semantic deficit? Educational Psychology Review.

Lamm O, Epstein R (1994) Dichotic listening performance under high and low lexical work load in subtypes of developmental dyslexia. Neuropsychologia 32: 757-785.

Lapidot M, Tubul G, Wohl A (1995-96) Mivchan eranut fonologit kekli nibui lerechishat hakri'a (A test of phonological awareness as a predictor of reading acquisition). Chelkat Lashon 19-20: 169-188.

Levin I, Korat O (1993) Sensitivity to phonological, morphological and semantic cues in early reading and writing in Hebrew. Merrill-Palmer Quarterly 39: 213-232.

Levin I, Ravid D, Rapaport S (1998) Developing morphological awareness and learning to write: a two-way street. In T Nunes (ed) Integrating research and practice in literacy. Amsterdam: Kluwer.

Manis FR, Seidenberg MS, Doi LM, McBride-Chang C, Peterson A (1996) On the bases of two subtypes of developmental dyslexia. Cognition 58: 157-195.

Meyler A, Breznitz Z (1998) Developmental associations between verbal and visual short-term memory and the acquisition of decoding skill. Reading and Writing 10: 519-540.

Navon D, Shimron Y (1984) Reading Hebrew: how necessary is the graphemic representation of vowels? In L Henderson (ed) Orthographies and reading: perspectives from cognitive psychology, neuropsychology, and linguistics. London: Lawrence Erlbaum Associates.

Ravid D (1996) Accessing the mental lexicon: evidence from incompatibility between representation of spoken and written morphology. Linguistics 34: 1219-1246.

Rayner K, Pollatsek A, Bilsky A (1995) Can a temporal processing deficit account for dyslexia? Psychonomic Bulletin and Review 2: 501-507.

Rothschild-Yakar L (1989) Bedikat tahalichei kri'a be'ivrit mitoch perspectiva hitpatchutit etsel talmidim halomdim beshtei shitot hora'a shonot (A study of reading processes in Hebrew from a developmental perspective among children learning in two different instructional methods). Unpublished doctoral dissertation, University of Haifa.

Share DL (1995) Phonological recoding and self-teaching: sine qua non of reading acquisition. Cognition 55: 151-218.

Share DL, Levin I (1999) Learning to read and write in Hebrew. In M Harris, G Hatano (eds) Learning to read and write: a cross-linguistic perspective, pp 89-111. Cambridge: Cambridge University Press.

Shatil E (1997) Predicting reading ability: evidence for cognitive modularity. Unpublished doctoral dissertation, University of Haifa.

Shaywitz SE, Escobar MD, Shaywitz BA, Fletcher JM, Makuch R (1992) Distribution and temporal stability of dyslexia in an epidemiological sample of 414 children followed longitudinally. New England Journal of Medicine 326: 145-150.

Shimron J (1993) The role of vowels in reading: a review of studies of English and Hebrew. Psychological Bulletin 114: 52-67.

Shimron J, Navon D (1981) The distribution of information within letters. Perception and Psychophysics 30: 483-491.

Shimron J, Navon D (1981-82) The dependence on graphemes and on their translation to phonemes in reading: a developmental perspective. Reading Research Quarterly 17: 210-228.

Shimron J, Sivan T (1994) Reading proficiency and orthography: evidence from Hebrew and English. Language Learning 44: 5-27.

Siegel LS, Share DL, Geva E (1995) Dyslexics have orthographic skills that are superior to normal readers. Psychological Science 6: 250-254.

Stanovich KE (1980) Toward an interactive-compensatory model of individual differences in the development of reading fluency. Reading Research Quarterly 16: 32–71.

Stanovich KE (1991) Discrepancy definitions of reading disability: has intelligence led us astray? Reading Research Quarterly 26: 7–29.

Stanovich KE, Siegel LS (1994) Phenotypic performance profile of children with reading disabilities: a regression-based test of the phonological-core variable-difference model. Journal of Educational Psychology 86: 24–53.

Stanovich KE, Cunningham AE, Cramer BB (1984) Assessing phonological awareness in kindergarten children: issues of task comparability. Journal of Experimental Child Psychology 38: 175–190.

Stanovich KE, Siegel LS, Gottardo A (1997) Converging evidence for phonological and surface subtypes of reading disability. Journal of Educational Psychology 89: 114–127.

Tolchinsky L, Teberosky A (1998) The development of word segmentation and writing in two scripts. Cognitive Development 13: 1–25.

Yanay Y, Porat S (1987) Haktav ha'ivri vehaktiv ha'ivrit: Ba'aya atika vehatza'at pitaron (An ancient problem and a proposed solution). Mada 31: 18–23. (Hebrew script and Hebrew spelling)

Yopp HK (1988) The validity and reliability of phonemic awareness tests. Reading Research Quarterly 23: 159–177.

CHAPTER 12

Reading difficulties in Indian languages

SONALI NAG-ARULMANI

The past several decades have produced extensive work in languages that use the Latin script. However, there is a second alphabet system, the spread of which is almost as extensive. This is the Brahmi script, and approximately 20 languages, spoken by close to one-third of the world's population, have their roots in the Brahmi script (Breton, 1997). India is the home for many of these languages. This chapter considers orthographic features that are typical of these Indian scripts and explores the links between these scripts and phonological skills, reading development and dyslexia. The first part of the chapter briefly presents the realities of a multilingual language environment, the Indian education system and reading programmes that are prevalent in India. The second section considers the unique features of the Indian orthographies and investigates the links with phonological skills and reading development in these scripts. The final part presents a case study of a child learning to read in Kannada, an Indo-Dravidian language to throw further light on the possible relationship between orthography and phonology.

Reading acquisition in the Indian context – a predominantly multilingual population

Language and literacy research in India presents unique challenges. According to the 1961 census, more than 1600 mother tongues were reported. Noted linguists in India place the number of languages in the country, not including the dialects, at anywhere between 105 and 486 (Singh, 1993). The Indian language systems are broadly divided into the Indo-Aryan group of languages (e.g. Hindi, Marathi, Gujarathi and Bengali) and the Indo-Dravidian group of languages (e.g. Kannada, Tamil, Malayalam and Telugu). The Indo-Aryan languages are native to the north of India while the Indo-Dravidian languages are spoken in the south.

235

In India, people from different linguistic backgrounds live in cosmopolitan communities, especially in the larger cities. In smaller towns and the rural areas, the native languages continue to be predominant, but it is becoming increasingly difficult to find 'pure monolinguals'. Let us consider the effect of English for example. In Nimberdoddi, a distant village in Karnataka (a South Indian state) unconnected by railways, village ladies intersperse their Kannada sentences with English words such as 'compound walls' for 'schools' and 'safety pins' to be bought at the village fair. Children in a village school in the state of Goa, on the east coast, start the day by singing the Indian National Anthem, which is in Bengali, the native language from the land of Tagore, on the west coast.

Let us consider a typical child who will enter a school in an Indian city, and see what languages she is exposed to.

Spoorthi is 4 years old. At home she speaks with her parents and grandparents in Kannada. When she talks with the household help, she switches to Tamil (another South Indian language). Every evening she goes to the playground near her home. Most of her friends know only Hindi (a North Indian language). Spoorthi now knows enough Hindi to teach her friends the rules of 'Node, Node, Thimmaiah', a local game of running and catching. Listening to Spoorthi chatting happily with her friends, you may pick up English words such as 'bus', 'TV', 'comic', 'chocolate'. Spoorthi's predominant language is Kannada, but she is a budding multilingual, like many other 4-year-olds across India.

Literacy in more than one language

Linguistic heterogeneity has led to several unique developments in India's language education policy (see Singh, 1993). One of the most far-reaching of these policies has been the three-language 'formula', which promotes literacy in three languages. Families choose what the L1, L2 and L3 will be in school. It is important to note that the L1 in school (the first language the child learns to read) may not be the mother tongue. In fact, there are children in our schools for whom L1, L2 and L3 are all languages other than their mother tongue.

Spoorthi's parents chose an English medium school for Spoorthi. Here she will listen to stories in English, learn English rhymes and practise pattern drawings that will lead to the letter families of the English alphabet. She will receive instruction in the Hindi alphabet, for about six hours a week. By the time Spoorthi is 8, she will start receiving reading instructions for a third language. Spoorthi's parents say she can choose Kannada, her mother tongue, as the third language in school. However, if Spoorthi's father shifts jobs and moves to say, Goa, the neighbouring state, Spoorthi may not be able to study Kannada as L3. She will probably have to choose Marathi, Konkani or Sanskrit (L3 commonly available in Goa).

The language a child speaks and the language in which the child receives reading instruction can be entirely different in the early school years. Consequently, researchers in India need to make careful inquiries about the child's linguistic background before interpreting research data. For clinicians and special needs teachers looking at children with language and reading difficulties, sensitivity to the interplay of different oral and written languages known to the child becomes essential.

Reading instruction

Reading instruction in the early years in the Indian languages promotes letter naming and learning the various permutations and combinations of consonants with vowels. Some schools have a rich tradition of spoken language activities through word play and songs with nonsense words and rhymes that promote awareness of sounds in each language. Other schools emphasize extensive exposure to the alphabet system through copy work. Exposure to print experiences in the early school years is incidental and rarely planned through display boards and exploring print in books. The first few years of reading instruction that Spoorthi may receive in Hindi will be something like this.

The teacher will introduce the first list of Hindi syllable sequences, which are CV clusters of 36 consonants along with the vowel /ə/. Spoorthi and her friends will recite the list in a singsong manner. Soon they will recite how each consonant will sound when wedded to other vowels (/ka:/, /mu/ or /bi:/). The teacher will ensure that Spoorthi does a lot of copywriting of the vowels and consonant–vowel clusters. Prescribed books will promote single word and simple sentence reading. By the time Spoorthi is in grade 2, her textbook will consist of short paragraphs.

The Indian orthographies

Let us now look at the unique features of the Indian orthographies. As already mentioned, the writing systems of the Indian language families have a common source in the Brahmi script. Given their common heritage, Indian scripts share certain orthographic similarities.

Transparent and regular

Orthographies may be placed on a continuum based on the mapping between the speech sounds and the letters used to represent them. On one end of the continuum are opaque languages with unreliable correspondence between the sound and symbol systems (a single sound may be represented through more than one symbol and vice versa). On the other end of the continuum are the transparent languages with a high degree of one-to-one correspondence between the speech sound and symbol system.

Most Indian orthographies fall at the transparent end of the continuum. Among the Indo-Dravidian languages for example, Kannada and Telugu are at the transparent end. Tamil, however, is more opaque. Barring a few exceptions for each language, there is a one-to-one grapho-phonological link. A given symbol is specifically linked to one distinct sound.

Semi-alphabetic and semi-syllabic

Orthographies may also be classified depending on the nature of the smallest written unit used. In alphabetic orthographies, the phoneme is the basic written unit. In logographic orthographies the visual notation is the smallest unit, representing either a morpheme or word. Finally there are orthographies where the basic written unit is not only phonemes but also syllables. Indian scripts belong to this category of orthography. A limited number of alphabet symbols represent phonemes (for example vowels in the word initial position). The predominant orthographic representation is, however, syllabographs. A syllabograph is a symbol that represents a syllable. Thus embedded in each syllabograph is more than one phoneme and more than one grapheme unit. Changing specific graphemic units in a syllabograph would lead to symbols representing other syllables in the language. The study of syllabographs is of interest, especially since comparatively little research has been directed to this form of orthography when compared to the alphabet and the logograph. The role of the syllabic symbol system during phonological processing and reading acquisition is not fully understood. Of particular relevance is research that explores the links between the orthographic characteristics of a syllabary (a language with syllabographs as symbols) and reading difficulties.

Vowels in the Indian languages have both a primary and a secondary form. For each vowel the primary and secondary written forms are completely different. Examples of primary vowels in Hindi are आ /aː/ and उ /u/. Vowels retain their primary form when they appear in the word initial position. For example the primary form of the vowel /iː/ in the Hindi and Kannada languages respectively is ई in ईश्वर (/iːʃvər/ – God) and ಈ in ಈಟಿ (/iːti/ – spear). Vowels in their primary forms also appear as a morpheme (for example ए /ae/ in Hindi means 'Hey' as in 'Hey look!' and ಈ /iː/ in Kannada means 'this'). Vowels take on a secondary form when they are preceded by consonants (CV, CCV, CCCV). The pattern of ligaturing of the secondary vowel form to a consonant is systematic and follows regular position rules. Examples of vowels ligatured to a consonant are given in Table 12.1.

Consonants may also have a primary and a secondary form. The primary form of the consonant is used in CV clusters. Table 12.1 shows syllabographs with the consonant /b/ common to all symbols. As is evident, the consonant in its primary form occupies a predominant position in the syllabograph. The

Table 12.1 Secondary forms of vowels ligatured to the consonant /b/ in Bengali and Kannada

	baa /baː/	be /bi/	bee /biː/	bu /bu/	buu /buː/
Bengali	বা	বি	বী	বু	বূ
Kannada	ಬಾ	ಬಿ	ಬೀ	ಬು	ಬೂ

ligatured vowel is the additional orthographic feature that makes each syllabograph a unique symbol for the particular syllable sound. When the consonant is part of a consonant cluster (CCV, CCCV) the secondary form is used. The number of consonants that have a secondary form differs among the Indian languages. In principle, the entire consonant system can be joined to form distinct graphemic representations of CCV and CCCV combinations. Examples of some CCV combinations are given in Table 12.2.

Table 12.2 CCV syllable representations in Bengali and Kannada

	swaa /swaː/	shnaa /ʃnaː/	ddaa /ððaː/	klaa /klaː/
Bengali	স্বা	শ্না	দ্দা	ক্লা
Kannada	ಸ್ವಾ	ಶ್ನಾ	ದ್ದಾ	ಕ್ಲಾ

Like the vowels, the secondary consonants follow specific ligaturing rules. In Kannada, for example, barring a few exceptions, ligaturing rules follow a downward extension of the syllabograph. Table 12.3 shows the step-by-step extension of the syllabograph /sthra/ (used in words like (shasthra – /ʃaːsθrə/ – ritual) and (asthra – /ʌsθrə/ – weapon).

The number of syllabographs that need to be mastered depends on the number of vowels and consonants in the language. Kannada, for example, has 16 vowels and 34 consonants. Children in grade 1 are first taught 50 introductory symbols of 16 primary vowels and 34 syllabographs, which represent consonant–vowel-'a' clusters. They then very quickly move on to learn the other CV derivations (how the other vowels are joined to each of the different consonants), amounting to 510 in all (examples given in Table 12.1). The CV derivations are available as charts, worksheets and ready reckoners. In grade 2, mastery continues through exposure to syllables embedded in words. Complex consonant clusters where the secondary form of the conso-

Table 12.3 The downward extension of a complex syllabograph in Kannada

Syllable	In Kannada	In English
CV	ಸ	sa
CCV	ಸ್ಥ	stha
CCCV	ಸ್ಥ್ರ	sthra

nant is used may sometimes be taught through separate lists. However, in many reading classrooms, children pick up the rich symbol system of CCV and CCCV clusters on encountering them in text, always embedded in a word.

Orthographic representations: phonemic or syllabic?

The predominance of syllabographs in the Indian languages raises the issue of whether the pattern of orthographic processing is different in these languages when compared to the alphabetic languages. It may be argued that the syllabographs promote orthographic representations at the syllabic level rather than at the phonemic level. However, one plausible hypothesis is that children taught syllable units will extrapolate phonemic knowledge in the course of learning to read and will be able to apply phonemic skills to their reading and spelling. Access to the phonemic level can be inferred if children spontaneously subdivide syllabographs into the constituent graphemes. Some examples of children using grapheme units are presented below.

- Analysis of spelling errors shows that when such errors occur, only part of the syllabograph is usually incorrect. Thus there may be errors in only the vowel or the consonant segment of the syllable. Such spelling errors appear to be of a higher frequency than errors of complete syllable substitutions (Nag-Arulmani, 1997; Pai, 1998).
- Analysis of errors in reading also shows that the highest percentage of errors occurs due to misreading of either the consonant or the vowel components of a syllabograph. Complete syllable substitutions are far fewer in number (Ramaa, 1993; Purushothama, 1994; Nag-Arulmani, 1997).
- One of the ways teachers cue children who have misread syllabographs is to transcribe (write) each part of the syllabograph and ask the child to read the graphemes and identify the error. Alternatively, the teacher may sound out the phonemes in the syllable and ask the child to correct the incorrect segment. This phonemic segmentation strategy enables the

learner to identify the requisite speech sound and associated grapheme. Purushothama (1994) reported that proficient readers who were given this form of cueing could correct 86% of their mis-readings. Among poor readers gains were only 39%.

It is possible that some children become more proficient at identifying syllabic units as wholes when compared to others. To test this hypothesis, teachers were asked to identify five to eight proficient readers and poor readers in grade 3, in three schools (ages 7 years 6 months to 8 years 9 months). As all children were multilingual, a Kannada listening comprehension test was given to ensure that all children showed grade-level proficiency in Kannada. At the next level of screening a list of 20 consonants and vowels were given in their primary forms, in a letter-naming task. This was to ensure that any errors in subsequent testing were not due to letter naming deficits of the primary form. Only those who could correctly name all letters were taken into the study. Ten students each were recruited for the study. The same list of 20 consonants and vowels from the letter naming task was used to develop two lists of 10 nonsense syllabographs. One list was of legal CCV nonsense syllables found in the Kannada language (*shchi* – /ʃtʃi/, *dya* – /ðjə/, *kki* – /kki/). The second was CCV nonsense syllables not native to the Kannada language (*jlaa* – /dzlaː/, *gsaa* – /gsaː/, *kcho* – /ktʃou/). Test instructions specifically mentioned that the child could read out any part of the syllable that she was uncertain of, before giving the final answer. This was to reduce guessing and to enable the tester to record grapheme level confusions. Syllable decoding was recorded for both lists under the following headings:

- Intrasyllabic processing: sounding out all components of the syllable.
- Intrasyllabic processing: sounding out only the primary consonant.
- Intrasyllabic processing: sounding out only the secondary vowel.
- Intrasyllabic processing: sounding out only the secondary consonant.
- Intrasyllabic processing: sounding out both the secondary letters (C and V).
- Fluent decoding.

Performance on the syllabograph-naming test is given in Table 12.4.

The proficient readers group performed better than the poor readers group on both lists. Proficient readers read illegal syllables less well than legal syllables. Seventy-two percent of all responses in both lists were fluent, suggesting decoding at the syllabograph level. Grapheme-level decoding was also noted and was most commonly used for naming the secondary consonant (10% for legal syllables and 19% for illegal syllables). Poor readers, on the other hand, performed poorly in both tasks. Fluent reading of the syllables

Table 12.4 Percentage of use of syllable decoding strategies on the Kannada syllabograph naming test

Syllable decoding strategy	Syllables used in Kannada		Syllables not found in Kannada	
	Proficient readers	Poor readers	Proficient readers	Poor readers
Intrasyllabic processing by sounding out:				
all components of the syllable	–	15%	–	65%
only the primary components	–	18 %	–	23%
only the secondary vowels	4%	–	8%	3%
only the secondary consonants	10%	10%	19%	18%
both the secondary letters (C & V)	3%	50%	7%	38%
Fluent decoding	79%	11%	65%	9%

was noted in only 10% of the total responses for the two lists. Grapheme-level decoding strategies were used most often. The main decoding strategy recorded was of sounding out the secondary forms of both consonants and vowels (50% for legal nonwords and 38% for illegal nonwords).

It is of interest that none of the proficient readers used the intrasyllabic decoding strategy of sounding out the primary consonant. Among the poor readers, 18% of the decoding strategies used for legal nonwords and 23% for illegal nonwords were by sounding out the primary consonant. A closer examination of responses shows a high error rate (76%), with responses preserving the first consonant in the syllable clusters but 'guessing at' the rest of the syllable.

The data suggest that there is a link between proficiency in reading and proficiency in syllabograph decoding and eventual automatic recognition of syllabographs as wholes. It would be interesting to follow up both groups as they gain mastery over the syllable inventory and check if their fluency in naming the syllabographs also improves. A related area that needs to be explored is whether there are stages through which orthographic representations progress and whether children with reading difficulties and dyslexia take longer to pass through these stages or whether their development is deviant. The influence of the semi-alphabetic and semi-syllabic nature of the Indian orthographies will be addressed further in a later section on links with phonological skills.

Reading phonetically

With mastery over the primary and secondary forms of the grapheme system, the advantage of reading a regular script begins to show. This is because it is possible to read most Indian orthographies phonetically. As words are regular there is no need to 'guess' which speech sound the symbol represents, as would occur in an opaque language. A given syllabograph can map on to only one sound in the Indian languages and vice versa. Reading in most Indian languages is, therefore, a matter of accurate identification of orthographic representations, translating them into their phonological correlates and assembling the sound competently.

There are a few exceptions to the direct, regular links between the sound and symbol systems highlighted above:

- Certain symbols have more than one sound (for example in Tamil the symbol க /kə/ has the two sounds of /kə/ and /gə/).
- Certain phonemes have more than one grapheme in the secondary form. For example in a CCV cluster the Hindi /r/ can be represented as क्र - /krə/, र्क - /rkə/, कृ - /kri/ (the other consonant in the CCV cluster is /kə/ - क).

It is at these points, when the orthographies become somewhat opaque, that interesting contrasts are picked up about reading and spelling processes. For example, the anuswaraa (a substitute for nasal sounds) is particularly opaque because of the variety of phonemes it maps on to. Mastery over this particular grapheme–phoneme link appears to take longer for good readers (Nag-Arulmani, 1997) and may be a point of significant difficulty for poor readers and dyslexics (Prakash et al., 1993; Ramaa, 1993; Pai, 1998).

Links with phonological skills

Evaluation of phonological skills has yielded some of the most interesting breakthroughs in reading research (see Goswami and Bryant, 1990). We now understand that skills such as awareness of the different sound units in a word, being able to manipulate these sound units and being able to segment a word into finer levels of sublexical units, are all critical phonological skills that promote reading acquisition. The phonological deficit hypothesis has been one of the most influential causal explanations for understanding the reading difficulties seen among dyslexics across the life span (Rack et al., 1992; Morton and Frith, 1995; Snowling, 2000). Cross-linguistic research in the various alphabetic languages has highlighted the unique ways in which individual language characteristics can impact the development of phonological and orthographic processing skills (Goswami et al., 1997, 1998). It would appear that 'finely grained' phonological representations promote ease in connecting with the alphabet (orthographic representations), with coarser phonological representations making reading difficult (Snowling and Nation, 1997).

Let us consider the phonology of the Kannada language. The vowel system in Kannada has five long and five short vowels. Diphthongs /ai/ and /ao/ are represented in the vowel inventory. Syllables within words have clear boundaries. All syllables are equally stressed. Within a syllable the Kannada intonation stresses the first part of the syllable, the primary consonant. Syllable clusters typically found in Kannada are CV and CCV clusters. Kannada has both reduplicated (repeated) CCV clusters (ಅಕ್ಕ (akka – /əkkə/ sister), ಹಳ್ಳಿ (halli – /həlli/ village)) and conjunct (different) CCV clusters (ಸ್ವರ (svaraa – /swərə/ pitch), ಸ್ಪೂರ್ತಿ (spoorthi – /spu:rθi/ enthusiasm)). Another complex consonant cluster, the CCCV cluster, is also found in Kannada but is relatively rare and seen in loan words, mainly from Sanskrit. Mono-syllabic words are rare. Most words are either bisyllabic (ಮಗು magu – /mʌgu/ child, ಊಟ uuta – /u:tə/ food) or polysyllabic (ಕೆಲಸ kelasa – /keləsə/ work, ಹದಿನೈದು hadinaidu – /hʌðinaiðu/ fifteen). Word endings are mainly open syllable. Even loan words from English may have a vowel added and become open syllable words in Kannada (bus+u, rail+u).

The phonological structure of the Kannada language may be expected to promote syllable segmentation, a phonological skill documented in beginning readers in other syllable-timed languages such as French (Cutler et al., 1986). The predominance of bisyllabic and polysyllabic words, along with the syllables performing the contrastive function more often than the phonemes, may be expected to promote syllable awareness. Research on phonological development in Kannada (and all Indian languages) is in its infancy, and relatively little is known about the pattern and rate of development.

A study by Prakash et al. (1993) with children from grades 1 to 3 addressed the issue of phonological processing in the early stages of Kannada reading development. The phonological tasks used in the study were:

- rhyme recognition using familiar trisyllabic words (CVCVCV pattern)
- syllable deletion of initial, medial and terminal targets, using familiar trisyllabic words (CVCVCV pattern)
- phoneme oddity task of bisyllabic nonsense words (CVCV) with an equal number of target phonemes in each of the four positions in the word
- phoneme deletion of bisyllabic and trisyllabic familiar words with both CV and CCV clusters and deletion targets as either C1, C2 or V.

The authors report average performance in grade 1 to be at 84.3% on the rhyme detection task and 92.6% on the syllable deletion task, improving further over grades 2 and 3. Performance on the phoneme manipulation tasks was poor (51.8% on the phoneme oddity task and 44.2% on the phoneme deletion task), improving over the following years. No correlation was found between performance on all four tasks and oral reading skills in grade 1. By grade 2, rhyme recognition ($r = 0.56$, $p < 0.05$), phoneme oddity ($r = 0.7$, $p < 0.01$) and phoneme deletion ($r = 0.58$, $p < 0.05$) showed significant correlations to reading performance. In grade 3, only phoneme deletion ($r = 0.57$, $p < 0.05$) retained a significant correlation with reading. Interestingly, the study reports that on the phoneme deletion tasks, an average accuracy rate of 70% was recorded from grade 1 through grade 3, when the target phoneme was a consonant. All subsequent gains were with vowel targets.

The authors interpret these results as suggestive of differences in phonological development in Kannada when compared to alphabetic languages. They conclude that phoneme awareness is not a 'critical factor' in the earliest stages of reading acquisition in Kannada. Two methodological issues, however, make interpretation of these findings difficult. Differences in performance between the large and the small sublexical units may, at least in part, have been because the stimuli were sometimes words and sometimes nonwords. Thus performance may have been influenced by differences in the lexicality level of the items and not the size of the sublexical units alone. Second, interpretations of differences in phonological development between Kannada and alphabetic languages like English have been made in the absence of a comparison group. It is only when a similar set of phonological tasks are tested on a matched group of children reading in the two orthographies that conclusions can be firmly drawn on differences in patterns and rates of phonological development.

In spite of these methodological shortcomings the study highlights some very interesting trends:

- Syllable manipulation did not correlate significantly with reading performance. However, a significant relationship was found between phoneme manipulation and reading performance. These linkages are similar to the linkages that have been reported in alphabetic languages (Goswami and Bryant, 1990; Rack et al., 1992).
- Children were able to manipulate consonant phonemes earlier than vowels. This finding once again demonstrates the role played by language-specific features in shaping phonological development. In Kannada phonology and orthography, the consonant occupies a dominant position. In a syllable, it is the consonant that is stressed. In a syllabograph, the consonant has a primary position with the vowel and all additional consonants ligatured to it. These features in the Kannada phonology and orthography may encourage the earlier mastery of consonant manipulation skills.

Phonological deficits in children with reading difficulties in Kannada have also been reported. Ramaa (1993) reports a syllable-level phonological deficit in dyslexics and poor readers. Children with reading difficulty were grouped into two, based on their discrepancy score. Children with a reading age discrepancy of more than 24 months were the dyslexic group. Those with lower discrepancy scores comprised the poor readers group. Of particular interest are the two syllable-manipulation tasks called word analysis (syllable segmentation) and word synthesis (syllable blending). Dyslexics showed significantly poorer performance on both tasks when compared to the proficient readers and poor readers. Poor readers were significantly poorer than the proficient readers on the syllable segmentation task, performing relatively better on the syllable blending task. The data suggest that the differences in deficits between the dyslexics and poor readers are not of quality but quantity. That is, both groups have a syllable manipulation difficulty, but in dyslexics the deficits are more extensive and across more than one sublexical exercise. The Ramaa study did not include phoneme level manipulations and therefore interpretation of associated phoneme level deficits is not possible.

Assessing the phonological skills of children learning to read in more than one language is an interesting new area of study (Nag-Arulmani, 1998). Are phonological skills the same for all languages known to the child? Will there be differences in phonological skills when the child has exposure to the orthography of the language? Will there be differences in phonological skills for languages that are supported by orthographic representations (the child has received reading instruction) and languages not supported by orthographic representation (the child has not received reading instruction)? The following case study further highlights the need to explore these questions.

Karthik, a 9-year-old child with developmental dyslexia, was assessed on a phoneme substitution task in English and Kannada, the two languages in which he was receiving reading instruction. Since Kannada, unlike English, is predominantly an open-syllable language with mainly bisyllabic and polysyllabic words, parity was not sought on the parameters of syllable length and CV combination patterns. The Kannada list consisted of bisyllabic CVCV words, whereas the English list consisted of monosyllabic CVC or CVVC words. In both languages, the child was required to substitute the initial phoneme with the phoneme /p/. The end product of the phoneme manipulation was a nonsense word.

Karthik's performance on the phoneme substitution task in the two languages is presented in Table 12.5. When we compared his performance to an age-matched control group of proficient readers, a global phonological deficit, spanning across both languages became evident. But Karthik's dominant language, his mother tongue, was Tamil – not English or Kannada. We decided to explore his skills in phonological manipulations in the Tamil language. He was asked to give a list of 40 Tamil words. From this list, 20 bisyllabic words were short-listed. Karthik's phoneme substitution performance on the Tamil list is also given in Table 12.5.

Table 12.5 Karthik's performance on a phoneme substitution task (maximum score = 20)

Language	Karthik's score	Control group (n =10)	
		Average	Range
Kannada	2	19	17–20
English	3	17	15–18
Tamil	9	–	–

At first glance it would appear that Karthik's phonological skills are much better in his mother tongue when compared to the languages in which he is receiving reading instruction. We need to be cautious about this interpretation because the difficulty level of the Tamil word list is not known. Therefore direct comparison with performance on the Kannada and English battery is inappropriate. Karthik's profile of performance, however, does raise certain questions.

First is the issue of whether children may have difficulties in making connections between orthographic representations and phonological representations. Could such difficulties affect efficiency in performing word segmentation, deletion and other phonological tasks? It is possible that Karthik was using a 'visual strategy' to work on the Kannada and English tasks. In Tamil, however, where he has no orthographic representations, he probably used a purely phonological strategy. Karthik's difficulties with phonological tasks could, at least in part, be located at the point where connections are made between phonology and orthography.

A related issue is whether deficits in either orthographic-processing skills or phonological skills would impact all languages in the same way. Further research is needed to understand which specific characteristics of the Indian languages play a significant role in the development of these skills.

Links with reading development

In English, letter naming is an excellent predictor of reading success (Adams, 1990). In the Indian languages, syllabographs have critical visual features that need to be recognized. Decoding a word would therefore require mastery not only of the primary forms of the vowels and consonants but also the ligatured, secondary forms. This section looks first at the time it takes for children to master the extensive syllabograph inventory and then presents data that suggest that reading failure may be directly linked to gaining this mastery.

A study was designed to investigate how long it takes to gain mastery over the extensive syllabary of the Tamil language. We were also concerned with how reliably we could use mastery of the syllabographs to predict reading development.

In a study of reading development in grades 2-4, a syllabograph-naming task was given to 300 children receiving reading instruction in the Tamil language. Twenty Tamil syllables (CV) were short-listed after checking for frequency of syllable occurrence in grade 2-4 textbooks. Three 100-word texts were extracted from the textbooks for each of the three classes tested. The 20 syllable clusters appeared at least five times across all of these samples of texts. The syllables were printed on 6" by 6" flash cards and presented in a random order at the rate of one every five seconds. The number of syllables correctly named was computed for every child. Analysis by grade of the number of children with different levels of mastery on the syllable-naming task is given in Table 12.6.

The data suggest that mastery of the extensive CV syllabary continues to develop well into grade 4 (age 9). When teachers were asked to suggest children who should be referred to our reading intervention programme, we found most of the children in grades 2 and 3 had mastered 40% or fewer of the symbols tested. In grade 4, children who had not mastered 75% of the symbols tested were referred for intervention. It should be noted that, in Tamil, children need to learn approximately 300 symbols, many of which are visually confusing. The acquisition of the entire symbol system is, therefore, protracted for all learners when compared to the 26 letters in the English alphabet. Poor mastery of the extensive syllabary is related to poor reading skills in Tamil.

The reading programme developed for these children targeted mastery over syllable names and synthesis of syllable sequences. Children in groups of 15 or 20 attended a minimum of 30 sessions. Segmentation and blending activities included both words and nonwords. At the end of the reading intervention, mastery of Tamil syllabographs for grade 2 children had increased to the 60–80% mastery level (which is within the range of performance of proficient grade 2 Tamil readers). Grade 3 and 4 children also showed consistent gains in syllabograph naming skills. Associated with these gains was improvement in reading accuracy and reading speed, as tested on a graded sentence reading task, across all three grades.

Other researchers have also reported that the mastery phase of the letter and syllable system extends over the first four years of schooling. Ramaa (1993) found that even good readers were misreading specific segments of Kannada syllabographs embedded in words. Among the 14 proficient readers

Table 12.6 Percentage of children attaining different levels of mastery on a Tamil syllabograph-naming task by grade (maximum score = 20)

Level of mastery	> 80%	60–80%	40–60%	20–40%	< 20%
Grade 2	12%	46%	16%	16%	10%
Grade 3	51%	26%	8%	12%	3%
Grade 4	84%	8%	2%	3%	3%

at grade 3, mastery of 93% of the alphabet system was noted. In the poor readers group, mastery dropped to 80%. The dyslexic group showed the most dramatic drop to less than 50% mastery – a difficulty with more than 30 of the 50 syllabographs tested.

Purushothama (1994) reports mastery levels for Kannada syllabographs presented individually. Ten proficient readers and ten poor readers in grade 3 were given a letter-recognition task. Fifty Kannada primary vowels and syllabographs were randomly presented for approximately half a second each, on individual flash cards. Error rate was 8% for proficient readers and 22% for poor readers. Interestingly, when the misread syllabographs were presented again with no time constraint, both groups were able to correct about 40% of their errors. Mastery level, however, continued to remain less than perfect for the proficient readers and significantly low for poor readers.

While mastery of the orthography is fundamental to reading, it is particularly so in a system with a large inventory of syllabographs. Processes that may be involved have been variously called symbol processing (Ramaa, 1993) and knowledge of rules of orthography (Purushothama, 1994). Further studies of orthographic representations are needed first to understand the norms of mastery of the syllabographs and to ascertain whether the difficulties seen in children with dyslexia and reading difficulties are due to a developmental lag or deviant development. Some of the questions that we are now looking at are given below:

- Are there stages through which orthographic representations get more and more discrete?
- Are children with dyslexia slower in moving through these stages?
- Would fluency at the syllabic level of orthographic representation imply reading proficiency?
- Do children with dyslexia have considerably more difficulty developing orthographic representations of syllables?

Reading in Kannada: are there protective features in the connections between orthography and phonology?

In this section, I present a case study that suggests that certain features in the Kannada orthography may play a protective role for dyslexics.

Aditya was referred to our centre with complaints of academic underperformance. He was 8 years old and studying in grade 3. Aditya's dominant language at home was Tulu, a South Indian language. Tulu is an Indo-Dravidian language belonging to the same family of South Dravidian languages as Kannada (Krishnamurthi, 1998). Tulu doesn't have its own script and uses the Kannada orthography for literary writings. Aditya was also fluent in Kannada and English. He had begun receiving reading instruction in Kannada and English since the age of 5. At the time of referral, Aditya's school day was roughly divided into four hours of work in English and one hour in Kannada.

On the Coloured Progressive Matrices (Raven, 1965), Aditya was at the 95th percentile, placing his performance in the intellectually superior range. His performance on the Weschler Objective Reading Dimensions (WORD; Rust et al., 1993), however, highlighted his reading and spelling difficulties in English. Age equivalents for his score on the basic reading subtest was 6 years 3 months, reading comprehension was 6 years 3 months and spelling was 6 years 9 months. To check Aditya's grasp of the English language he was also assessed using the Test for Reception of Grammar (TROG; Bishop, 1983). His raw score of 16 indicated that his language comprehension was at approximately the 9-year level. On clinical examination, Aditya was found to have no emotional or behavioural problems. The marked discrepancy in his English reading and spelling skills could not be explained as due to lack of exposure to the language or opportunity for reading instruction. Further testing was initiated to understand Aditya's orthographic and phonological processing skills.

The orthographic skills battery consisted mainly of letter naming in both languages and a syllabograph-naming task only for Kannada. In an English letter-recognition task, Aditya showed complete mastery of letter names and letter sounds. In the Kannada primary consonants and vowels list (letter names and sounds are the same in Kannada), Aditya's performance was 94%. In the Kannada syllabograph-naming test, described earlier, Aditya attained an accuracy score of 90% on the legal Kannada syllables list and 60% on the illegal syllable list. Fluent decoding was noted in nine out of 10 syllables in the legal syllables list and seven out of 10 in the illegal syllables list. The intrasyllabic decoding strategy of sounding out the secondary consonant was noted for the four syllables in which errors were recorded.

Aditya was also given a Kannada and English phonological battery consisting of several phoneme and syllable manipulation tasks. Table 12.7 gives Aditya's performance on the syllable segmentation, syllable blending and phoneme substitution tasks for both English and Kannada. His performance was compared to that of age- and grade-matched control groups. In English, the control group had an average reading age of 8 years 6 months in the WORD basic reading. For Kannada, the control group consisted of students rated as proficient readers in Kannada by their teachers and who had scored 50 and above on a Kannada listening comprehension test comprising 65 questions.

As can be seen from Table 12.7, Aditya performed poorly on all the phonological tasks when compared to the age-matched controls in both languages. Aditya's scores demonstrate that he has a core deficit in phonological skills, manifested both in Kannada and English sublexical manipulation tasks. His reading of letters and syllables in both Kannada and English, however, is age-appropriate. We studied the impact of this skill profile on a specific reading task in the two languages. It was hypothesized that even though Aditya had a core phonological deficit, adequate letter naming (in Kannada and English) and syllabograph naming (necessary for Kannada only) would enable Aditya to read nonwords in Kannada but not in English. For English, a nonword list consisting of 30 monosyllabic, bisyllabic and trisyllabic regular and irregular items developed by Hatcher et al. (1994) was used. A parallel Kannada nonword list consisting of bisyllabic and trisyllabic words with CV and CCV syllables was constructed. The nonwords were created by changing one or more phonemes in familiar words (for example ಊಟ (uuta – /uːtə/ - food) changed to ಊಗ (uuga – /uːgə/)). Aditya's performance when compared to age-matched controls is given in Table 12.8.

Aditya's performance on the Kannada nonword reading test was within the range of the age-matched control group. However, on the English nonword reading test, his performance was much poorer than the age-matched control group. The results suggest that adequate orthographic

Table 12.7 Aditya's performance on a phonological tasks battery compared to age and grade-matched control groups (maximum score = 10)

Phonological task	Aditya's score	Control group (n = 10)	
		Average	Range
Syllable manipulations			
Kannada syllable segmentation	4	9	7–10
Kannada syllable blending	3	8	7–10
English syllable segmentation	4	8	7–10
English syllable blending	4	9	7–10
Phoneme manipulations			
Kannada phoneme substitution	5	9	7–10
English phoneme substitution	4	7	5–9

Table 12.8 Aditya's performance on nonword reading task (maximum score = 30)

Phonological task	Aditya's score	Normal group (n = 10)	
		Average	Range
Kannada nonwords	24	26	21–30
English nonwords	4	19	11–26

knowledge of letters and syllables was a sufficient prerequisite for reading nonwords in Kannada. This was not the case in English. The impact of Aditya's phonological deficit was far less devastating for Kannada reading than English reading. The regular, transparent and phonetic nature of the orthography enabled Aditya to read nonwords. The opaque nature of English, however, appeared to play no such protective function, with reading and spelling progress for English being more than 18 months below grade level. Similar differences in reading and spelling skills development in the Indian languages versus English have been reported in other biliterate dyslexics as well (Karanth, 1992).

Conclusion

This chapter has considered three types of difficulties that children learning to read in the semi-alphabetic Indian languages can experience:

- in orthographic processing
- in phonological processing
- in making the connections between phonology and orthography.

In the orthographic domain, well-defined representations of the extensive syllabograph inventory appear to be linked to reading proficiency. Mastery of the syllabographs continues to occur well into the fourth year of schooling, even for proficient readers. Case studies and small group studies suggest that mastery of syllabographs may be a sensitive measure of difficulties in making 'fine grained' orthographic representations. We also need to consider the possibility that some children experience difficulties in making connections between poorly defined orthographic representations and phonology.

In the phonology domain, there is a need to examine the pattern and rate of phonological development in the Indian languages. The role of language-specific phonological characteristics in shaping phonological development needs to be particularly addressed, given the salience of the syllable as a phonological unit in the Indian languages. Further clarification is needed about the sensitivity of syllable-manipulation tasks as well as the more powerful phoneme-level tasks for identifying phonological deficits among poor readers and dyslexics. Coming to the impact of the phonological deficit, we may speculate that there is a threshold beyond which phonological skills deficits will interfere with learning to read, the threshold being much higher for the more transparent languages like Kannada than for an opaque language like English. Of special interest is whether the specific opaque symbols in Tamil and other Indian languages would be more sensitive to picking up difficulties with phonological manipulations.

One area that has not been explored in this chapter is the role played by semantics in reading development. Future research would need to explore this dimension as well, to provide a more comprehensive understanding of how dyslexics use their knowledge of semantics, orthography and phonology to decode words in the Indian languages.

Acknowledgements

The author is thankful to The Promise Foundation and the staff of the Programme for Assisted Learning (PAL) for their continuous support in the various stages of this project. The research reported here was partly supported through grants made to The Promise Foundation by the Community of Schaan, Liechtenstein and the Infosys Foundation. I would particularly like to thank Roopa Kishen, Rathna Latha, Vanitha Dubey, Evangeline Sukumar and Dr Srinivasa Murthy for their inputs at various stages of the projects reported in this chapter.

References

Adams MJ (1990) Beginning to read: thinking and learning about print. Cambridge, MA: MIT Press.

Bishop DVM (1983) The Test for Reception of Grammar (TROG). Published by the author and available from the Age and Cognitive Performance Research Centre, University of Manchester, M13 9PL.

Breton RJL (1997) Atlas of the languages and ethnic communities of South Asia. New Delhi: Sage Publications.

Cutler A, Mehler J, Norris D, Segui J (1986) The syllable's differing role in the segmentation of French and English. Journal of Memory and Language 25: 385–400.

Goswami U, Bryant PE (1990) Phonological skills and learning to read. London: Lawrence Erlbaum Associates.

Goswami U, Porpodas C, Wheelwright S (1997) Children's orthographic representations in English and Greek. European Journal of Psychology of Education 12: 273–292.

Goswami U, Gombert JE, de Barrera F (1998) Children's orthographic representations and linguistic transparency: nonsense word reading in English, French and Spanish. Applied Psycholinguistics 19: 19–52.

Hatcher PJ, Hulme C, Ellis AW (1994) Ameliorating early reading failure by integrating the teaching of reading and phonological skills: the phonological linkage hypothesis. Child Development 65: 41–57.

Karanth P (1992) Developmental dyslexia in bilingual-biliterates. Reading and Writing, pp 297–306. Netherlands: Kluwer.

Krishnamurthy Bh (1998) Patterns of sound change in Dravidian. In R Singh (ed) The year book of South Asian languages and linguistics. New Delhi: Sage Publications.

Morton J, Frith U (1995) Causal modelling: a structural approach to developmental psychopathology. In D Cicchetti, DJ Cohen (eds) Manual of developmental psychopathology, pp 357–390. New York: Wiley.

Nag-Arulmani S (1997) Difficulties in reading, spelling, writing and number work in Kannada and Tamil medium schools. Bangalore: The Promise Foundation.

Nag-Arulmani S (1998) Dyslexia: exploring the multilingual question. Paper presented at the National Conference on Learning Disabilities, Bangalore, India.

Pai PV (1998) Hinditar bhashao ke karan honevali barthni ki thrutiya. Paper presented at the Department of Hindi, University of Bombay, Mumbai, India.

Prakash P, Rekha D, Nigam R, Karanth P (1993) Phonological awareness, orthography and literacy. In R Scholes, B Willis (eds) Literacy: linguistic and cognitive perspectives, pp 55-70. London: LEA.

Purushothama G (1994) A framework for testing Kannada reading on the basis of automaticity, rules of orthography and segmental processing. Manasagangotri, Mysore: Central Institute of Indian Languages.

Rack JP, Snowling MJ, Olson K (1992) The nonword reading deficit in developmental dyslexia: a review. Reading Research Quarterly 27: 29-53.

Ramaa S (1993) Diagnosis and remediation of dyslexia: an empirical study in Kannada, an Indian language. Mysore: Vidyasagar Printing and Publishing House.

Raven JC (1965) The Coloured Progressive Matrices. London: Lewis.

Rust J, Golombok S, Trickney G (1993) Weschler Objective Reading Dimensions. The Psychological Corporation.

Singh UN (1993) Foreword in P Dasgupta, The otherness of English: India's auntie tongue syndrome, pp 13-43. New Delhi: Sage Publishers.

Snowling MJ (2000) Dyslexia. Oxford: Blackwell Publishers.

Snowling MJ, Nation K (1997) Language, phonology and learning to read. In C Hulme, MJ Snowling (eds) Dyslexia: biology, cognition and intervention, pp 153-166. London: Whurr.

CHAPTER 13

Dyslexia in Japanese and the 'Hypothesis of granularity and transparency'

TAEKO NAKAYAMA WYDELL

This chapter presents a cross-linguistic study of developmental dyslexia in English and Japanese, with special emphasis on the occurrence of developmental dyslexia in different writing systems. To account for the possible differences in the prevalence of developmental dyslexia in the quasi-regular English alphabet and the two non-alphabetic writing systems of Japanese – morphological Kanji and syllabic Kana – the hypothesis of granularity and transparency postulated by Wydell and Butterworth (1999) will be introduced.

Much research with English dyslexics has revealed that the impairments experienced in childhood persist into adulthood, even though their reading skills may fall within the normal range (e.g. RE studied by Campbell and Butterworth, 1985; Louise studied by Funnell and Davison, 1989; M-J studied by Howard and Best, 1994, 1996). For these individuals, reading continues to be relatively slow and laborious. Furthermore, performance in a variety of spoken language tasks (e.g. verbal short-term memory (STM), phonological awareness, rapid object or word naming, etc.) continues to be impaired (e.g. Elbro et al., 1995). RE, for example, was a compensated phonological dyslexic and a university student at the time of testing. Her ability to read real words accurately was within the normal range for her age and level of education, but she was poor at phonological tests that required awareness of the phonemic structure of words (e.g. rhyme or homophone judgements). She was also poor at segmenting heard words into their component sounds. She had a restricted STM, and her ability to read nonwords was very poor. Consequently she was unable to use letter–sound correspondences to decode. RE compensated for her inability to use mappings from letters to phonemes by painstakingly acquiring a 'sight vocabulary' of new words, their meanings and pronunciations on a whole-word basis as she came across them.

The underlying cognitive process that is common to all the tasks described above is phonology (Frith, 1995, 1997). Indeed, an unusually high proportion of English-speaking developmental dyslexics fall into the 'developmental phonological dyslexia' category. The phonological deficit hypothesis of dyslexia has thus gained particular prominence in recent years (see Chapter 1). Many researchers have tested its theoretical claims and implications, and their research findings over a wide range of tasks lend empirical support to the hypothesis (e.g. Snowling et al., 1986; Snowling, 1987; Snowling and Hulme, 1989; Brady and Shankweiler, 1991; Frith, 1995, 1997; Frith et al., 1995). The phonological deficit is particularly in evidence in English, where the orthographic system is quasi-regular and the learning of complex orthographic-to-phonological mappings (e.g. *ea* in *bead* and *neat* versus *bread* and *head*) is taxing even for normal readers (Landerl et al., 1997; Wydell and Butterworth, 1999). As discussed by Wydell and Butterworth (1999), learning to read English is a matter of learning how phonemes (speech sounds) map on to graphemes (the letter(s) that correspond to one phoneme). In English, acquiring this knowledge is particularly problematical because one grapheme may represent a number of alternative phonemes (e.g., *ough* in *through* versus *thorough* versus *bough* versus *cough* versus *though*). Failure to acquire appropriate subsyllabic skills is characteristic of developmental phonological dyslexia.

In contrast to the numerous studies on dyslexia in English, little research has thus far been carried out on developmental dyslexia in Japanese. It is hoped this chapter will shed light on why this is the case. However, before tackling the topic of dyslexia in the Japanese language, I will give a brief introduction to Japanese orthography so that the reader can have a clearer understanding of how dyslexia may manifest itself in the Japanese writing system.

Japanese orthography

The Japanese writing system consists of two qualitatively different scripts: logographic, morphographic Kanji, derived from Chinese characters; and two forms of syllabic Kana, Hiragana and Katakana, which are derived from Kanji characters (see Sampson, 1985; Wydell et al., 1993 for further discussion). These three scripts are used to write different classes of words, as shown in Table 13.1. Kanji characters are used for nouns and for the root morphemes of inflected verbs, adjectives and adverbs. Hiragana characters are used mainly for function words and the inflections of verbs, adjectives and adverbs, and for some nouns with uncommon Kanji representations. Katakana characters are used for the large number of foreign loan words in contemporary Japanese. Therefore, a sentence in Japanese can normally be written in a mixture of these three scripts.

Table 13.1 Japanese Kanji, Hiragana and Katakana

Word class	Word	English translation
noun	学生 GA-KU-SE-I	student
verb	学ぶ MA-NA-bu	to learn
adjective	美しい U-TSU-KU-shi-i	beautiful
function word	しかし shi-ka-shi	but
foreign loan word	テレビ te-re-bi	television

Note: Kanji pronunciation is transcribed in upper case, while both Hiragana and Katakana pronunciations are transcribed in lower case.

Japanese Kana

There is an almost perfect one-to-one relationship between a Kana character (print) and its pronunciation (sound). That is, one character always represents one particular syllable or mora (syllable-like unit) of the Japanese language, and its pronunciation does not change whether the character appears in the first, the middle or at the end of a multi-syllable word. This is different from English, where orthographic units (graphemes) not only map on to subsyllabic phonological units (phonemes), but the precise phoneme also depends on context – the location within the word (e.g. *ea* may be read as /i:/ in *beak* or /e/ in *bread*, as /ei/ in *steak* or as /ɛ/ in *learn*). For both Hiragana and Katakana, there are 46 basic Kana characters (Takebe, 1979), but with diacritical marks (either " or °) and others, all the 110 syllabic or moraic sounds which exist in the Japanese language can be transcribed either in Hiragana or Katakana.

Children in the first year of primary school education (6–7 years old) are taught Hiragana first, and then Katakana. Because of the transparent relationship between a Kana character and its pronunciation, children master both

Kana scripts very quickly (Makita, 1968; Muraishi, 1972; Sakamoto and Makita, 1973; Gibson and Levin, 1975).

Japanese Kanji

In contrast, the relationship between character and pronunciation in Kanji is very opaque. Kanji characters are at the other extreme end of the print-to-sound transparency continuum. This is because each Kanji character is a morphographic element that cannot be decomposed phonetically in the way that an alphabetic word can be. There are no separate components of a character that correspond to the individual phonemes (see Wydell, 1998, and Wydell et al., 1995, for further discussion).

Words in Kanji have one to five characters, with two being the modal number and 2.4 the mean (Yokosawa and Umeda, 1988). Also, most Kanji characters have one or more ON-readings, (pronunciations that were imported from spoken Chinese along with their corresponding characters) as well as a KUN-reading from the original Japanese spoken language. Some characters have no KUN-reading, but for those which have, the KUN-reading is almost always the correct reading when this character constitutes a word on its own (e.g. the character 花 pronounced as /hana/ in KUN-reading is a single-character word meaning 'flower'. Also the same KUN-reading can be seen in two-character words such as 花束 /hanataba/ meaning 'bouquet' or 花屋 /hanaya/ meaning 'florist'. However, the same character is also pronounced as /ka/ in ON-reading as in 花瓶 /kabin/ meaning 'vase' or 花粉 /kafun/ meaning 'pollen').

Kanji is essentially learned by rote. Children are introduced to new Kanji characters in texts, and are not taught analytical ways of looking at Kanji characters in terms of phonetic and semantic radicals until they are at junior high school level (age 13–15). Some of the more complex Kanji characters have, as part of their structure, phonetic radicals giving 'some' indication of their sound values. Similarly, they have semantic radicals giving general information on their meaning. The children first learn simple characters without these radicals. Even when they learn complex Kanji characters with these radicals in them, the phonetic radicals give no clue at all to the KUN-reading, and in a sample of 1668 most commonly used Kanji characters analysed by Saito et al. (1995), only 32% have ON-readings identical to their phonetic radicals. Therefore, Kanji learning is at the level of whole characters, if not at the whole-word level. The learning method that is in dominant use is repeated writing (Kusumi, 1992) or rehearsal by writing (Naka and Naoi, 1995), including KUSHO – literally meaning 'write in the air' (Sasaki, 1987). Children are encouraged to write new Kanji characters repeatedly (often page after page) until they also acquire (almost automatic) motor sequences of the Kanji characters. This is because children also have to learn the sequences of each constituent stroke in a character; for example strokes in a character mostly start from the left uppermost position. During the six years of primary school education, children are introduced to 996 different Kanji characters, which are prescribed in the list GAKUNENBETSU KANJI HAITO HYO by the Japanese Ministry of Education. By the end of compulsory education at the age of 15, a total of about 2000 Kanji characters have been taught. It should be noted, though, that adults usually acquire some 3000 characters for most everyday activities.

Thus, the two different types of scripts, syllabic/moraic Kana and logographic Kanji, require Japanese children to use different strategies. For Kana, where the relationship between a Kana character and its sound is one-to-one and transparent, children use simple (sublexical) script-to-sound translation during reading. On the other hand, since for Kanji the character-to-sound relationship is often one-to-many and opaque, and the correct pronunciation is determined at the word level, Japanese children learn Kanji characters and words by rote, essentially by repeated writing.

Dyslexia in Japan

Having to cope with not just one but three different scripts, it might be reasonable to assume that Japanese children would experience greater difficulty in learning to read and write than native English-speaking children learning the English alphabet. However, the concept of developmental dyslexia is relatively unknown in Japan, and some research (e.g. Makita, 1968) revealed that in Japan fewer than 0.1% of children have a reading disability. Makita (1968), Muraishi (1972) and Sakamoto and Makita (1973) all presented evidence for the ease with which the Japanese writing system is learnt. More recently, in order to identify school children with learning disability (LD) in Japan, a longitudinal nationwide survey across 325 primary schools was conducted between 1993 and 1996 by Kokuritsu Tokushu-Kyouiku Kenkyujyo (the National Research Institute of Special Education) (1996). The children with LD were defined as those with at least 24 months of delay in any subject area, including the Japanese language (i.e. receptive language, speech, reading and writing). The survey results showed that for reading, the percentages of the children with reading impairments and delay decreased as the children progressed to higher grades – 2.28%, 1.80%, 1.56%, 1.39% and 1.08% for the 2nd, 3rd, 4th, 5th and 6th grade, respectively. For writing, they were 4.45%, 3.13%, 2.85%, 2.19% and 1.81% for the 2nd, 3rd, 4th, 5th and 6th grade respectively. By the time the children reached sixth grade, the final grade in primary school education, only 1% of the children showed reading delay or impairment. This figure is higher than those found in the earlier studies (e.g. Makita, 1968), but is still far lower than that reported in the English-speaking world.

As described above, Japanese-speaking children acquire two different reading strategies because the two types of Japanese scripts have different processing requirements. A simple and transparent character-level decoding strategy (assembled phonology) for Kana is acquired first, which gives the Japanese children the basis for literacy. Subsequently, and gradually, the whole-word level of reading strategy (addressed phonology) for Kanji is acquired, essentially by rote. The Kana writing system with its transparent print-to-sound mappings ensures fast and accurate learning of Kana characters, which helps children to subsequently learn the Kanji writing system with its opaque print-to-sound mappings. This is because the whole-word pronunciation of a Kanji word is initially given in Kana, and children learn a Kanji symbol and its pronunciation by rote. Are these characteristics of Japanese orthography the reason why many fewer Japanese children suffer from reading disabilities? Can one thus attribute the high rate of literacy in Japan to the writing system? To test the validity of these proposals, Stevenson et al. (1982) conducted reading tests on fifth grade primary school children in the US, Japan and Taiwan. The tests consisted of reading meaningful textual material presented in clauses, sentences and paragraphs, rather than single-word reading. The children were asked to respond to true or false and multiple choice questions. It was found that there were children in all three countries (6.3% in the US, 5.4% Japan and 7.5% Taiwan) who were performing at least two grade levels below average fifth graders. The performance of the Chinese and Japanese children in these tests was consistently related to cognitive abilities, in particular general information (i.e. common knowledge that a child has accumulated through everyday experience) and verbal memory. Their study, however, did not include any single-word reading tests where no contextual information can be utilized. Since single-word reading tests are generally used to diagnose children with reading impairments, their study does not permit any conclusions to be made about the occurrence of phonological dyslexia in any of the countries.

More recently, single case studies of children with reading disorders in Japanese have started to emerge. For example, Kaneko et al. (1997, 1998) reported a case study of KA, a second grade primary school boy (7 years old) who showed severe difficulty in reading Kana and Kanji. He could read only 50% of the basic set of Kana characters and his accuracy in writing-to-dictation for the same set was only 60%, while normal 7-year-old children would have fully mastered the reading and writing of all of the Kana characters. He also showed a deficit in visuospatial perceptual tasks (e.g. copying a drawing of a cube or on the Block Design subtest of the Wechsler Intelligence Test for Children (1987), a test requiring the child to reconstruct two-dimensional patterns using blocks). Further, his SPECT (single photon emission computed tomography) revealed reduced cerebral blood flow in the left inferior parietal lobules, including the angular gyrus, compared to normals. For such reported cases, there is often an identifiable neurological cause for the reading difficulty. The majority of children in Japan who are classified as having a learning disability have both reading and writing difficulties, and often the writing impairment is more severe than the reading impairment. Significantly, in Japan there are very few reported cases of children with reading impairments only. The Japanese researchers usually attribute these reading and writing impairments among children to 'visual' or 'visuospatial' processing problems (e.g. Kaneko et al., 1997, 1998) rather than phonological processing problems. Similarly, the more recent survey of the National Research Institute of Special Education (1996) also revealed that even when the children are identified as having reading disabilities, they tend to have other (specific) cognitive deficits as well. Therefore, these children are different from the developmental dyslexic children described in the majority of English studies (but see, for example, Lovegrove (1986) or Stein (1994) for the hypotheses that reading difficulties may be caused by visual processing impairments).

Hypothesis of granularity and transparency

To account for differences in the prevalence of developmental dyslexia and differences in the nature of the reading problems between Japan and English-speaking countries, Wydell and Butterworth (1999) postulated the hypothesis of granularity and transparency. Failure to acquire appropriate subsyllabic skills is characteristic of developmental phonological dyslexia. The hypothesis of granularity and transparency maintains that orthographies can be described according to two dimensions – 'transparency' and 'granularity'. They argue that any orthography where the letter–sound mappings are one-to-one or transparent will not produce a high incidence of phonological dyslexia (characterized by a defective print-to-sound conversion mechanism) regardless of the level of translation (i.e. phoneme, syllable, character, etc.). This is the 'transparency' dimension. They also argue that even when this letter–sound relationship is opaque and not one-to-one, if an orthography's smallest orthographic unit represents coarse or large sound units (i.e. a whole character or whole word), there will not be a high incidence of phonological dyslexia. This is the 'granularity' dimension. Figure 13.1 (taken from Wydell and Butterworth, 1999) illustrates that any orthography used in any language can be placed in the transparency–granularity orthogonal dimension described by this hypothesis.

The hypothesis argues that any orthography that falls into the shaded area in the table should not produce a high incidence of phonological dyslexia. Given the characteristics of Japanese orthography, both Japanese Kana and Kanji can be placed in the shaded area. The granularity of the smallest Kana orthographic unit representing phonology is finer than the whole word, but

GRANULAR SIZE

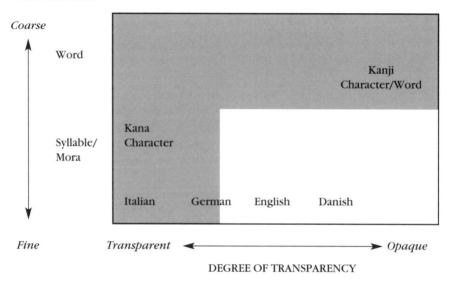

Note: The shaded area on the – 'transparency' dimension represents almost 100% transparency

Figure 13.1 Hypothesis of granularity and transparency and orthography-to-phonology correspondence

coarser than the grapheme, and its orthography-to-phonology translation relationship is at the level of syllables and one-to-one. On the other hand, the unit of granularity for Kanji is much coarser at the character/whole-word level, and the relationship between orthography and phonology is very opaque, hence Kanji too can be placed in the shaded area. Thus, by this hypothesis of granularity and transparency, neither of the two orthographies used in Japanese should lead to a high incidence of phonological dyslexia. With this categorization, however, English can be placed outside the shaded area, because the granularity for English is fine (at the level of the phoneme), but the mapping between orthography and phonology is not consistently one-to-one and is not transparent. According to this hypothesis, therefore, English orthography may lead to a high incidence of phonological dyslexia in people who have phonological-processing deficits.

Landerl et al.'s (1997) study lends support to the 'transparency' dimension of the hypothesis. They examined reading and phonological-processing skills in English and German dyslexic children against their normal age-matched and reading-level-matched controls. They found that although the same underlying phonological processing deficit might be present in both German and English dyslexic groups, there were differences in the severity of reading impairment, with English dyslexic children showing a marked adverse effect on acquisition of reading skills compared to German dyslexic children. These differences were also apparent between the normal German and English control subjects in reading performance. Landerl et al. suggested that these differences were due to differences in orthographic 'consistency'. That is, different orthographies have different mapping rules, and there is a wide range in the degree of consistency with which alphabets represent phoneme by grapheme. 'Consistency' here is interchangeable with 'transparency'. For orthographies such as Italian or Spanish, the grapheme-to-phoneme mapping is, in general, one-to-one and consistent/transparent. In contrast, for others such as English, the grapheme-to-phoneme mapping is often one to many and less consistent/transparent (e.g. Parkin, 1982; Seidenberg et al., 1984). Thus it was assumed that orthographic consistency/transparency affects both the nature and degree of reading difficulties.

Landerl et al. further argued that phonological recoding or decoding may not necessarily be a demanding task. When grapheme-to-phoneme mappings are consistent/transparent, children can easily acquire the grapheme–phoneme correspondence rules and use these to assemble pronunciations for novel letter strings (e.g. Italian or Spanish children). Phonological recoding becomes a demanding task only when the grapheme–phoneme correspondences in an orthography are inconsistent/opaque (e.g. English). Therefore, if the grapheme–phoneme correspondences are consistent, even children with phonological deficits may be able to learn to map print on to sound without showing a delay in reading acquisition. The hypothesis of granularity and transparency makes similar predictions. Also, the granularity dimension of the hypothesis predicts that developmental phonological dyslexia should not manifest itself in a writing system where the unit of granularity is coarse at a whole-character or whole-word level.

AS: An English–Japanese bilingual with monolingual dyslexia

Given the differences between the two orthographies used in Japanese and English, the hypothesis of granularity and transparency predicts that it might be possible to find an English–Japanese bilingual individual with monolingual dyslexia in English. Wydell and Butterworth (1999) reported such a case, AS.

AS was an adolescent boy born to highly literate Anglo-Australian parents, but was educated in Japan until the age of 18. On the standard IQ test in Japanese (Suukenshiki Chinou-Kensa) he was in the top 31 percentile. His spoken language at home was strictly English. Despite his appearance (a tall blond with blue eyes) his ability to read and write in Japanese was superior to that of his Japanese contemporaries. However, in contrast to his fluent spoken English, his ability to read and write in English was poorer than that of his Japanese contemporaries. His reading and writing problems in English were first noticed by his parents, in particular by his father, who claimed that he had similar problems when he was a child, although he has now compensated for his difficulties. This is consistent with the literature on the genetic origins of dyslexia in English (e.g. Stevenson et al., 1987; Pennington, 1990, 1994; DeFries, 1991).

The results of a selection of tests carried out on AS are presented here to highlight the dissociation between his ability to read Japanese at a superior level and his inability to read English even at the same level as his Japanese contemporaries. These are taken from the detailed case study on AS by Wydell and Butterworth (1999).

AS's reading in Japanese

Kanji

Table 13.2 shows the accuracy data of AS together with those of normal Japanese adults. Also shown are AS's median RTs for each word condition together with the median RTs of the two youngest subjects (age 20 and 22) from Wydell et al. (1997).

Table 13.2 AS's performance on two-character Kanji word naming test

Word Type	AS (Control) High frequency (n = 20)			AS (Control) Low frequency (n = 20)		
		S.7	S.14		S.7	S.14
Consistent	95%	(99.2%)		95%	(97.9%)	
RT (ms)	880	814	924	800	786	776
Inc-ON	100%	(98.7%)		90%	(89.2%)	
RT (ms)	883	813	812	802	760	810
Inc-KUN	100%	(97.9%)		80%	(87.2%)	
RT (ms)	965	919	1377	838	791	916
Jukujikun	85%	(89.2%)		60%*	(81.7%)	
RT (ms)	1070	1119	1215	843	960	1052

Note: The stimuli were evenly divided into four different word types: (1) Consistent-ON (those in which each constituent character has a single ON-reading and no KUN-reading); (2) inconsistent-ON (those in which either one or both characters has a KUN-reading, but a target word takes a typical ON-reading); (3) inconsistent-KUN (those in which each character has both an ON-reading and a KUN-reading, but a target word takes an atypical KUN-reading); and (4) Jukujikun (a limited and unusual set of Kanji words, in which a whole word has a unique pronunciation that does not correspond to any standard ON- or KUN-reading of the component character (see Wydell (1998) for more details).

His accuracy in reading two-character Kanji words was equivalent to the Japanese undergraduate level except for low-frequency/familiarity Jukujikun (z = -3.63, p < 0.0009). The latter might be due to the fact that he had not had enough exposure to low-familiarity Jukujikun (Japanese exception words, analogous to English *bough, through, thorough*, etc.). When AS was tested with these words, he was 16 years old, while the youngest subject who participated in Wydell et al.'s (1997) experiment was 20 years old (mean age: 31). Kanji learning is essentially a life-long continuous learning process. If he were continuously educated within the Japanese educational system, he would most probably be able to read these low-familiarity Jukujikun by the time he graduated from a Japanese university. AS's naming latency is also comparable to those of the two young adults from Wydell et al.'s (1997) experiment. His shorter latency for low-frequency Jukujikun words suggests a sort of speed and accuracy trade-off, that is he only knew a small set of these words, but those he knew he could access and pronounce quickly.

Kana

AS's performance on the Kana test is shown in Table 13.3, together with the performance of 10 normal Japanese adult subjects.

His ability to read Katakana strings was again equivalent to that of any accomplished reader. Note especially that he had no problem reading nonwords that sounded like real words (similar to English pseudohomophones, e.g. *phox* for 'fox') as well as those that did not. This is in marked contrast to phonological dyslexics in English, such as RE (Campbell and Butterworth, 1985), and to AS's reading in English, which will be discussed now.

Table 13.3 AS's performance on Katakana word naming test

Word type	AS	(Control)	AS	(Control)
	High frequency (n = 40)		Low frequency (n = 40)	
Katakana word	100%	(99.75%)	100%	(96.25%)
Kanji in Katakana	97.5%	(97.25%)	97.5%	(95%)
Nonword in Katakana	91.3% (92.1%)			

Note: There were three types of stimuli: (1) Kanji words transcribed into Katakana; (2) Katakana proper words; and (3) word-like nonwords where the second syllable (mora) of three syllables was changed. Altogether, there were 240 Katakana stimulus strings: 40 high-frequency and 40 low-frequency words for each word condition, and 80 Katakana nonwords.

AS's performance on tests in English

Compared to his superior reading ability in Japanese, AS showed marked impairments in reading English. Some of his erroneous responses are shown in Table 13.4.

Table 13.4 Examples of AS's errors in reading words (Schonell and NART) and nonwords (Glushko)

Target word	AS's response
Schonell	
ANGEL	angry
BISCUIT	/'bɪskɔːt/
CEILING	killing
CONSCIENCE	/kɒnsɪ'kens/
DOWNSTAIRS	/daʊnes'trʌs/
FASCINATE	/'fæsiːent/
ORCHESTRA	/ɒtreɪ 'stɔɪ/
PHYSICS	/'peɪsɪks/
PNEUMONIA	/seɪ'menuə/
SOLOIST	/'səʊlɪt/
TERRESTRIAL	/'triːzəntrɪl/
UNIVERSITY	/ʌnɪn'vestriː/
NART	
ACHE	archer
BOUQUET	/'blækuːet/
CAMPANILE	/klæmpə'næliː/
DEBT	/'debet/
GOUGE	/'gəʊgəʊ/
HEIR	/'hiːrɪə/
IDYLL	/'ɪdjuːl/
NAIVE	nervy
PLACEBO	/'plækəbləʊ/
SIDEREAL	/'siːdɜː - e'rɒl/
Glushko's nonwords	
BROBE	broad
CATH	/tʃæs/
DOON	dawn
GODE	god
HEEF	/hɜːθ/
LOLE	lowly
MUNE	/'hænɜː/
MOOP	mock
TAZE	/'tezʊ/
WOTE	/hɔːt/

On the Schonell Reading List he scored 42.5%, while for the National Adult Reading Test (NART; Nelson, 1983) he gave only one correct response out of 50 items (i.e. 'simile'). Yet his actual responses were always spontaneous, as if he knew the words very well, and never laborious. Correctly pronounced words tend to be high-frequency and very familiar words (e.g. *book, school, little, postage*). Some of these words are irregular words, such as *island*, but these tended to be fairly high-frequency/familiar words that were probably well established in his orthographic lexicon.

AS compared to the English control subjects

Table 13.5 summarizes the results of AS's performance on various tests in English together with the results from English age-matched pupils in London.

AS also showed marked impairments in the tasks that required phonological manipulation. For example, he was severely impaired on the nonword repetition task compared to the English normally developing readers. Some researchers argue that impaired nonword repetition is a hallmark of developmental dyslexia, and that the task can be used as a diagnostic tool for identi-

Table 13.5 The results of AS's performance on various tests in English with English control data where available

Task			Performance level		
			AS	Control	
Digit span					
English	Forward		5		
	Backward		5		
Japanese	Forward		5		
	Backward		5		
Phonological tasks					
(1) Gathercole & Baddeley's (1996)					
nonword repetition			34/40 (85%)	38.4/40 (96%)	sig.
(2) Spoonerizing					
			10/20 (50%)	18.7/20 (93.5%)	sig.
(3) Stuart's consonant deletion:					
	Word		34/40 (85%)	95%	sig.
	Nonword		36/40 (90%)	91%	n.s.
(4) Stuart's consonant-cluster deletion:					
	Word		24/40 (60%)	92.5%	sig.
	Nonword		31/40 (77.5%)	86%	sig.
(5) Reading Glushko's (1979)					
nonwords aloud			12/43 (43%)	42/43 (97.7%)	sig.

Note: The above data were extracted from Wydell & Butterworth (1999).

fying those children who might develop a reading impairment (e.g. Gathercole, 1995). He was also impaired on the 'spoonerism' task (where the initial phonemes of a pair of words are exchanged, e.g. 'car park' → 'par cark'), as were the well-compensated adult phonological dyslexics studied by Paulesu et al. (1996). His responses were laborious and took considerably longer than his English control subjects. His forward and backward digit span was 5 in English, as well as in Japanese. These scores are more than 1 s.d. below the norms for age-matched controls and at the lower end of the normal range. STM is often impaired in developmental phonological dyslexics and their memory span is shorter than normal subjects (e.g. Campbell and Butterworth, 1985; Funnel and Davison, 1989). Rack (1994) noted that 'one of the most reliable and often quoted associated characteristics of developmental dyslexia is an inefficiency in short term memory'. AS's reduced STM span is thus indicative of AS being dyslexic in English.

Why then does his STM span not affect his reading in Kanji and Kana? According to Baddeley's working memory hypothesis (Baddeley, 1986), during reading, the visual form is translated into an articulatory sequence, which then generates a phonological representation to be held in the phonological store, which Baddeley calls the phonological loop. Furthermore the phonological loop appears to be critical only in tasks requiring relatively complex analysis of the sound structure of printed material (Gathercole and Baddeley, 1993). The sound-structure analysis of Kana is certainly simpler than English, since a single Kana character represents a whole syllable/mora, while for English, phoneme blending is often required. This analysis for Kanji is also qualitatively different from English, as discussed earlier, since each character is a morphographic element that cannot be phonetically decomposed in the way an English word can. Thus AS's ability to read both Kana and Kanji is unimpaired.

AS compared to the Japanese and the English control subjects

In the next assessment, 10 of AS's Japanese classmates were included as his Japanese control subjects. This was to eliminate the possibility that AS's phonological dyslexia was the consequence of his limited exposure to English. These Japanese subjects had little exposure to English, especially when compared to AS. These classmates started to learn English at junior high school at the age of 12 as part of their school curriculum, and apart from learning English at school, they had no exposure to English except for occasional television programmes and films. It was hypothesized that the performance levels for these tests by his Japanese classmates would be similar to or perhaps lower than AS's. Certainly these children had far less exposure to English than AS, both aurally and visually.

Table 13.6 shows the results of AS's performance together with those of both the Japanese and English control subjects on the selected tests.

Table 13.6 Comparison of the performance levels of AS on reading, spelling, and phonological tests with those of English and Japanese control subjects

(i) Rhyme judgements	Mean	Range	
Words (n = 60)			
(Howard & Franklin, 1996)			
English subjects (n = 23)	57 (95%)	40–60	sig.
AS	26 (43%)		
Japanese subjects (n = 10)	42.2 (70%)	35–54	sig.
Nonwords (n = 50)			
(Best, 1996)			
English subjects (n = 24)	46.8 (94%)	36–50	sig.
AS	28 (56%)		
Japanese subjects (n = 10)	31.7 (63%)	22–48	n.s.
(ii) Lexical decisions (Frith, in preparation)			
Phonological lexical decisions (n = 90)			
English subjects (n = 25)	82.8 (92%)	63–89	sig.
AS	46 (52%)		
Japanese subjects (n = 10)	57.0 (63%)	47–66	sig.
Orthographic lexical decisions (n = 90)			
English subjects (n = 25)	85.6 (95%)	74–90	sig.
AS	52 (57.8%)		
Japanese subjects (n = 10)	59.5 (66%)	54–65	sig.
(iii) Reading and spelling (NART by Nelson, 1983)			
Reading (n = 50)			
English subjects (n = 25)	46 (92%)	34–50	sig.
AS	20 (40%)		
Japanese subjects (n = 10)	27.67 (55%)	23–39	(p = 0.058)
Spelling (n = 50)			
English subjects (n = 25)	43.7 (87%)	26–50	sig.
AS	11 (22%)		
Japanese subjects (n = 10)	12.8 (26%)	9–18	n.s.

Note: The above data were extracted from Wydell & Butterworth (1999).

In general, AS's performance on rhyme judgements (Howard and Franklin, 1996), lexical decisions (Frith, in preparation), and reading and spelling (Schonell and Schonell, 1960) were not only worse than those of the English controls, but also the Japanese controls. On visual word rhyme judgements (e.g. *train/crane*; *tough/fluff*), he was significantly worse than the English control subjects and even the Japanese control subjects. On nonword rhyme judgements (Best, 1996) (e.g. *nayes/taze*), however, he was significantly worse than the English subjects but no worse than the Japanese subjects, although his score was towards the lower range of the Japanese subjects. This is possibly because the nonword rhyme judgements were somehow more taxing for the Japanese subjects than the English subjects. The discrepancy between the word and nonword rhyme judgements, i.e. a sort of lexicality effect, was greater for the Japanese subjects than the English subjects or AS. AS's score on nonword rhyme judgements was in fact slightly better than that on word rhyme judgements.

For both the orthographic (i.e. spelling test) and phonological (i.e., YES to *brane* or *phox*) lexical decisions, AS was significantly worse than both the English and Japanese subjects. If lack of exposure to English is the cause of AS's poor performance on these phonological manipulation tasks, then the Japanese subjects who had had far less exposure to English than AS should not have performed better than he did. The fact that AS was worse than the Japanese subjects on these tasks might be another indication that AS was dyslexic in English. There is a strong link between impaired phonological processing and phonological dyslexia. For example, Paulesu et al. (1996) showed that their adult well-compensated dyslexics still showed residual phonological deficits on tests of phoneme deletion and spoonerisms (see Snowling et al., 1997 for a further discussion on phonological processing skills of dyslexia).

On reading and spelling, AS was significantly worse than the English control subjects. His reading score was also worse than that of the Japanese subjects, although this difference failed to reach significance. His spelling score was no worse than that of the Japanese subjects, although it was towards the lower range of the Japanese score. Given the fact that he was taught English at home, no matter how informal and imperfect the teaching might have been, he should perform better than his control subjects who only started to learn English at the age of 11 to 12. Further, the qualitative analysis of errors revealed that the errors made by the Japanese subjects tended to be regularization errors (e.g. *pint* read as rhyming with *hint*), indicating that they had some grasp of grapheme-to-phoneme translation, while the errors made by AS showed almost no regularization errors. Also, on reading, there seemed no apparent pattern in his errors apart from word substitution. This suggests that AS's ability to map graphemes and phonemes in English was impaired and hence he could not make generalizations (e.g., Manis et al., 1996). The qualitative differences between his spelling and reading errors and those of his Japanese control subjects are shown in Table 13.7.

Discussion

Wydell and Butterworth (1999) described the case of AS, a well-balanced, intelligent and well-educated English–Japanese bilingual boy born into a caring and highly literate English-speaking family. However, there was a clear

Table 13.7 Qualitative differences between AS's spelling and reading errors and those of his Japanese control subjects

Target word	AS	Control
Reading		
university	/ʌn-ˈjʊnɪsitiː/	all correctly pronounced
nourished	/ˈnɔːðɜːd/	/-ʃeəd/; /- ɔː -/
beguile	/bɪˈgʊl/	/- gʊiːl/
grotesque	/grɑʊˈtɛskəl/iɪ	/- kjuː/; / - kʊ/
homonym	harmony	/hɒˈmaʊnɪn/
campaign	/ˈkæmpeg/	/- eɪ -/
situated	/ˈstuːtəd/	/- stuːæ -/
judicature	/dʒekɪˈkæntra/	/dʒæ-/; /ˈkætuː/
Spelling		
audience	ordience	oudience (majority); ordience
antique	antiece	anteek (majority); antic
attractive	atrɛctinv	atractiv (majority); atlactiv
nephew	nefaie	nefeu; nephue; nepue
physics	fisicth	physicks; physicse; fisix; figgix
preferential	prefrrencall	plefarental; preferanthele; prephalentul
fascinate	fasanait	facinate (majority); fatsimate

dissociation between AS's ability to read (and write) English and Japanese. AS was a phonological dyslexic in English who was probably more similar to JM (Snowling et al., 1994) than RE (Campbell and Butterworth, 1985) or Louise (Funnell and Davison, 1989), because he was not a compensated dyslexic at the time the case was reported. In contrast, he was a skilled reader in Japanese. This dissociation was predicted by the hypothesis of granularity and transparency, which was introduced earlier in this chapter, with two orthogonal dimensions as postulated in the introduction. The orthographic 'transparency' dimension of the hypothesis would predict that AS should not have problems reading syllabic (moraic) Kana, since the character-to-sound translation is highly transparent and has an almost perfect one-to-one correspondence. The 'granular' dimension of the hypothesis predicted that AS should not have problems in reading logographic/morphographic Kanji either. This is because the grain-unit for Kanji is coarse, and is at the whole-character or the whole-word level.

AS was also dysgraphic. The nature of his errors in spelling is quite different from those of his Japanese contemporaries, who showed a better knowledge of grapheme–phoneme mappings.

General discussion

The objective of this chapter is to consider why there are so many English-speaking developmental (phonological) dyslexics, while there are hardly any reported cases of developmental dyslexia in Japan. It is said that up to 10% of the population of the English-speaking word fall into this group (e.g. Rodgers, 1983; Snowling, 2000). One of the explanations that Wydell and Butterworth (1999) offered is that the process of phonological recoding may be organized differently for English and Japanese. This was similar to what Landerl et al. (1997) suggested in their cross-linguistic study of German- and English-speaking children. According to Landerl et al., the different organization of phonological recoding may be triggered by the key orthographic feature distinguishing the two orthographies, that is the difference in the consistency or 'transparency' of grapheme–phoneme relations for vowels: '...the high consistency of the German grapheme–phoneme relations for single vowels allows for the immediate on-line assembly of syllables' (p 328). Indeed Treiman et al. (1995) showed that in English, the consistency between the vowel graphemes and phonemes for monosyllabic CVC words with the same vowel graphemes was only 60%. Therefore, the correct pronunciations of the vowels in English are determined by graphemic context, which prevents immediate on-line assembly of syllables. In contrast, in German, the immediate on-line assembly of syllables is possible as it is in Italian or Spanish and Japanese Kana.

In Japanese Kana, phonological recoding is essentially at the level of syllables/morae rather than phonemes. Moreover, there is almost a perfect one-to-one mapping between a Kana character and its pronunciation, and thus Kana orthography is very transparent. What this means is that unlike English, but similar to German, Italian and Spanish, for Kana reading 'no sequence of isolated phonemes has to be retained in working memory' (Landerl et al., 1997, p 329). This is particularly interesting, as AS's digit span in English was identical to that in Japanese. Yet his impoverished STM appears to be detrimental only when he is reading English and not when reading Japanese. Further, the smallest grain-unit required for reading a Kanji word is at least at the individual character level making up words, if not at the word level, which is even coarser than the level of syllables/morae.

As discussed earlier, Kanji learning is essentially by rote, remembering whole characters as words. Indeed, studies with Kanji (e.g. Morton et al., 1992; Wydell et al., 1995) suggest that phonological processing in Kanji relies primarily on a whole-word level.

Wydell and Butterworth (1999) further suggested that AS's reading and writing problems in English were essentially due to English orthography requiring a finer processing of the orthography-to-phonology mapping. They then speculated that the occurrence of developmental phonological dyslexia should be equally high in other orthographies that are similar to English in the two orthogonal dimensions of the hypothesis. Danish is such a candidate. Danish orthography also requires a finer-'grain' processing of the orthography-to-phonology mapping (Jensen, 1973), and Denmark reports in UNESCO's Handbook in Reading (1972) a high level of reading problems among children. A recent national study further revealed that approximately 12% of adults in Denmark have difficulties in reading at least half of the text types in the study (e.g. Elbro et al., 1995). Thus, the hypothesis of granularity and transparency predicts that it would be possible to find a Danish/Japanese bilingual individual who was dyslexic only in Danish.

It was also suggested that AS's reading and writing problems might have a genetic origin, as Pennington and his colleagues (e.g. Cardon et al., 1994) proposed. Also AS may suffer from neuroanatomical anomalies, just like the developmental phonological dyslexics described by Paulesu et al. (1996). Despite the possible existence of these genetic and neuroanatomical problems, Wydell and Butterworth demonstrated that developmental dyslexia is not a general deficit that will apply to any orthography the reader has learned, as theories of visual deficits (e.g. Lovegrove et al., 1986) or STM deficit (e.g. Baddeley, 1986) would suggest. Rather this is an interaction between a cognitive deficit and the specific demands of the orthography to be learned. It may be the case that AS has some cognitive deficit, but this deficit only affects the reading processes (demands) required for English. That is, English requires a finer-'grain' processing of the orthography-to-phonology mapping, while Japanese requires a much coarser-grain processing.

Acknowledgement

Part of this work was supported financially by a fellowship to the author (042023/Z/94/GM/HA/JAT) from the Wellcome Trust.

References

Baddeley A (1986) Working memory, reading and dyslexia. In E Hjelmquist, L Nilsoon (eds) Communication and handicap: aspects of psychological compensation and technical aids. Amsterdam: Elsevier Science.

Best W (1996) Nonword rhyme judgement test. Unpublished test. Birkbeck College, London.

Brady S, Shankweiler D (1991) Phonological processes in literacy. New Jersey: Lawrence Erlbaum.

Campbell R, Butterworth B (1985) Phonological dyslexia and dysgraphia in a highly literate subject: a developmental case with associated deficits of phonemic processing and awareness. Quarterly Journal of Experimental Psychology 37A: 435–475.

Cardon LR, Smith FD, Fulker DW, Kimberling WJ, Pennington BF, DeFries JC (1994) Quantitative trait locus for reading disability on chromosome 6. Science 265: 276–279.

DeFries JC (1991) Genetics and dyslexia: an overview. In M Snowling, M Thomson (eds) Dyslexia: integrating theory and practice. London: Whurr.

Elbro C, Moller S, Nielsen EM (1995) Functional reading difficulties in Denmark. A study of adult reading of common text. Reading and Writing: An Interdisciplinary Journal 7: 257–276.

Frith U (1995) Dyslexia: can we have a shared theoretical framework? In N Frederickson, R Reason (eds) Phonological assessment of specific learning difficulties. Educational and Child Psychology 12: 1.

Frith U (1997) Brain, mind and behaviour in dyslexia. In C Hulme, M Snowling (eds) Dyslexia: biology, cognition and intervention, pp 1–19. London: Whurr.

Frith U (in preparation) Orthographic and phonological lexical decision tests for children.

Frith U, Landerl K, Frith C (1995) Dyslexia and verbal fluency: more evidence for a phonological deficit. Dyslexia 1: 2–11.

Funnell E, Davison M (1989) Lexical capture: a developmental disorder of reading and spelling. Quarterly Journal of Experimental Psychology 41A: 471–487.

Gathercole SE (1995) Nonword repetition: more than just a phonological output task. Cognitive Neuropsychology 12: 857–861.

Gathercole SE, Baddeley AD (1993) Phonological working memory: a critical building block for reading development and vocabulary acquisition. European Journal of Psychology in Education 8: 259–272.

Gathercole SE, Baddeley AD (1996) The children's test of nonword repetition. London: The Psychological Corporation.

Gibson EJ, Levin H (1975) Psychology of reading. Cambridge, MA: MIT Press.

Glushko RJ (1979) The organisation and activation of orthographic knowledge in reading aloud. Journal of Experimental Psychology: Human Perception and Performance 5: 674–691.

Howard D, Best W (1994) Impaired nonword reading with normal word reading: a case study. Journal of Research in Reading 20: 55–65.

Howard D, Best W (1996) Developmental phonological dyslexia: real word reading can be completely normal. Cognitive Neuropsychology 13: 887–934.

Howard D, Franklin S (1996) Missing the meaning? Cambridge, MA: MIT Press.

Jensen AR (1973) Spelling errors and the serial-position effect. Journal of Educational Psychology 53: 105–109.

Kaneko M, Uno A, Kaga M, Matsuda H, Inagaki M, Haruhara N (1997) Developmental dyslexia and dysgraphia – a case report. NO TO HATTATSU (Brain and Child Development) 29: 249–253. (In Japanese)

Kaneko M, Uno A, Kaga M, Matsuda H, Inagaki M, Haruhara N (1998) Cognitive neuropsychological and regional cerebral blood flow study of a developmentally dyslexic Japanese child. Journal of Child Neurology Brief Communications 13: 9.

Kokuritsu Tokushu-Kyoiku Kenkyujyo (Japanese National Research Institute of Special Education) (1996). Report C-28: Kyouka-gakushuu-ni tokuina-konnan-wo shimesu jidou-seito-no ruikeika-to shidouhou-no kenkyu (Categorisation of primary school children with LD and a study on remediation methods).

Kusumi T (1992) Meta memory. In Anzai Y, Ishizaki S, Otsu Y, Hatano G, Miozoguchi H (eds) Handbook of cognitive science (in Japanese), Kyoritsu Shuppan: Tokyo.

Landerl K, Wimmer H, Frith U (1997) The impact of orthographic consistency on dyslexia: a German–English comparison. Cognition 63: 315–334.

Lovegrove W, Martin F, Slaghuis W (1986) A theoretical and experimental case for a visual deficit in specific reading disability. Cognitive Neuropsychology 3: 225-267.

Lovegrove W (1994) Visual deficits in dyslexia: Evidence and implications. In Fawcett A, Nicolson RI (eds) Dyslexia in Children: Multidisciplinary Perspectives. New York: Havester Wheatsheaf.

Makita K (1968) The rarity of reading disability in Japanese children. American Journal of Orthopsychiatry 38: 599-614.

Manis FR, Seidenberg MS, Doi LM, McBride-Chang C, Peterson A (1996) On the bases of two subtypes of developmental dyslexia. Cognition 58: 157-195.

Morton J, Sasanuma S, Patterson K, Sakuma N (1992) The organisation of lexicon in Japanese: single and compound Kanji. British Journal of Psychology 83: 517-531.

Muraishi S (1972) Acquisition of reading Japanese syllabic characters in pre-school children in Japan. Paper presented at 20th International Congress of Psychology, Tokyo.

Naka M, Naoi H (1995) The effect of repeated writing on memory. Memory and Cognition 23: 201-212.

Nelson H (1983) National Adult Reading Test (NART). Windsor: NFER.

Parkin A (1982) Phonological recoding in lexical decision: effects of spelling-to-sound regularity depend on how regularity is defined. Memory and Cognition 10: 43-53.

Paulesu E, Frith U, Snowling M, Gallagher A, Morton RSJ, Frackowiak R, Frith CD (1996) Is developmental dyslexia a disconnection syndrome? Evidence from PET scanning. Brain 119: 143-157.

Pennington BF (1990) The genetics of dyslexia. Journal of Child Psychology and Psychiatry 31: 193-201.

Pennington BF (1994) Genetics of learning disabilities. Journal of Child Neurology 10 (Supplement): s69-s76.

Rack JP (1994) Dyslexia. The phonological deficit hypothesis. In Nicolson R, Fawcett A (eds) Dyslexia in children: multidisciplinary perspectives. London: Harvester Wheatsheaf.

Rodgers B (1983) The identification and prevalence of specific reading retardation. British Journal of Educational Psychology 53: 369-373.

Saito H, Kawakami M, Matsuda H (1995) Kanji-kousei-ni okeru buhin (bushu)-on'in taiou-hyo (Variety of phonetic components of radical types in complex left-right Kanji). Jouhou-Kagaku-Kenkyu 2: 89-115.

Sakamoto T, Makita K (1973) Japan. In J Downing (ed) Comparative reading. New York: Macmillan.

Sampson G (1985) Writing systems. Stanford, CA: Stanford University Press.

Sasaki M (1987) Why do Japanese write characters in space? International Journal of Behavioural Development 10: 135-149.

Schonell FJ, Schonell PE (1960) Diagnostic and attainment testing. Edinburgh: Oliver & Boyd.

Seidenberg MS, Walters GS, Barnes MA, Tanenhaus MK (1984) When does irregular spelling or pronunciation influence word recognition? Journal of Verbal Learning and Verbal Behaviour 23: 383-404.

Snowling M (1987) Dyslexia: a cognitive developmental perspective. Oxford: Basic Blackwell.

Snowling M (2000) Dyslexia. Oxford: Blackwell.

Snowling M, Hulme C (1989) A longitudinal case study of developmental phonological dyslexia. Cognitive Neuropsychology 6: 379-401.

Snowling M, Hulme C, Goulandris N (1994) Word recognition in developmental dyslexia: a connectionist approach. Quarterly Journal of Experimental Psychology 47A: 895–916.

Snowling M, Stackhouse J, Rack J (1986) Phonological dyslexia and dysgraphia: a developmental analysis. Cognitive Neuropsychology 3: 309–339.

Snowling M, Nation K, Moxham P, Gallagher A, Frith U (1997) Phonological processing skills of dyslexic students in higher education: a preliminary report. Journal of Research in Reading 20: 1, 31–41.

Stein J (1994) A visual defect in dyslexics? In A Fawcet, R Nicolson (eds) Dyslexia in Children. Hemel Hempstead: Harvester Wheatsheaf.

Stevenson HW, Stigler JW, Lucker, GW, Lee S in collaboration with Hsu C, Kitamura S (1982) Reading disabilitites: the case of Chinese, Japanese, and English. Child Development 53: 1164–1181.

Stevenson J, Graham AA, Fredman G, McLoughlin V (1987) A twin study of genetic influences on reading and spelling ability and disability. Journal of Child Psychology and Psychiatry 28: 229–247.

Takebe T (1979). NIHONGO NO HYOKI (The Japanese orthography, in Japanese).Tokyo: Kadokawa.

Treiman R, Mullenix J, Bijeljac-Babic R, Richmond-Welty ED (1995) The special role of rimes in the description, use and acquisition of English orthography. Journal of Experimental Psychology: General 124: 107–136.

UNESCO (1972) Handbook in reading. In EJ Gibson, H Levin (1975) Psychology of reading. Cambridge, MA: MIT Press

Wechsler D (1987) Wechsler Intelligence Scale for Children – Revised (in Japanese). San Antonio, TX: The Psychological Corporation.

Wydell TN (1998) What matters in Kanji word naming: consistency, regularity, or ON/KUN-reading difference? Reading and Writing: An Interdisciplinary Journal 10: 359–373.

Wydell TN, Butterworth BL (1999) A case study of an English–Japanese bilingual with monolingual dyslexia. Cognition 70: 273–305.

Wydell TN, Patterson K, Humphreys GW (1993) Phonologically mediated access to meaning for KANJI: Is a ROWS still a ROSE in Japanese KANJI? Journal of Experimental Psychology: Learning, Memory and Cognition 19: 491–514.

Wydell TN, Butterworth B, Patterson K (1995) The inconsistency of consistency effects in reading: the case of Japanese Kanji. Journal of Experimental Psychology: Learning, Memory and Cognition 21: 1155–1168.

Wydell TN, Butterworth B, Shibahara N, Zorzi M (1997). The irregularity of regularity effects in reading: the case of Japanese Kanji. Paper presented at the meeting of the Experimental Psychology Society, Cardiff.

Yokosawa K, Umeda M (1988) Process in human Kanji word recognition. In Proceedings of the 1988 IEEE International Conference on Systems, Man and Cybernetics, pp 377–380.

CHAPTER 14

Reading acquisition and developmental dyslexia in Chinese: a cognitive perspective

CONNIE SUK-HAN HO

Is dyslexia only a Western problem?

In the 1960s and 1970s, dyslexia was widely believed to be a problem that affected readers in alphabetic languages only (e.g. Makita, 1968; Rozin and Gleitman, 1977). Based on early informal observations or surveys, readers of Asian languages (e.g. Chinese, Japanese and Korean) were reported to have a low incidence of reading disability (Makita, 1968; Kuo, 1978; Sheridan, 1983). Frith (1985) suggested that the low prevalence of developmental dyslexia in Japan was probably due to the fact that the Japanese script involved logographic and syllabic skills rather than alphabetic skills. Similarly, Liberman et al. (1974) elaborated this orthographic hypothesis by saying that for young children, explicit phoneme segmentation was harder than syllable segmentation. They expected syllable-based writing systems (e.g. Chinese and Japanese) to be easier to learn to read than those based on an alphabet (e.g. English) (see Chapter 13). If this is the case, dyslexic alphabetic readers may try to tackle their reading problems by learning to read a syllable-based script. Rozin et al. (1971) had designed such an innovative project to teach American children with reading problems to read English represented by Chinese characters. Their project was successful in teaching the children to read 30 Chinese characters and some Chinese sentences in their English translation. They suggested that these children failed to read English well because they had poor phonemic representations, but they could read Chinese well because of the absence of grapheme–phoneme mappings in Chinese. However, Stevenson (1984) rightly pointed out that by teaching the participants 30 Chinese characters in English, Rozin et al. had only demonstrated a simple form of paired-associate learning without confronting the complex, abstract nature of the Chinese writing system.

Contrary to the common belief mentioned above, Stevenson and his colleagues (1982) demonstrated that the prevalence of dyslexia is comparable among American, Japanese and Chinese children. Hirose and Hatta (1988) have also reported that about 11% of fifth graders in Japan have two or more years delay in reading. It follows from these findings that no writing system appears to guarantee immunity from dyslexia. The underestimation of the incidence of dyslexia among Asian populations in the past was probably due to insufficient understanding of dyslexia and the absence of objective assessment instruments. For instance, dyslexic children are easily overlooked in the Chinese community. Low achievement in reading and spelling are often misconceived as being caused by poor learning motivation, laziness and low abilities.

In this chapter, I examine developmental dyslexia in relation to the Chinese orthography, which is a non-alphabetic script used by the largest population in the world. I consider whether there are different underlying cognitive deficits for dyslexia in Chinese as compared with dyslexia in alphabetic languages. To familiarize the reader with the Chinese language, I first describe its various linguistic characteristics and then review two closely related areas of research, namely reading acquisition in Chinese and developmental dyslexia in Chinese.

Linguistic characteristics of the Chinese language

Sound structure of the Chinese language

There are seven major dialect groups in Chinese. To promote national unity, a national language, Putonghua, has been used as the official spoken language in China since 1956. Putonghua is close to Mandarin and it is also the native language of about 70% of the Chinese population. The phonological structure of Chinese speech units is relatively simple. The basic speech unit is the syllable. It is conventional to dissect a Chinese syllable into two segments: initial (i.e. the onset) and final (i.e. the rime). For instance, there are 22 onsets and 38 rimes in Putonghua that make up about 400 syllables, whereas there are 19 onsets and 51 rimes in Cantonese (a southern dialect in China) that make up about 650 syllables.

Chinese is a tonal language. In other words, a change in the tone of a Chinese syllable changes the meaning of the morpheme. The number of tones in the Chinese language varies from one dialect to another. For instance, there are four tones in Putonghua and nine tones in Cantonese.

The Chinese orthography

Graphic features of the Chinese script

A Chinese writing reform began in China in 1956, and over 2000 Chinese characters were simplified. These simplified characters are used in China and

Singapore, while people in Taiwan and Hong Kong still use the traditional script.

The basic graphic unit in Chinese is a character. There are about 3000 Chinese characters in daily use in China (Foreign Language Press Beijing, 1989) and about 4500 frequently used characters in Taiwan (Liu et al., 1975). Chinese characters are made up of different strokes. Each stroke is written in one movement of a brush or pen. One stroke is usually a single line (e.g., ⼀ , ⼁ , ⼃ or ⼂) or a dot (e.g. ⼂), but it can also involve an angle (e.g. ⼅). Some characters can have just one stroke (e.g. 一 'one') while others can have as many as 24 strokes (e.g. 靈 'spirit'). The average number of strokes of 2000 commonly used characters is 11.2 for the traditional script and 9.0 for the simplified script (Chan, 1982).

In orthographic structure, Chinese characters can be divided into integrated forms and compound forms. Integrated form is a single complete character, such as 人 'person' and 中 'middle', which cannot be further decomposed into smaller meaningful stroke patterns. Compound form is a character that is formed from two or more stroke patterns. An integrated character can appear as a stroke pattern in a compound character (e.g. 中 'middle' in the character 沖 'flush'). The stroke patterns in a compound character may serve different semantic or phonological functions (see the next section). Chen (1993) reported that the number of stroke patterns in a character is a better indicator of character complexity than the number of strokes in a character. For instance, both characters 需 'need' and 端 'end' have 14 strokes, but the former has two stroke-patterns while the latter has three. According to Chen, the character 'end' is more complicated than the character 'need'.

How the Chinese script represents its spoken language

Different orthographies in the world represent their spoken languages differently. In alphabetic languages, the graphic units are made to represent more or less the elementary units in speech (i.e. phonemes). In the Chinese language, graphic units represent basic units of meaning (i.e. morphemes) and characters are monosyllabic. One obvious advantage of this logographic and morphosyllabic nature of Chinese is that the same script can be used in a large population where people speak different dialects.

In fact, Chinese is not as logographic as people expect because only a small percentage (about 10%) of Chinese characters convey meaning by pictographic or ideographic representation. According to Zhu (1987), about 90% of Chinese characters are ideophonetic compounds, each comprising a meaning-based component (the semantic radical) and a sound-based component (the phonetic radical). There are about 200 semantic radicals and 800 phonetic radicals in Chinese (Hoosain, 1991).

Semantic radicals can be characters in their own right, or unpronounce-able graphic units. In general, the semantic radical in a character signifies the semantic category of the character. Sometimes the semantic implication of the semantic radical is transparent (e.g. the semantic radical 氵 stands for 'water', and characters with this semantic radical such as 溪 'small river', 河 'river' and 海 'sea' are often related to 'water'), but sometimes it is opaque (e.g. the semantic radical 女 stands for 'female'; characters with this semantic radical such as 奶 'milk', 姓 'surname' and 嫖 'visiting prostitutes' are only indirectly related to 'female'), or sometimes the semantic radical is irrelevant (e.g. the semantic radical 糸 stands for 'silk' or 'thread', characters with this semantic radical such as 紅 'red', 終 'end' and 級 'class' are totally unrelated to 'silk' or 'thread'). Thus, the semantic cueing function of the semantic radical is limited to signifying a broad category of meaning, which does not always provide reliable information. The exact, rich, complex and subtle meaning of each Chinese character has to be learned individually.

The phonetic radical provides sound cues to an ideophonetic compound. Again phonetic radicals can be characters in their own right or unpronounce-able graphic units. In principle, there are at least two possible ways that the pronunciation of a Chinese ideophonetic compound can be reached via the phonetic radical: by direct derivation or analogy. First, a Chinese reader can directly derive the pronunciation of a compound character from the sound of its phonetic radical, for instance, if a reader does not know the character 碼 [ma]5 'yard'[1] but he or she knows the sound of its phonetic radical 馬 [ma]5 'horse'. Since 馬 and 碼 are homophones, the reader can derive the sound of 碼 from the sound of 馬. Like the phonological regularity of English words, the sound information provided directly by the phonetic radical varies in reliability or regularity. Second, a reader can deduce by analogy the sound of a character from the sound of other characters having the same phonetic radical (e.g. the sound of 碼 [ma]5 'yard' can be deduced from that of 螞 [ma]5 'ant' and 瑪 [ma]5 'agate'). This is similar to the neighbourhood effect and consistency effect in English (e.g. Laxon et al., 1994).

We called the above script-sound regularities in Chinese orthography-phonology correspondence (OPC) rules (Ho and Bryant, 1997a). These OPC rules are different from the grapheme-phoneme correspondence (GPC) rules in English in that the method of phonetic notation in reading English is atomistic, whereas it is part-to-whole in reading Chinese (Chen, 1993). For words in alphabetic languages, each orthographic unit (i.e. a letter) has a unique phonetic value, e.g. *f* is pronounced /f/. The pronunciation of a regular word is arrived at by assembling the phonetic values of all

---

[1] In the syllable [ma]5, /m/ is the onset and /a/ is the rime of the syllable. '5' means that the syllable is in the 5th tone, i.e. a low rising tone.

the orthographic units in a word. This is what we call atomistic. On the other hand, the pronunciation of a Chinese character can be derived from the phonetic value of just one orthographic component, i.e. the phonetic radical of the character. Thus, the phonetic radical, as a part of the character, encodes or specifies the syllabic pronunciation of the whole character.

Based on some linguistic analyses, Zhu (1987) suggested that the semantic cueing function of the semantic radical in a Chinese character is stronger than the phonological cueing function of the phonetic radical. For instance, in the 3756 frequently used Chinese characters, there are 184 characters with the semantic radical ' 扌 '. Of these 184 characters, only a few are not related to the meaning of 'hand' or 'motion' (Zhu, 1987). On the other hand, the predictive accuracy of the pronunciation of an ideophonetic compound character from its phonetic radical is about 40% (Zhou, 1980; Zhu, 1987). In other words, about four out of 10 ideophonetic compounds have the same onsets and rimes as those of their phonetic radicals, although tones may be different.

If tone is taken into consideration, only 26% of ideophonetic compounds have the same onsets, rimes and tones as those of their phonetic radicals (Fan, 1986). If frequency of usage is taken into consideration, the predictive accuracy drops to only 19% (Zhu, 1987). This implies that ideophonetic compounds are more regular phonologically in the low-frequency range than in the high-frequency range. However, this is only an intra-character regularity index (i.e. an index of how reliable a phonetic radical is in providing sound cues to a Chinese character consisting of that particular phonetic radical); an index of inter-character consistency (i.e. an index of how consistent are the pronunciations of Chinese characters sharing the same phonetic radical) is not reported. These researchers seem to assume that Chinese readers only derive sound information directly from the phonetic radical (i.e. direct derivation is the only rule for decoding), and they have neglected the possible impact of orthographic neighbours enabling derivation by analogy.

The reader can refer to the writings of Leong (1989), Hoosain (1991), Tzeng (1994), Taylor and Taylor (1995) and Chen (1996) for further details about the linguistic characteristics of the Chinese language.

Research in reading acquisition in Chinese

Understanding how ordinary Chinese children acquire reading skills will help us understand why some children have difficulties in learning to read Chinese. In this section, I first consider some educational practices in three Chinese populations and then discuss which cognitive skills are important in learning to read Chinese and why.

Educational practices in three Chinese populations

In mainland China, Putonghua is the medium of instruction in school. Children first learn Pin-Yin (an alphabetic phonetic system in which each letter stands for one phoneme) and then use it to help them learn to read simplified Chinese characters. People in Taiwan speak Mandarin. Children learn to read Chinese traditional script with the help of Zhu-Yin-Fu-Hao (a subsyllabic phonetic system in which each graphic unit stands for either an onset or a rime of a Chinese syllable). In Hong Kong, children speak Cantonese and learn to read Chinese traditional script without the help of any phonetic system. Pin-Yin or Zhu-Yin-Fu-Hao symbols are printed along-side the Chinese characters in junior elementary grades but these phonetic symbols are removed from Chinese text in senior grades. In all three regions, Chinese characters are commonly taught with a whole-word approach without much emphasis on the significance of intra-character components. Although semantic radicals are taught systematically at about grade 3, they are mainly used as units for looking up characters in Chinese dictionaries instead of providing semantic information in reading. In recent years, a modern teaching method called 'concentrated character learning' has been introduced in China. Chinese characters are taught systematically in groups. Characters that share either a phonetic or a semantic radical are learned together. Children learn about 2600 to 2800 Chinese characters in their elementary grades.

Cognitive skills that are important in learning to read Chinese

There is ample evidence to show that phonological skills, especially phono-logical awareness, are important predictors of children's beginning reading success in alphabetic scripts (e.g. Lundberg et al., 1980, 1988; Bradley and Bryant, 1983, 1985; Frith and Snowling, 1983; Mann and Liberman, 1984; Perfetti et al., 1987; Wagner and Torgesen, 1987; Gathercole et al., 1991; Wagner et al., 1994, for review). People often suggest that the importance of phonological skills in learning to read alphabetic scripts such as English is related to their alphabetic nature. The script of an alphabetic system basically maps on to the sound of its language and phonological awareness has been demonstrated as essential for the acquisition of the letter–sound correspon-dence rules (e.g. Byrne, 1992).

An important theoretical question arises as to whether phonological skills are universally important in learning to read any orthography. In this chapter, I examine Chinese as an example of a non-alphabetic script. The great number of visually distinct and complicated Chinese characters and the absence of GPC rules in Chinese often lead people to suggest that Chinese characters are learned as logograms (e.g. Baron and Strawson, 1976) and, as such, visual skills rather than phonological skills are likely to be important in learning to read Chinese. There seems to be some supporting evidence for this hypothesis. For instance, Lee et al. (1986) have reported a significant correlation between spatial relations score and Chinese reading score for first graders in Taiwan. Hung (1999) also reported that visual sequential memory correlated significantly with Chinese children's reading performance. Similarly, Huang and Hanley (1995) found that a combined visual score (visual form discrimination and visual paired-associate) was a better predictor of Chinese word reading than a combined phonological score (odd man out and phoneme deletion) in Chinese third graders in Taiwan and Hong Kong. However, their visual paired-associate learning task, which was the best predictor of Chinese word reading in their study (r > 0.70), might not be a pure measure of visual skills. In this task, the children were asked to learn the associations of colours with some abstract line drawings. It was highly likely that the third graders used colour names as phonological codes to aid their learning, as this task closely resembles a visual–verbal association task. In another study, Huang and Hanley (1997) reported that the performance in the same visual paired-associate learning task before entering school corre-lated significantly with children's reading performance one year later among first graders in Taiwan. However, the same correlation was not significant when the effect of differences in IQ was controlled. The study had employed Raven's Coloured Progressive Matrices as a measure of general intelligence. This visual measure of intelligence might have tremendously weakened the association between reading and the visual paired-associate learning score. Future research should further examine the role of visual–verbal association skills in learning to read Chinese.

Contrary to the above findings, there is other evidence showing that visual discrimination skills (e.g. Ho, 1997) and visual memory skills (e.g. McBride-Chang and Chang, 1995; Ho, 1997; Hu and Catts, 1998) do not correlate significantly with Chinese reading performance in children, but phonological processing skills such as phonological awareness (e.g. Ho, 1997; Ho and Bryant, 1997b; Huang and Hanley, 1997; Hu and Catts, 1998), phonological memory (e.g. Stevenson et al., 1985; McBride-Chang and Chang, 1995; Ho, 1997; Hu and Catts, 1998) and phonological retrieval (e.g. Hu and Catts, 1998; McBride-Chang and Ho, 2000) are important contribu-tors to early reading success in Chinese. The same types of phonological processing skills that are important in learning to read alphabetic scripts are found to be important in learning to read Chinese. However, these studies are only simultaneous correlational studies with no control of extraneous variables such as IQ. In Huang and Hanley's (1997) longitudinal study conducted in Taiwan, they reported that after controlling for the effects of differences in IQ and vocabulary ability, a combined phonological awareness score (odd man out and phoneme deletion) of first graders significantly predicted their Chinese word-reading performance one year later.

Interestingly, when they partialled out the effect of differences in reading performance before entering school, phonological skills no longer predicted later Chinese character reading. Since their early phonological score correlated significantly with the initial reading score, controlling for the effect of initial reading skills might have artificially weakened the predictive power of the early phonological score. A better research design would therefore be to test children's phonological skills before they can read. Ho and Bryant (1997b) conducted a four-year longitudinal study of such a design in Hong Kong. In this study, we found that after controlling for the effects of age, IQ and socioeconomic background, Chinese children's pre-reading visual perceptual skills significantly predicted their reading performance one and two years later and visual memory skills predicted reading performance only two years later. On the other hand, children's pre-reading phonological awareness skills significantly predicted their reading performance two and three years later. We propose that learning to read Chinese progresses from a visual phase to a phonological phase, similar to the developmental pattern in learning to read alphabetic scripts (Frith, 1985).

The next question one may ask is why phonological skills are important in learning to read Chinese, as they are in learning to read alphabetic scripts. There are at least two possible reasons. The first is that learning the OPC rules in Chinese requires the same sort of sensitivity to one's speech sounds as learning the GPC rules in alphabetic scripts. The second is that phonological skills are involved in learning to read any orthography (including Chinese) because of the close connection between spoken and written languages. I would like to stress that these two possibilities are not mutually exclusive and I will examine each of them in turn in the following sections.

The association between learning the Chinese OPC rules and phonological skills

Despite the predominance of ideophonetic compounds in Chinese, some researchers do not appear to think that these OPC rules are regular enough to help reading (e.g. Wang, 1973; Hoosain, 1991). However, many recent studies have shown that Chinese readers, both adults (e.g. Chen and Allport, 1995; Feldman and Siok, 1997; Taft and Zhu, 1997) and children (e.g., Ho and Bryant, 1997a,b; Shu and Anderson, 1997; Yang and Peng, 1997; Chan and Nunes, 1998; Ho et al., 1999; Wu et al., 1999) do use the phonetic radical for sound cues and the semantic radical for meaning cues in reading and writing Chinese characters. For instance, Ho and Bryant (1997a) found that Chinese first and second graders in Hong Kong named phonologically regular Chinese characters more accurately than irregular ones. They also reported that phonetic-related errors (i.e. errors in using the phonetic radical as sound cues in reading irregular Chinese characters, such as the character怕 [pa]3 being incorrectly read as its phonetic radical白[baak]9) were the most dominant type in reading Chinese characters and words. Similarly, Yang and Peng (1997) reported that Chinese third graders in mainland China named regular characters faster than irregular ones only in the low-frequency range. They also reported significant consistency effects (i.e. characters having the same phonetic radicals and same pronunciations, e.g. 爸 [ba]1, 疤 [ba]1, 笆 [ba]1, 芭 [ba]1, were named better than characters having the same phonetic radicals but different pronunciations, e.g.汁 [dzap]7, 計[gai]3, 針 [dzam]1, 什[sam]6) for both third and sixth graders. These findings seem to show that Chinese children tend to read familiar compound characters holistically and unfamiliar compound characters analytically.

What then are the skills that are important in learning and applying these OPC rules in reading Chinese? Ho and Bryant's (1997a) study suggested that awareness of subsyllabic units may be crucial for Chinese beginning readers to make orthographic analogies between Chinese characters having the same phonetic components and similar pronunciations (e.g. partial homophones or rhyming syllables), just as the awareness of onset and rhyme is important for the use of orthographic analogies by English beginning readers (e.g. Goswami, 1990, 1991). In other words, phonological awareness may be important in learning the OPC rules in Chinese. Ho and Bryant's (1997b) findings supported this suggestion, and found that rhyme awareness correlated significantly with Chinese ideophonetic compound reading and pseudocharacter reading (a measure of the knowledge of the OPC rules) in first graders. Rhyme awareness ceased to predict Chinese ideophonetic compound reading when the effects of differences in IQ and pseudocharacter reading were partialled out. It appears that phonological awareness is important in the acquisition of the OPC rules, and the OPC rules are important in learning to read Chinese.

Ho et al. (1999) conducted another study to examine directly the association between the making of orthographic analogies and phonological awareness, using a training paradigm similar to the one developed by Goswami (1986). We first taught some Chinese first and third graders the pronunciations of some unknown Chinese characters that later served as clue characters. We then asked the children to read some analogous characters (which shared common phonetic radicals with the clue characters) and some control characters. We found that the children read the analogous characters significantly better than the control characters, and phonological awareness did not correlate significantly with the magnitude of improvement in character naming after the phonological analogy training. Since only phonologically consistent characters were employed in this study (i.e. the clue characters and the analogous characters represented identical syllables rather than similar syllables, e.g. rhyming ones), awareness of subsyllabic units might not be necessary in making such analogies. Thus, the connection between phonological awareness and the learning of OPC rules in Chinese is not conclusive. Future research is needed to clarify these inconsistent findings.

Relationship between spoken and written languages

There is common agreement that there is a close relationship between a writing system and its spoken language. A writing system represents the syntax, sound and meaning of its spoken language. Reading is considered as a secondary linguistic activity (e.g. Mattingly, 1972) in that learning to read depends on some primary linguistic skills, which are acquired through spoken language development (e.g. Bowey and Patel, 1988). Therefore, the processing of written language is expected to utilize elements in the processing system for spoken language, such as phonology.

A study by McBride-Chang and Ho (2000) found that phonological processing skills (phonological awareness, phonological memory and phono-logical retrieval) significantly predicted Chinese word reading in preschoolers even after controlling for the effects of age and vocabulary. In the same study, we reported that speech perception correlated significantly with Chinese word reading, and also significantly predicted syllable deletion (a measure of phonological awareness) after controlling for the effects of differences in age, vocabulary and verbal memory. These results suggest that spoken language development (such as speech perception) may contribute directly to the development of phonological awareness and indirectly to the development of reading skills. It seems that the association between phono-logical awareness and early reading performance in Chinese found in this and other studies is due to the close connection between spoken and written languages. Apart from phonology, reading also requires similar processing components of the spoken language, such as syntax and meaning. Future research is needed to expand our knowledge in this area.

Research in developmental dyslexia in Chinese

Research in Chinese developmental dyslexia has been rather limited, probably because of the early belief that it had a low prevalence among Chinese communities. Based on the available research evidence, I will first outline the cognitive deficits of Chinese children with developmental dyslexia and then describe some of my own attempts at training these children. One needs to bear in mind that different studies may use different selection criteria for participants and their results may also be affected by the different educational practices in their countries. For those studies conducted in my laboratory, all the participants were Chinese primary school children in Hong Kong. The children with dyslexia were referred by the local education authority. All of them had at least average intelligence (i.e. with IQ 90 or above) and their reading achievement was at least one year backward (as measured by a standardized Chinese word reading test). The children were carefully screened to ensure they did not have any suspected brain damage, uncorrected sensory impairment, serious emotional or behavioural problems.

The cognitive deficits of Chinese children with developmental dyslexia

The problem of developmental dyslexia can be examined at different perspectives/levels, e.g. neurological, biological, behavioural and cognitive (Manis et al., 1996; Dalby et al., 1998; Fagerheim et al., 1999). A person's perspective determines to a large extent the types of data he or she will collect. In the present analysis, I take a cognitive approach and will focus on examining the underlying cognitive deficits of Chinese children with developmental dyslexia.

Visual skills

Research on the cognitive deficits of Chinese dyslexic children focuses mainly on two aspects: their visual and phonological skills. Because of the logographic nature of the Chinese script, many people think that visual skills are important in learning to read Chinese. From the studies reviewed in previous sections, we know that some visual discrimination and visual memory skills are important in learning to read Chinese at the initial stage (e.g. Ho and Bryant, 1997b). If that is the case, children who have poor visual skills may have reading problems in Chinese.

Woo and Hoosain's (1984) study has provided some supporting evidence for the above hypothesis. They tested 13 Chinese dyslexic children (with a mean age of 8 years and 5 months) and found that these children made more visual-distractor errors in Chinese character recognition than the average readers of the same age but not more phonological-distractor errors. The Chinese dyslexic readers also showed inferior performance in all the subtests of the Frostig Developmental Test of Visual Perception, which contains tests of eye-motor co-ordination, figure-ground, constancy of shape, position in space and spatial relationships. Woo and Hoosain concluded that the Chinese dyslexic children had a disability in basic visual perceptual functions. It is noteworthy that the Frostig test used in their study is in fact a visual-motor test, which involves both visual perception and fine motor co-ordination. It was possible that these children had poor visual perceptual skills, or fine motor skills, or both. Future studies may examine these possibilities.

Phonological skills

There is increasing research evidence to show that phonological processing skills are as important in learning to read Chinese as in learning to read alphabetic scripts. Dyslexic readers of alphabetic scripts exhibit deficits in processing phonological information. Is this phonological deficit hypothesis also applicable to the case of Chinese? I will now review some studies that were designed to examine the phonological deficit hypothesis in Chinese developmental dyslexia, and consider whether Chinese dyslexic children have deficits in phonological awareness, phonological memory and phonological retrieval – the three primary phonological processing skills suggested by Wagner and Torgesen (1987).

Phonological awareness deficits

To test the phonological awareness deficit hypothesis, Huang and Zhang (1997) tested 32 Chinese dyslexic second graders and 32 average readers of the same age. They reported that the dyslexic group performed significantly worse than the control group on initial phoneme deletion, sound categorization and tone detection. This study shows that Chinese dyslexic children are poor in phonological awareness skills. However, one could not tell whether these children had phonological awareness deficits or whether their weakness in phonological awareness was a result of their poor reading skills. To address this issue, we conducted a study with a reading-level match design (Ho et al., 2000). We found that the Chinese dyslexic children performed significantly worse than their age controls in onset detection and rhyme detection, but performed significantly less well than the reading-level controls only in rhyme detection. These results suggest that Chinese dyslexic children are not very sensitive to the structure of speech sound, and they have particular deficits in rhyme awareness. Other researchers have suggested that phonological awareness deficits may reflect the problem that alphabetic dyslexic readers have in constructing low-level phonological representations (e.g. Crain et al., 1990; Gathercole and Baddeley, 1993; Elbro et al., 1998). Consistent with this suggestion, Lam and Cheung (1996) reported some clinical findings based on a sample of 30 Chinese children with a mean age of 4 years 8 months referred to a regional child assessment centre. Over one-third of those having early phonological problems (35%) or language problems (50%) were found to have reading and writing disabilities later. However, we need more systematic research to establish firmly this connection among early language/phonological problems, phonological awareness deficits and reading disabilities.

Phonological memory deficits

Aaron (1989) has suggested that the main problem children with developmental dyslexia face is phonological memory, and that this applies to any orthographic system. Hulme and Roodenrys (1995) argue that the short-term memory (STM) problems of poor or dyslexic readers are not causally related to their poor reading but are an index of other phonological deficits that are a cause of reading difficulties. As in reading alphabetic scripts, research evidence has shown that phonological memory is also important for reading acquisition in Chinese (e.g. Ho, 1997; Hu and Catts, 1998). Thus, I expected that Chinese dyslexic children might also have poor phonological memory. In their large-scale cross-cultural study, Stevenson et al. (1982) reported that those cognitive skills that best discriminated low and average Chinese readers of fifth grade were general information, verbal memory and memory for words. Similarly, Zhang et al. (1997) reported that Chinese dyslexic children aged 11 to 13 performed significantly worse than normally achieving children of the same age in digit memory and memory for text. Consequently, we employed a reading-level match design in two studies to examine the phonological memory deficit hypothesis in Chinese developmental dyslexia (Ho and Lai, 1999; Ho et al., 2000). We found that the 8-year-old Chinese dyslexic children performed significantly worse than both the age controls and the reading-level controls on digit repetition, word repetition and nonword repetition. These results suggest that Chinese children with dyslexia have difficulties in maintaining phonological representations in STM. As with alphabetic readers, these memory deficits are likely to adversely affect Chinese dyslexic children's acquisition of vocabulary and their development of stable graphic–sound associations, which will in turn hinder their normal reading development (e.g. Gathercole and Baddeley, 1989, 1990, 1993; Gathercole et al., 1991).

Phonological retrieval deficits

Research findings show that phonological retrieval skills (as often measured by rapid naming) are a significant predictor of early reading success in Chinese (Hu and Catts, 1998; McBride-Chang and Ho, 2000). We conducted a study to examine the phonological retrieval deficit hypothesis in Chinese developmental dyslexia (Ho and Lai, 1999). To the best of my knowledge, this is the only study conducted on this topic. We tested three groups of children – dyslexic, age control and reading-level control – with 20 in each group. We found that in both the discrete-trial format (with naming stimuli presented one at a time through a computer) and the continuous format (with naming stimuli presented all together on a piece of cardboard) the dyslexic group named digits, colours, pictures and Chinese characters significantly more slowly than the age-control group, but similarly to the reading-level control group. It appeared that the dyslexic children had difficulties both at the basic level of name retrieval (as tested in the discrete-trial format) and at the complex level that requires scanning and sequencing strategies (as tested in the continuous format). We concluded that Chinese dyslexic children may have some generalized difficulties in speed of access to the lexicon.

The various research findings reviewed above demonstrate that Chinese dyslexic children also have phonological deficits in line with those of their alphabetic counterparts.

Knowledge of the OPC rules

Several studies have shown that children make use of the phonetic radical in a Chinese character for sound cues, and knowledge of such OPC rules is important in learning to read Chinese. One may ask whether Chinese dyslexic children acquire knowledge of the OPC rules as other average readers. Ho et al. (2000) found that Chinese dyslexic children read regular Chinese characters significantly better than irregular ones of similar frequencies. In addition, the dyslexic children read as many regular characters as did the reading-level control group, but the dyslexics read fewer irregular characters than the controls. These findings suggested that the Chinese dyslexic children made use of the phonetic radical for sound cues but they tended to remember fewer exceptions than did normally achieving children. These results suggest that apart from phonological deficits, Chinese dyslexic children may also have other cognitive deficits (e.g. deficits in orthographic processing) that need further investigation. In any case, the research findings obtained so far have already provided some useful information to guide early identification and remediation of developmental dyslexia among Chinese communities.

Training studies

The two small-scale training studies outlined below, conducted in our laboratory, were designed on the basis of previous research findings in areas of reading acquisition and reading problems in Chinese, especially those related to knowledge of the OPC rules and phonological skills.

Training in OPC rules

In the first training study (Ho and Ma, 1999), we investigated Chinese dyslexic children's efficiency in employing phonological strategies (i.e. the use of OPC rules) in reading and the effectiveness of training in phonological strategies in improving their reading performance. An experimental group of 15 Chinese dyslexic children received five days of intensive training in phonological strategies, while a comparable control group did not. The training involved the teaching of the basic structure of Chinese characters, the different functions of semantic and phonetic radicals, and how phonetic radicals sometimes provide reliable sound cues and sometimes do not. The results showed that before training the Chinese dyslexic children did not use the phonological strategies as efficiently as the Chinese average readers, and the training programme was effective in significantly improving the experimental group's reading performance. The improvement was mainly in reading more phonologically regular Chinese characters. In other words, the dyslexic children made better use of the phonetic radicals for sound cues after training. However, this study failed to put enough emphasis on teaching irregular characters. Future remediation should focus on teaching irregular and exceptional characters and the sound of individual phonetic radicals.

Training in phonological awareness

In view of the phonological awareness deficits experienced by Chinese dyslexic children, we conducted a second training study to examine the effectiveness of phonological awareness training in improving their reading performance (Ho and Cheung, 1999). An experimental group of 15 Chinese dyslexic children in Hong Kong received five sessions of training in phonological awareness skills through computers, while a comparable control group received no training. The results showed that the experimental group improved significantly in their performance in the Chinese word reading test after training, but the control group did not. Interestingly, the experimental group showed significant improvement in the computer version of the rhyme awareness tasks but not in the experimental version of the same tasks. This may be partly due to the fact that the computer tasks included pictures that reduced the memory load substantially, while the experimental tasks were purely auditory. In other words, the phonological awareness training may have improved the phonological sensitivity of the dyslexic children in this study but not their phonological memory. I also observed that the dyslexic children responded very well to the computer-mediated learning tasks. Their learning motivation and attention were greatly enhanced with computer training.

Many studies have indicated that the best approach to help alphabetic poor readers or dyslexic children is to combine phonological training with teaching of letter knowledge (e.g. Blachman, 1987, 1997; Blachman et al., 1996). Blachman (1997) has suggested that once children are aware that speech can be segmented and the segmented units can be represented by letters, they should be taught to utilize these insights in reading and spelling. Similarly, we can consider combining phonological training with teaching of OPC rules to see whether this approach produces better results than either phonological training or OPC training alone for Chinese dyslexic children.

Conclusion

In this chapter, I have reviewed studies relating to reading acquisition and developmental dyslexia in Chinese. There is convergent research evidence showing that phonological processing skills are important contributors to early reading success and reading failure in Chinese, as they are in alphabetic scripts. I conclude that there seem to be similar causes of reading problems in Chinese and alphabetic languages. However, research data on developmental dyslexia in Chinese are very limited at this stage. More research is needed to consolidate this tentative conclusion.

References

Aaron PG (1989) Orthographic systems and developmental dyslexia: a reformulation of the syndrome. In PG Aaron, RM Joshi (eds) Reading and writing disorders in different orthographic systems, pp 379–400. Dordrecht: Kluwer.

Baron J, Strawson C (1976) Use of orthographic and word-specific knowledge in reading words aloud. Journal of Experimental Psychology: Human Perception and Performance 2: 386–393.

Blachman BA (1987) An alternative classroom reading program for learning disabled and other low-achieving children. In R Bowler (ed) Intimacy with language: a forgotten basic in teacher education, pp. 49-55. Baltimore, MD: Orion.

Blachman BA (1997) Early intervention and phonological awareness: a cautionary tale. Foundation of reading acquisition and dyslexia. London: LEA.

Blachman BA, Ball E, Black S, Tangel P (1996) Promising practices for improving beginning reading instruction. Unpublished raw data.

Bowey JA, Patel RK (1988) Metalinguistic ability and early reading achievement. Applied Psycholinguistics 9: 367–383.

Bradley L, Bryant PE (1983) Categorizing sounds and learning to read – a causal connection. Nature 301: 419–421.

Bradley L, Bryant PE (1985) Rhyme and reason in reading and spelling. IARLD Monographs, No.1. Ann Arbor, MI: University of Michigan Press.

Byrne B (1992) Studies in the acquisition procedure for reading: rationale, hypotheses, and data. In PB Gough, LC Ehri, R Treiman (eds) Reading acquisition. New Jersey: Lawrence Erlbaum Associates.

Chan L, Nunes T (1998) Children's understanding of the formal and functional characteristics of written Chinese. Applied Psycholinguistics 19: 115-131.

Chan MY (1982) Statistics on the strokes of present-day Chinese script. Chinese Linguistics 1: 299–305. (In Chinese)

Chen HC (1996). Chinese reading and comprehension: a cognitive psychology perspective. In MH Bond (ed) The handbook of Chinese psychology, pp 43–70. New York: Oxford University Press.

Chen Y-P (1993) Word recognition and reading in Chinese. Unpublished doctoral dissertation, University of Oxford, Britain.

Chen Y-P, Allport A (1995) Attention and lexical decomposition in Chinese word recognition: conjunctions of form and position guide selective attention. Visual Cognition 2: 235-268.

Crain S, Shankweiler D, Macaruso P, Bar-Shalom E (1990) Working memory and comprehension of spoken sentences: investigations of children with reading disorder. In G
Vallar, T Shallice (eds) Neuropsychological impairments of short-term memory, pp
477-508. Cambridge: Cambridge University Press.

Dalby MA, Elbro C, Stodkilde-Jorgensen H (1998) Temporal lobe asymmetry and dyslexia:
an in vivo study using MRI. Brain and Language 62: 51-69.

Elbro C, Borstrom I, Petersen, DK (1998) Predicting dyslexia from kindergarten: the
importance of distinctness of phonological representations of lexical items. Reading
Research Quarterly 33: 36-60.

Fagerheim T, Raeymaekers P, Tonnessen FE, Pedersen M, Tranebjaerg L, Lubs HA (1999)
A new gene (DYX3) for dyslexia is located on chromosome 2. Journal of Medical
Genetics 36: 664-669.

Fan HY (1986) Some discussion on the orthography of modern Chinese characters. Paper
presented in the National Conference of Chinese Character Research, China. (In
Chinese)

Feldman LB, Siok WWT (1997) The role of component function in visual recognition of
Chinese characters. Journal of Experimental Psychology 23: 776-781.

Foreign Language Press Beijing (1989) Chinese characters. Beijing: Foreign Language
Press.

Frith U (1985) Beneath the surface of developmental dyslexia. In KE Patterson, JC
Marshall, M Coltheart (eds) Surface dyslexia. London: Lawrence Erlbaum Associates.

Frith U, Snowling M (1983) Reading for meaning and reading for sound in autistic and
dyslexic children. British Journal of Developmental Psychology 1: 329-342.

Gathercole SE, Baddeley AD (1989) Evaluation of the role of phonological STM in the
development of vocabulary in children: a longitudinal study. Journal of Memory and
Language 28: 200-213.

Gathercole SE, Baddeley AD (1990) Phonological memory deficits in language disordered
children: is there a causal connection? Journal of Memory and Language 29: 336-360.

Gathercole SE, Baddeley AD (1993) Working memory and language. Hove: Lawrence
Erlbaum Associates.

Gathercole SE, Willis C, Baddeley AD (1991) Differentiating phonological memory and
awareness of rhyme: reading and vocabulary development in children. British Journal
of Psychology, 82: 387-406.

Goswami U (1986) Children's use of analogy in learning to read: a developmental study.
Journal of Experimental Child Psychology 42: 73-83.

Goswami U (1990) A special link between rhyming skill and the use of orthographic analogies by beginning readers? Journal of Child Psychology and Psychiatry 31: 301-311.

Goswami U (1991) Learning about spelling sequences: the role of onsets and rimes in
analogies in reading. Child Development 62: 1110-1123.

Hirose T, Hatta T (1988) Reading disabilities in modern Japanese children. Journal of
Research in Reading 11: 152-160.

Ho CS-H (1997) The importance of phonological awareness and verbal short-term
memory to children's success in learning to read Chinese. Psychologia 40: 211-219.

Ho CS-H, Bryant PE (1997a) Learning to read Chinese beyond the logographic phase.
Reading Research Quarterly 32: 276-289.

Ho CS-H, Bryant PE (1997b) Phonological skills are important in learning to read Chinese.
Developmental Psychology 33: 946-951.

Ho CS-H, Cheung C-K (1999) Does training in phonological awareness skills improve Chinese dyslexic children's reading performance? Educational Research Journal 14: 209-228.

Ho CS-H, Lai DN-C (1999) Naming-speed deficits and phonological memory deficits in Chinese developmental dyslexia. Learning and Individual Differences 11: 173-186.

Ho CS-H, Ma RN-L (1999) Training in phonological strategies improves Chinese dyslexic children's character reading skills. Journal of Research in Reading 22:131-142.

Ho CS-H, Wong W-L, Chan W-S (1999) The use of orthographic analogies in learning to read Chinese. Journal of Child Psychology and Psychiatry 40: 393-403.

Ho CS-H, Law TP-S, Ng PM (2000) The phonological deficit hypothesis in Chinese developmental dyslexia. Reading and Writing 13: 57-79.

Hoosain R (1991) Psycholinguistic implications for linguistic relativity: a case study of Chinese. Hillsdale, NJ: Lawrence Erlbaum Associates.

Hu C-F, Catts HW (1998) The role of phonological processing in early reading ability: what we can learn from Chinese. Scientific Studies of Reading 2: 55-79.

Huang HS, Hanley JR (1995) Phonological awareness and visual skills in learning to read Chinese and English. Cognition 54: 73-98.

Huang HS, Hanley JR (1997) A longitudinal study of phonological awareness, visual skills, and Chinese reading acquisition among first graders in Taiwan. International Journal of Behavioural Development 20: 249-268.

Huang HS, Zhang HR (1997) An analysis of phonemic awareness, word awareness and tone awareness among dyslexia children. Bulletin of Special Education and Rehabilitation 5: 125-138.

Hulme C, Roodenrys S (1995) Verbal working memory development and its disorders. Journal of Child Psychology and Psychiatry 36: 373-398.

Hung LY (1999) A study on the visual perceptual skills of Chinese primary school children in Taiwan. Paper presented at the Conference of Reading Difficulties in Chinese, Taiwan, January.

Kuo WF (1978) A preliminary study of reading disability in the Republic of China. National Taiwan Normal University's Collected Papers 20: 57-58.

Lam CCC, Cheung PSP (1996) Early developmental problems as indicators for specific learning disabilities among Chinese children. Paper presented at the 47th Annual Conference of the Orton Dyslexia Society, Boston, November.

Laxon V, Masterson J, Moran R (1994) Are children's representations of words distributed? Effects of orthographic neighbourhood size, consistency and regularity of naming. Language and Cognitive Processes 9: 1-27.

Lee S-Y, Stigler JW, Stevenson HW (1986) Beginning reading in Chinese and English. In BR Foorman, AW Siegel (eds) Acquisition of reading skills: cultural constraints and cognitive universals. Hillsdale, NJ: Lawrence Erlbaum Associates.

Leong CK (1989) Reading and reading difficulties in a morphemic script. In PG Aaron, RM Joshi (eds) Reading and writing disorders in different orthographic systems, pp 267-282). Dordrecht: Kluwer.

Liberman IY, Shankweiler D, Fischer FW, Carter B (1974) Explicit syllable and phoneme segmentation in the young child. Journal of Experimental Child Psychology 18: 201-212.

Liu IM, Chuang CJ, Wang SC (1975) Frequency count of 40,000 Chinese words. Taipei: Lucky Books.

Lundberg I, Olofsson A, Wall S (1980) Reading and spelling skills in the first school years predicted from phonemic awareness skills in kindergarten. Scandinavian Journal of Psychology 21: 159-173.

Lundberg I, Frost J, Peterson O-P (1988) Effects of an extensive program for stimulating phonological awareness in preschool children. Reading Research Quarterly 23: 263-284.

Makita K (1968) The rarity of reading disability in Japanese children. American Journal of Orthopsychiatry 38: 599-614.

Manis FR, Seidenberg MS, Doi LM, McBride-Chang C, Petersen A (1996) On the bases of two subtypes of developmental dyslexia. Cognition 58: 157-195.

Mann VA, Liberman IY (1984) Phonological awareness and verbal short-term memory. Journal of Learning Disabilities 17: 592-599.

Mattingly IG (1972) Reading, the linguistic process, and linguistic awareness. In JF Kavanagh, IG Mattingly (eds) Language by ear and by eye. Cambridge, MA: MIT Press.

McBride-Chang C, Chang L (1995) Memory, print exposure, and metacognition: Components of reading in Chinese children. Journal of Psychology 30: 607-616.

McBride-Chang C, Ho CS-H (2000) Developmental issues in Chinese children's character acquisition. Journal of Educational Psychology 92: 50-55.

Perfetti CA, Beck I, Bell LC, Hughes C (1987) Phonemic knowledge and learning to read are reciprocal: a longitudinal study of first grade children. Merrill-Palmer Quarterly 33: 283-319.

Rozin P, Gleitman LR (1977) The structure and acquisition of reading 2: The reading process and the acquisition of the alphabetic principle. In AS Reber, DL Scarborough (eds) Toward a psychology of reading. Hillsdale, NJ: Lawrence Erlbaum Associates.

Rozin P, Poritsky S, Sotsky R (1971) American children with reading problems can easily learn to read English represented by Chinese characters. Science 171: 1264-1267.

Sheridan EM (1983) Reading disabilities: can we blame the written language? Journal of Learning Disabilities 16: 81-86.

Shu H, Anderson RC (1997) Role of radical awareness in the character and word acquisition of Chinese children. Reading Research Quarterly 32: 79-89.

Stevenson HW (1984) Orthography and reading disabilities. Journal of Learning Disabilities 17: 296-301.

Stevenson HW, Stigler JW, Lee S-Y, Lucker GW (1985) Cognitive performance and academic achievement of Japanese, Chinese and American children. Child Development 56: 718-734.

Stevenson HW, Stigler JW, Lucker GW, Lee SY, Hsu CC, Kitamura S (1982) Reading disabilities: the case of Chinese, Japanese and English. Child Development 53: 1164-1181.

Taft M, Zhu X (1997) Submorphemic processing in reading Chinese. Journal of Experimental Psychology 23: 761-775.

Taylor I, Taylor MM (1995) Writing and literacy in Chinese, Korean and Japanese. Amsterdam: John Benjamins Publishing Company.

Tzeng OJL (1994) Chinese orthography and reading: a clarification. In N Bird (ed) Language and learning, pp 52-72. Hong Kong: Institute of Language in Education, Hong Kong Education Department.

Wagner RK, Torgesen JK (1987) The nature of phonological processing and its causal role in the acquisition of reading skills. Psychological Bulletin 101: 192-212.

Wagner RK, Torgesen JK, Rashotte CA (1994) Development of reading-related phonological processing abilities: new evidence of bidirectional causality from a latent variable longitudinal study. Developmental Psychology 30: 73-87.

Wang WS-Y (1973) The Chinese language. Scientific American 228: 50-63.

Woo EYC, Hoosain R (1984) Visual and auditory functions of Chinese dyslexics. Psychologia 27: 164-170.

Wu N, Zhou X, Shu H (1999) Sublexical processing in reading Chinese: a developmental study. Language and Cognitive Processes 14: 503-524.

Yang H, Peng D-L (1997) The learning and naming of Chinese characters of elementary school children. In H-C Chen (ed), Cognitive processing of Chinese and related Asian languages, pp 323-346. Hong Kong: The Chinese University Press.

Zhang CF, Zhang JH, Chang SM, Zhou J (1997) A study of cognitive profiles of Chinese learners' reading disability. Paper presented at the Second International Chinese Psychologists Conference, Hong Kong, December. (In Chinese)

Zhou YK (1980) Precise guide to pronunciation with Chinese phonological roots. Jilin, China: People's Publishing. (In Chinese)

Zhu YP (1987) Analysis of cuing functions of the phonetic in modern China. Unpublished paper, East China Normal University. (In Chinese)

Index